T0192152

Sports Medicine

Edited by

David Drez, Jr., M.D.

Clinical Professor of Orthopaedics
LSU School of Medicine
Department of Orthopaedics
New Orleans, LA
Director of Sports Medicine
McNeese State University and Lake Charles Memorial Hospital
Lake Charles, LA

Bernard R. Bach, Jr., M.D.

The Claude Lambert–Helen Thomson Professor
Department of Orthopaedic Surgery
Director, Sports Medicine Section
RUSH University Medical Center
Chicago, IL

Charles Nofsinger, M.D.

Assistant Professor
Department of Orthopaedics
University of South Florida
Tampa, FL
Attending Surgeon
Department of Orthopaedic Surgery
University Community Hospital
Tampa, FL

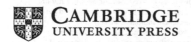

CAMBRIDGE
UNIVERSITY PRESS

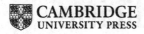

CAMBRIDGE
UNIVERSITY PRESS

Shaftesbury Road, Cambridge CB2 8EA, United Kingdom

One Liberty Plaza, 20th Floor, New York, NY 10006, USA

477 Williamstown Road, Port Melbourne, VIC 3207, Australia

314–321, 3rd Floor, Plot 3, Splendor Forum, Jasola District Centre, New Delhi – 110025, India

103 Penang Road, #05–06/07, Visioncrest Commercial, Singapore 238467

Cambridge University Press is part of Cambridge University Press & Assessment, a department of the University of Cambridge.

We share the University's mission to contribute to society through the pursuit of education, learning and research at the highest international levels of excellence.

www.cambridge.org
Information on this title: www.cambridge.org/9780521735261

First published 2008

A catalogue record for this publication is available from the British Library

Library of Congress Cataloging-in-Publication data
Sports medicine / edited by David Drez Jr., Bernard R. Bach Jr.,
Charles Nofsinger.
    p. ; cm.
ISBN 978-0-521-73526-1 (pbk.)
1. Sports medicine – Handbooks, manuals, etc.   I. Drez, David.
II. Bach, Bernard R.   III. Nofsinger, Charles.   IV. Title.
[DNLM: 1. Athletic Injuries – Handbooks.
2. SportsMedicine – Handbooks. QT 29 S76388 2008]
RC1211.S655   2008
617.1´027–dc22   2008025639

ISBN   978-0-521-73526-1   Paperback

NOTICE

Because of the dynamic nature of medical practice and drug selection and dosage, users are advised that decisions regarding drug therapy must be based on the independent judgment of the clinician, changing information about a drug (e.g., as reflected in the literature and manufacturer's most current product information), and changing medical practices.

While great care has been taken to ensure the accuracy of the information presented, users are advised that the authors, editors, contributors, and publishers make no warranty, express or implied, with respect to, and are not responsible for, the currency, completeness, or accuracy of the information contained in this publication, nor for any errors or omissions, or the application of this information, nor for any consequences arising therefrom. Users are encouraged to confirm the information contained herein with other sources deemed authoritative.

Ultimately, it is the responsibility of the treating physician, relying on experience and knowledge of the patient, to determine dosages and the best treatment for the patient. Therefore, the authors, editors, contributors, and publishers make no warranty, express or implied, and shall have no liability to any person or entity with regard to claims, loss, or damage caused, or alleged to be caused, directly or indirectly, by the use of information contained in this publication.

Further, the authors, editors, contributors, and publishers are not responsible for misuse of any of the information provided in this publication, for negligence by the user, or for any typographical errors.

Contents

Preface

A myriad of sports medicine textbooks have flooded the publishing marketplace in the past 20 years. *Sports Medicine*, and its first two iterations as *Pocket Sports Medicine*, was developed and marketed for the increasing demand of PDA users. The genesis of this concept evolved around the observation that many young physicians, residents, interns, and medical students need a quick way to access information "on the run." Relevant sports medicine topics were determined, an outstanding faculty of contributing authors was recruited, and 150 sports medicine topics were identified. *Pocket Sports Medicine* was organized in a fashion that would allow the reader or "accessor" an opportunity to learn or review basic information on topics as varied as neck injuries in athletes, ACL injuries, LisFranc fracture-dislocations, groin injuries, and "Little Leaguer's elbow." Although not designed to provide a comprehensive review, a single topic could be reviewed in less than 2 minutes. The consistent organizational structure follows a theme of 1) history, 2) physical examination, 3) imaging, 4) differential diagnosis, 5) treatment, and 6) pearls and pitfalls. Topics are organized in a bullet point outlined format. The editors believe that the printed format of the popular PDA derivative has a place in the lab coat pockets of residents, medical students, and ER physicians. When dealing with sports injuries, time management is at a premium. In the time that it takes to walk to the medical school library to read about hemarthrosis, you can read about the topic in *Sports Medicine*. We hope that you find this sports medicine contribution an asset to your education.

David J. Drez, Jr., M.D.
Bernard R. Bach, Jr., M.D.
Charles Nofsinger, M.D.

ACHILLES TENDINITIS

GEORGE B. HOLMES, JR., MD
REVISED BY CHARLES NOFSINGER, MD

HISTORY
- ■ Mechanism
  - ➤ Overuse, muscle imbalance, poor exercise biomechanics
- ■ Initial complaints
  - ➤ Pain, swelling, decreased activity tolerance
- ■ Chronic complaints
  - ➤ Pain with activity, difficulty running and jumping
  - ➤ Swelling
- ■ Common in runners

PHYSICAL EXAM
- ■ Acute
  - ➤ Diffuse swelling, pain with palpation, pain with dorsiflexion
  - ➤ Lateral pain – Associated with supination
  - ➤ Medial pain – Associated with pronation
- ■ Chronic
  - ➤ Pain, decreased dorsiflexion, atrophy
  - ➤ Longitudinal swelling rather than well localized
- ■ Classification
  - ➤ Insertional vs. noninsertional

STUDIES
- ■ Radiographs
  - ➤ AP, lateral, mortise views (lateral most important)
  - ➤ Radiographs generally normal
  - ➤ Calcifications, traction spurs – Degenerative changes, degenerative changes or partial tear
- ■ MRI
  - ➤ Tendinitis – Peritendinous fluid/edema, no tendinous signal changes
  - ➤ Differential diagnosis using MRI
    - • Tendinosis (intrasubstance signal changes)
    - • Partial tear
    - • Retrocalcaneal bursitis

DIFFERENTIAL DIAGNOSIS
- ■ Achilles tendinosis

- Partial tear
- Haglund's deformity
- Retrocalcaneal bursitis

TREATMENT
- Nonoperative
  - ➤ Types of nonoperative treatment
    - Immobilization (cast, walking boot)
    - Heel lift
    - Anti-inflammatory medications
    - Achilles stretching
    - Physical therapy (including ice massage)
    - Steroids contraindicated due to risk of rupture
- Operative
  - ➤ Debridement if refractory to conservative measures
  - ➤ Lysis of adhesions

DISPOSITION
N/A

PROGNOSIS
- Pure tendinitis without associated tendinosis usually responds well to conservative measures.
- Surgical results for insertional Achilles tendinitis are worse than those for noninsertional Achilles tendinitis.
- Long-term complications
  - ➤ Tendon ruptures after steroids by mouth or injection
  - ➤ Chronic swelling or pain can result even after debridement.

CAVEATS AND PEARLS
- MRI very useful in distinguishing between tendinosis and tendinitis

---

ACHILLES TENDON RUPTURE

GEORGE B. HOLMES, JR., MD
REVISED BY CHARLES NOFSINGER, MD

HISTORY
- Mechanism
  - ➤ Sudden contraction

➤ Susceptible tendons are weakened by degenerative disease such as obesity, diabetes, hypertension, and the effects of corticosteroids, all of which lead to vascular compromise

■ Acute rupture: complaints
  ➤ Stabbing pain in posterior calf
  ➤ Pts often complain that they were "kicked" in calf
  ➤ Pain, swelling, decreased or absent push-off

■ Chronic rupture: complaints
  ➤ Difficulty walking, inability to run, chronic weakness, altered gait, pain and swelling

PHYSICAL EXAM

■ Acute
  ➤ Palpable defect in posterior calf in area of Achilles tendon, along with ecchymosis and swelling
  ➤ Thompson test

■ Chronic
  ➤ ± palpable defect of posterior calf
  ➤ Weakness in pure plantarflexion of foot

■ Classification
  ➤ Acute ruptures
    • Diagnosis within 0–4 weeks of injury
  ➤ Chronic ruptures
    • Diagnosis 1–3 months after injury

STUDIES

■ Radiographs
  ➤ AP, lateral, mortise views (lateral most important)
  ➤ Radiographs generally normal
  ➤ Calcifications, traction spurs – Degenerative changes, degenerative changes or partial tear (indicative of longstanding disease of the tendon)

■ MRI
  ➤ Generally not necessary for diagnosis of acute ruptures
  ➤ May be useful in cases of suspected chronic ruptures
  ➤ Useful in differential diagnosis
    • Partial tendon tear
    • Localization of tear
    • Gastrocsoleus tear
    • Plantaris tear

DIFFERENTIAL DIAGNOSIS
- Achilles tendinosis
- Partial tear
- Avulsion
- Ankle sprain
- Isolated plantaris tear
- Gastrocsoleus muscle tear

TREATMENT
- Acute
  - Nonoperative for acute ruptures
    - Cast or brace immobilization (nonweight-bearing, 6–8 weeks)
  - Operative for acute ruptures
    - Open vs. percutaneous repair (Ma procedure)
      - Ma (lower incidence of wound problems)
      - Lower rate of rerupture with direct repair
- Chronic
  - Nonoperative for chronic ruptures
    - AFO or similar bracing (palliative care)
  - Operative for chronic ruptures
    - Achilles reconstruction using graft (salvage procedure)
      - Flexor hallucis longus
      - Fascial graft
      - Peroneus brevis
  - Rehabilitation
    - Goals of physical therapy: ROM and strengthening
    - 5–6 months before return to contact sports
    - Role of earlier ROM gaining greater popularity

DISPOSITION
N/A

PROGNOSIS
- Results of conservative or operative repair generally good (greater strength with repair)
- Results of treatment after chronic rupture not as good as with acute repair
  - Reconstruction generally does not allow for return to competitive sports
- Complications
  - Rerupture (greater with conservative treatment)

> Equinus (heel cord tightness)
> Skin slough, infection, painful scar

CAVEATS AND PEARLS
- Careful handling of the soft tissue is imperative to avoid wound complications.

ACROMIOCLAVICULAR SEPARATION

JAMES D. FERRARI, MD
REVISED BY CHARLES NOFSINGER, MD

HISTORY
- Direct force by far most common mechanism
- Fall onto point of shoulder
- Acromion gets driven downward and clavicle is stabilized by sternoclavicular (SC) ligaments
- Sequence of ligamentous injuries: acromioclavicular (AC) ligaments, coracoclavicular (CC) ligaments, deltoid and trapezial muscle attachments, skin
- Inferior dislocation (type VI separation) likely caused by downward force on clavicle
- Injury may also be caused by indirect force with humeral head being driven into acromion
  > Will cause no damage to CC ligaments
- A common athletic injury
  > Football
  > Hockey
  > Lacrosse
  > Bicycling (esp. mountain biking)
  > Snowboarding
- Motorcycle accidents
  > Tend to be complex with associated injuries
- Patients report pain, swelling at AC
- Chronically may have deformity, clicking, pain

PHYSICAL EXAM
- Inspection of deformity
  > Rule out posterior buttonholing of clavicle through delto-trapezial fascia
- Neurovascular and rotator cuff strength exam

- Palpation of AC and CC regions
- Cross-body adduction
- Injuries to rule out acutely
  - Clavicular shaft fracture
  - Acromion and coracoid fractures
  - Brachial plexus injuries
  - SC joint injuries
  - Pneumothorax
  - Scapulothoracic dissociation
- Chronically must rule out other sources of pain
  - SLAP tear
  - Cervical radiculopathy
  - Rotator cuff tear

STUDIES
- Preferably done standing
- AP (Zanca view)
  - 15° cephalic tilt to avoid superimposition of AC joint on scapula
  - Reduced exposure needed as in AP view of glenohumeral joint
- Axillary view
  - Rule out posterior displacement of clavicle
  - Rule out coracoid and acromion fractures
  - Film other side if questionable
- Standing AP view of both shoulders
  - Measure CC distances and calculate % increase on affected side
  - CC distance normally 1.0–1.3 cm
- Weighted views
  - Help distinguish type II from type III
  - Not needed, as they seldom change treatment plan or decision to perform surgery
- MRI
  - Can delineate ligamentous injury and arthritis, useful for surgical planning

DIFFERENTIAL DIAGNOSIS
- Lateral clavicle fracture
- Periosteal sleeve fracture
- Bipolar AC separation + SC joint injury
- Combined AC separation + coracoid process fracture
- Glenohumeral joint dislocation

TREATMENT

- Classification system based on injury to AC and CC ligaments and severity and direction of displacement of clavicle
  - I: Sprain of AC ligaments; CC ligaments intact; no increase in CC distance
  - II: Disruption of AC ligaments and sprain of CC ligaments; increase in CC distance <25%; weighted views would show equal CC distances
  - III: Disruption of AC and CC ligaments; CC distance 25–100%; deltotrapezial fascia is intact
  - IV: Disruption of AC and CC ligaments; clavicle is posteriorly displaced into deltotrapezial fascia; may not have significant superior displacement
  - V: Disruption of AC and CC ligaments; marked superior displacement of clavicle with CC distance of 100–300%; torn deltotrapezial fascia
  - VI: Disruption of AC ligaments +/– CC ligaments; inferior displacement of clavicle in either subacromial (CC ligaments intact) or subcoracoid (CC ligaments disrupted) location; subcoracoid dislocation associated with severe injury, rib fractures, and clavicle fracture
- Treatment
  - Types I and II
    - Ice and sling for comfort for 1–2 weeks
    - Return to activity when full pain-free range of motion present
    - May take longer in type II injuries
    - Kenny Howard brace – presses down on clavicle and pushes arm upwards
      - Must be worn 24 hours a day
      - Can cause skin breakdown over clavicle and anterior interosseous nerve palsy
    - Pts w/ type II may develop persistent symptoms in future secondary to posttraumatic degeneration, osteolysis of distal clavicle, loose cartilage fragments, or unstable meniscus
      - Treat with distal clavicle excision +/– CC stabilization
      - Distal clavicle excisions fare poorly if grade II injury present
  - Type III
    - Operative vs. nonoperative treatment remains controversial
    - Literature unclear on the matter, but careful review reveals that recent trend is to opt for nonoperative treatment

- Patients treated nonoperatively recover sooner, with no difference in strength or pain
- Exceptions to this are in overhead laborers and perhaps throwing athletes
- Nonoperative treatment
  - Sling for 2–4 weeks
  - Early pendulum and ROM exercises
  - Begin strengthening at 4–6 weeks
  - Avoid contact sports for 4–8 weeks
- Types IV and V
  - Operative treatment recommended
  - Early (first 2 weeks) surgery results are better than late surgery
  - Type IV tends to be more painful
  - Type V symptomatology generally relative to degree of displacement
- Type VI
  - Operative treatment recommended
  - Excision of distal clavicle facilitates reduction
- Operative treatment
  - Acute indications are grades IV, V, and VI separations
  - Relative indications include grade III separations in overhead laborers
  - >30 operative techniques described
  - Transfer of coracoacromial ligament with or without CC fixation (Weaver-Dunn)
    - Distal clavicle may or may not be resected
    - Late AC joint degeneration avoided with resection
    - CC fixation achieved with suture or synthetic material through a drill hole in the clavicle
    - Placing cerclage around clavicle causes abnormal anteriorization of clavicle and potential for material to cut through clavicle
    - Avoid use of permanent synthetic tapes (Dacron or Mersilene) due to foreign body reaction and late infection
  - CC fixation
    - Screw placed through clavicle into coracoid
    - Biomechanically strong
    - Perform in conjunction with repair of ligaments when done acutely
    - Requires removal at 8 weeks

- Technically difficult
- Easy to drill into coracoid but often screw can "blow out" the coracoid
- May abnormally anteriorize the clavicle
➤ AC fixation
  - Kirschner wires across AC joint
  - Can be done percutaneously without repair of CC ligaments or open with repair
  - Violates joint and can lead to arthritis
  - Requires second procedure for hardware removal
  - Pins can migrate!
  - Never use smooth pins
➤ Dynamic muscle transfer
  - Transfer of coracoid with short head of biceps to clavicle
  - Exchange of a dynamic constraint for a static one
  - Half have continued aching
  - Risk of injury to musculocutaneous nerve
■ Rehabilitation
  ➤ Sling for 6 weeks
  ➤ Daily pendulum exercises started at week 1
  ➤ No active forward flexion or abduction for 6 weeks
  ➤ No lifting of any kind for 6 weeks
  ➤ Start progressive active range of motion and strengthening at 6 weeks

DISPOSITION
N/A

PROGNOSIS
■ Nonoperative treatment of grade III injuries appears to be equivalent to surgery
  ➤ Earlier return with nonoperative treatment
■ Nonoperated athletes may return to play when range of motion full and strength normal
■ Operatively treated athletes should avoid contact for 6 months
■ Complications of surgery
  ➤ Loss of reduction
  ➤ Infection
  ➤ Deltoid dehiscence
  ➤ Calcification of CC ligaments (not a problem; seen also in nonoperative treatment)

> Erosion of fixation through clavicle
> Foreign body reaction to synthetic tapes

CAVEATS AND PEARLS
- Results of surgery done within a few weeks of injury are superior to those done chronically
- Grade IV separations don't always have superior displacement
- No need for aggressive rehabilitation
- A small amount of superior displacement can be expected after reconstruction
- Conoid ligament (medial) controls vertical stability
- Trapezoid ligament (lateral) controls axial load of joint
- Superior and posterior AC ligaments control anterior-posterior motion
- Only 5–8° of motion at AC joint
  > Clavicle does rotate 40–50° with full elevation of shoulder
  > Upward rotation of clavicle is combined with downward rotation of the scapula, controlled by CC ligaments (synchronous scapuloclavicular rotation)
  > AC or CC fixation has little effect on shoulder motion

ACUTE CARTILAGE INJURIES OF THE KNEE

KENT E. YINGER, MD
BERT R. MANDELBAUM, MD
REVISED BY CHARLES NOFSINGER, MD

HISTORY
- Work or recreational injury
- Mechanism
  > Landing impact injury with isolated chondral defect
  > Noncontact injury with sudden deceleration or cutting, associated meniscal or ligamentous injury
  > Contact injury with varus or valgus force, associated meniscal or ligamentous injury
- Painful
- May have mechanical symptoms (e.g., locking, catching) from chondral flap

PHYSICAL EXAM
- Moderate effusion

- May have hemarthrosis on aspiration if osteochondral fracture
- Tender over affected condyle, plateau, or patellofemoral joint ±
  joint line tenderness

STUDIES
- Radiographs
  - AP, lateral sunrise (three or four views)
  - Normal
- MRI
  - Will show signal changes at articular surface and possibly sub-
    chondral bone bruise
  - Necessary to detect associated meniscal or ligament pathology

DIFFERENTIAL DIAGNOSIS
- Meniscal tear
- Osteochondritis dissecans
- Atraumatic osteonecrosis/avascular necrosis

TREATMENT
- Evaluate alignment
  - If malalignment, consider osteotomy
- Arthroscopy to determine lesion:
  - Size
  - Containment
  - Depth
- Depth of lesion (Outerbridge classification)
  - Grade I – Softening of cartilage
  - Grade II – Fibrillations
  - Grade III – Fissuring
  - Grade IV – Full thickness to bone
- Grade I – No treatment
- Grade II and III
  - Arthroscopic debridement results in replacement with fibrocar-
    tilage – poor wear characteristics
- Grade IV
  - Mesenchymal stem cell stimulation
    - Microfracture or drilling into subchondral bone results in
      replacement with fibrocartilage
  - Substitution replacement
    - Replacement of defect with autograft or allograft plug(s); also
      known as mosaicplasty or OATS procedure

➤ Biologic replacement
- Requires two surgeries: autologous chondrocytes are harvested and cultured, then later placed into the defect and covered with periostium
- Results in hyaline cartilage – better wear characteristics

DISPOSITION
N/A

PROGNOSIS
- Acute cartilage injury results in release of degradative enzymes (stromelysin), which contributes to further cartilage breakdown.
- Treatment with thermal probe may cause death down to subchondral bone.
- Partial-thickness lesions do not heal without treatment
  ➤ May cause meniscal injury and cartilage injury to opposite side of joint
- Full-thickness defects 0–1 cm^2 that are well contained do well with drilling or microfracture
- Full-thickness defects 1–2 cm^2 that are well contained do well with drilling, microfracture, or OATS procedure
  ➤ 50–70% good results at 5 years
- Full-thickness defects >2 cm^2 that are well contained do well with autologous chondrocyte implantation
  ➤ Depending on location 70–90% good results at 8–10 years
  ➤ Can be treated with OATS procedure with minimal long-term data available
- Large poorly contained lesions have lower probability of regeneration success
  ➤ Result in lower levels of function that ultimately may require TKA
  ➤ Can be treated with large shell allografts (experimental)

CAVEATS AND PEARLS
- Early arthroscopy for classification and treatment will prevent additional chondral and meniscal injury.
- Meniscal pathology, ligamentous instability, and significant malalignment, if untreated, will all result in chondral injury.
- Advances in imaging technology are not yet sufficient to detect and classify these injuries.

ACUTE COMPARTMENT SYNDROME

JEFFREY GUY, MD
REVISED BY CHARLES NOFSINGER, MD

HISTORY

- *Definition:* Increased pressure in a confined tissue space that reduces capillary blood flow below a level necessary for viability of normal tissue
- *Etiology 1:* Increased volume within a closed space (i.e., trauma, hemorrhage, or reperfusion injury)
- *Etiology 2:* Decreased size of an enclosed space (i.e. cast, constrictive dressing, or MAST trousers)

Pathogenesis

- Muscle injury: edema/hemorrhage – Increased pressure in enclosed space – ischemia – further soft tissue damage
- Circulatory injury: Swelling with reperfusion – increased pressure in enclosed space – ischemia – further soft tissue damage
- Muscle ischemia reversible up to 4 hours, irreversible after 8
- Nerve ischemia results in reversible neuropraxia under 3 hours and irreversible after 8

Compartments

- Anterior
- Lateral
- Deep posterior
- Superficial posterior

PHYSICAL EXAM

- Five P's: Pain, Pallor, Paresthesias, Pulselessness, Paralysis
- Pain out of proportion to injury
- Pain with passive stretch of foot
- Pallor skin tone
- Loss of or decreased pulses (uncommon and/or a very late finding)
- Paralysis or sensory changes after ischemia >1 hour
- Tense, swollen compartments (most sensitive finding)
- Glossy appearance of skin

STUDIES
- Labs
  - Elevated CPK values are common with ischemia but also elevated in trauma
- **Compartment pressure measurement**
  - Indicated in polytrauma, obtunded patient, or with inconclusive clinical diagnosis
  - Direct measurement of involved compartments using needle catheter such as a Stryker STIC catheter, WICK catheter, or transducer from arterial line
  - Pressure threshold requiring fasciotomy is controversial.
  - Multiple sampling sites, with the highest value recorded and used to determine the need for fasciotomy
  - Fasciotomy recommended with a measured pressure >35 mmHg or a pressure 20 mmHg below the measured diastolic blood pressure (number varies)

DIFFERENTIAL DIAGNOSIS
- Compartment syndrome is a surgical emergency. If clinically suspected, then the diagnosis is compartment syndrome until proven otherwise.

TREATMENT
- Nonoperative
  - Remove compressive dressings, casts, etc.
  - Elevate leg to level of heart only.
  - Compartment measurements if clinically suspicious
- Operative
  - Two-incision fasciotomy to decompress compartments
  - Anterolateral incision – half the distance between fibula and tibial crest; used to decompress the anterior and lateral compartments
  - Beware exiting superficial peroneal nerve through fascial defect distally
  - Posterior medial incision – 2 cm posterior to medial tibia
  - Delayed primary closure at 4–7 days with possible skin graft if needed

DISPOSITION
N/A

PROGNOSIS
- Good if recognized and treated early
- Poor if delayed diagnosis and/or intervention

Complications
- Infection
- Claw toes
- Dysfunctional extremity
- Amputation

CAVEATS AND PEARLS
- Early recognition is the key to successful treatment.
- Remember the five P's.
- If you are thinking about checking the compartment pressures, check them!
- Acute compartment syndrome is a surgical emergency.

ACUTE FRACTURES OF THE FIFTH METATARSAL

SCOTT A. RODEO, MD
REVISED BY CHARLES NOFSINGER, MD

HISTORY
- Three distinctly different patterns
  - Avulsion fracture of styloid process
  - Transverse fracture of proximal diaphysis (Jones fracture)
  - Distal spiral fractures (Ballet fracture)
- Avulsion fractures occur by inversion mechanism.
- Jones fracture common in running, jumping sports
- May report prodrome of pain prior to presentation with Jones fracture, suggesting stress reaction in bone
- Lateral foot pain with weight-bearing

PHYSICAL EXAM
- Tenderness over base of fifth metatarsal
- Pain with active eversion of foot
- May have pain with passive inversion
- Be sure to examine lateral ankle ligament stability.

STUDIES
- Plain radiographs (AP, lateral, oblique)
  - Avulsion type is usually extra-articular
  - Three patterns Jones fracture: acute, delayed union, nonunion
- True acute Jones fracture will have sharp fracture line, no intra-medullary sclerosis.
- Delayed union: see some evidence of pre-existing fracture (wider fracture gap, some intramedullary sclerosis)
- Don't confuse avulsion type with two sesamoids: os peroneum (in peroneus logus) and os vesalianum (in peroneus brevis).
- Don't confuse avulsion type with unfused apophysis at base of fifth metatarsal (closes age 16).

DIFFERENTIAL DIAGNOSIS
- Stress fracture
- Lateral ankle ligament injury
- Injury to cuboid-metatarsal joint
- Peroneus brevis tendinitis/tenosynovitis

TREATMENT
- Avulsion fracture of styloid process
  - Short-leg walking cast 2–3 weeks
  - Weight-bear as tolerated
  - Even nonunion of this type of fracture can be left alone.
- Symptomatic nonunion (rare): excise fragment, repair peroneus brevis
- Displaced intra-articular avulsion fracture (rare): consider open reduction/internal fixation
- Jones fracture
  - Acute: nonweight-bearing cast immobilization 6–8 weeks
    - Consider surgical treatment in athlete
  - Delayed union: consider trial of nonweight-bearing cast, immobilization, may require surgery
  - Nonunion: surgery
    - Medullary curettage and inlay bone graft or closed intra-medullary screw fixation with 4.5-mm malleolar screw
    - Use largest screw diameter possible.
  - Postop: nonweight-bearing cast for 2 weeks, followed by progressive weight-bearing in hard-soled shoe
- Ballet fracture
  - Short-leg walking cast or Cam walker

DISPOSITION
N/A

PROGNOSIS
- Acute fractures heal in 6–8 weeks.
- Delayed union treated conservatively may take >1 year for full healing.
- Nonunion treated with surgery heals in average 3 months.
- Return to sports after surgery: approximately 8 weeks
- Complications of screw fixation
  - Screw fracture
  - Screw protrusion out of metatarsal
  - Tenderness over screw head
  - Refracture

CAVEATS AND PEARLS
- These fractures have propensity for nonunion due to poor blood supply.
- Refracture can occur if return to sports too early.
- Use of foot orthosis recommended for early return to sports
- Plain radiographs may not be sensitive enough to determine healing – Consider CT or tomograms.
- If refracture occurs after return to sports, consider exchange to larger screw or use of inlay bone graft.

ACUTE NAVICULAR FRACTURE

MAYO A. NOERDLINGER, MD

HISTORY
- History of trauma
- Midfoot pain and swelling

PHYSICAL EXAM
- Swelling and exquisite pain on dorsomedial aspect of midfoot
- Dorsal lip avulsion – two ligaments insert on dorsum of navicular
  - Dorsal talonavicular
    - Stressed with inversion and plantarflexion
  - Anterior aspect of deltoid ligament
    - Stressed with eversion

- Tuberosity fractures
  - ➤ Result of acute valgus or eversion injury increases stress on posterior tibialis tendon

STUDIES
- AP, oblique, and lateral radiographs
  - ➤ Examine closely for midtarsal joint (Lisfranc) injuries
- Bone scans, CT scan, MRI for occult fractures
- Differentiate acute tuberosity fracture from accessory navicular
  - ➤ Accessory navicular is smooth and regular

DIFFERENTIAL DIAGNOSIS
- Cuneiform and cuboid fractures
- Navicular stress fracture
  - ➤ Running or jumping athletes
- Navicular avulsion fracture

TREATMENT
- Dorsal lip avulsion
  - ➤ Conservative
    - Weight-bearing cast for 4–6 weeks
  - ➤ Open reduction and internal fixation if fragment is >25% of navicular
- Displaced acute fractures treated with anatomic and stable internal fixation
  - ➤ Anatomic reduction of talonavicular joint more critical
    - Mobility of this joint is important for function
  - ➤ Anatomic reduction of anterior and distal navicular not critical
    - Naviculocuneiform joints have little motion

DISPOSITION
N/A

PROGNOSIS
- Navicular is largely covered with articular cartilage
  - ➤ Not much room for nutrient vessels to enter
  - ➤ Makes the tarsal navicular subject to osteonecrosis

CAVEATS AND PEARLS
- Located in the uppermost part of the arch, the navicular is the keystone for vertical stress on the arch
- Anatomic reduction essential to restore talonavicular motion

ANTERIOR CRUCIATE LIGAMENT INJURY

BERNARD R. BACH, JR., MD

HISTORY

- Mechanism: sudden deceleration, cutting, valgus force contact or noncontact, hyperextension
- Patient may recall pop or tearing sensation – 80%
- Painful, inability to continue activity
- Rapid hemarthrosis within 3 hours – 80%
- If chronic may have history of recurrent instability
- Common sports: skiing, basketball, volleyball, football, soccer
- May be isolated or in conjunction with multiple ligament injuries – medial collateral (MCL), posterior cruciate (PCL), posterolateral or knee dislocation
- Often associated with meniscal pathology and/or articular cartilage injury
- Knee instability complaints: jumping, twisting, deceleration, cutting activities

PHYSICAL EXAM

- Acute: effusion, bloody hemarthrosis if aspirated
- Joint line tenderness suggestive of associated meniscal pathology
- Ligament laxity exam – compare to uninjured knee
- Abnormal Lachman test most sensitive test
- Increased anterior tibial translation @ 20–30° knee fusion
- Positive pivot shift test (Losee, Hughston, flexion rotator drawer variants)
- Pathognomonic of complete anterior cruciate ligament (ACL) injury
- Subluxation – Reduction phenomenon related to axial compression, valgus loading, and flexion/extension occurred at 15–30°
- Associated ligament laxity tests
  - ➤ MCL – Valgus laxity at 0°, 30°
  - ➤ Lateral collateral ligament – Valgus laxity at 0°, 30°
  - ➤ PCL – Increased posterior translation at 90° (posterior drawer), posterior sag test (gravity flexion test)
  - ➤ Posterolateral – Increased posterolateral rotation, increased external tibial rotation, asymmetric dial test
- Locked knee – Displaced bucket handle meniscal tear, rule out associated ACL injury

STUDIES

- Radiographs
  - AP, lateral, tunnel, Merchant (four views)
  - Generally normal
  - Lateral capsular sign (Segond fracture): marginal avulsion fracture from anterolateral tibial plateau pathognomonic
  - Lateral notch sign (chronic ACL): accentuation of indentation of sulcus terminalis in lateral femoral condyle; rarely seen with PCL/posterolateral corner (PLC) injury
  - Chronic ACL deficiency: periarticular osteophytes, tibial eminence peaking, intercondylar notch narrowing
- MRI
  - Highly sensitive/specific for ACL injury
  - Generally does not differentiate between partial or complete ACL injury
  - Associated meniscal pathology common
  - Bone bruise noted (80%), lateral femoral condyle, lateral tibial condyle most common
  - Effusion frequently noted
  - MRI value: detecting associated meniscal pathology and articular cartilage pathology
- KT-1000
  - Instrumented laxity testing device
  - Measures side-to-side differences (SSD) and absolute translation
  - Dx: maximum manual SSD >3 mm; 30-pound anterior translation >10 mm

DIFFERENTIAL DIAGNOSIS

- Hemarthrosis
  - ACL, patellar dislocation, peripheral meniscal tear, intra-articular fracture, PCL injury, popliteus tendon avulsion
- Instability
  - Patellar instability
  - Meniscal tear (e.g., bucket handle)
  - Posterolateral
  - Quad weakness – giving way with level walking/standing

TREATMENT

- Acute
  - Establish diagnosis

- ➤ Ice, resolution of swelling, closed-chain quad motion recovery
- ➤ Avoid immobilization
- ➤ Physical therapy
- ➤ Consider MRI
- ■ Treatment considerations
  - ➤ Age
  - ➤ Activity level
    - Category I sports (e.g., basketball, football, soccer, volleyball)
  - ➤ Associated injuries (e.g., meniscus, MCL)
  - ➤ Amount of pathologic laxity (e.g., Grade 2 or 3 pivot)
  - ➤ Sports participation
  - ➤ Expectation
  - ➤ KT-1000 maximum manual (>6 mm SSD, poor prognosis)
- ■ Treatment options
  - ➤ Nonsurgical
    - Activity modification mandatory
    - ACL brace – Low-level activities
      - Does not prevent instability
      - Reduces severity and frequency of instability
    - May require arthroscopy for meniscal pathology
  - ➤ Surgical: tissue options
    - Patellar tendon autograft
    - Hamstrings
    - Quadriceps tendon
    - Allograft
      - Irradiated vs. nonirradiated
      - Patellar tendon vs. Achilles tendon

DISPOSITION
N/A

PROGNOSIS
- ■ Nonsurgical treatment
  - ➤ Low probability of high-level sports participation
  - ➤ High likelihood of recurrent injuries – meniscal, articular
  - ➤ Subjective satisfaction generally low
  - ➤ 50% function due to ACL functional brace
- ■ Surgical treatment
  - ➤ Preferred for most individuals
  - ➤ Stability success 85–90%
  - ➤ Patient satisfaction 95%

➤ Patellar pain testing variable (10–40%)
➤ Side-to-side functional testing: 40–90% normal
■ Return to play
➤ Nonoperative
• Should be braced
• Usually 4–6 weeks
• Caution that reinjury common
➤ Reconstructive
• Graft and sport dependent
• 4–6 months most surgeons; others recommend 6–9 months
• Criteria – Normal stability, motion functional testing within 10–15%
■ Complications of surgical treatment
➤ Infection (1%)
➤ Deep venous thrombosis, pulmonary embolus (1%)
➤ Patellar fracture, patellar tendon rupture (1%)
➤ Loss of motor (extension and/or flexion)
➤ Recurrent laxity (micro/macrotraumatic)
➤ Reinjury (5–10%) – Time-dependent
➤ Opposite side ACL injury – More common than graft disruption

CAVEATS AND PEARLS
■ Suspect ACL injury in athlete with hemarthrosis.
■ A patient with a displaced bucket handle meniscal tear (locked knee) has an ACL injury until proven otherwise.
■ "Partial" ACL injuries are extremely uncommon (<5%); athlete has an ACL-deficient knee until proven otherwise.
■ ACL diagnosis is established by history and exam; MRI should not be used to establish diagnosis.
■ ACL reconstructive surgery is not a surgical emergency.
■ Postop motion complications reduced with delayed surgical treatment
■ Beware of associated MCL injury, which may contribute to delayed motion recovery.
■ Medial meniscal tears more common in chronic ACL knees; lateral meniscal tears more common in acute injuries
■ Postoperative ACL bracing controversial
■ ACL injuries three to four times more common in females (multifactorial)
■ Accelerated rehab programs for patellar tendon graft current standard

- Surgical results similar for patellar tendon vs. hamstring autograft
- Surgical results of single- vs. double-incision arthroscopic techniques similar
- Current graft choices: patellar tendon autograft, hamstring, quadriceps tendon, nonirradiated patellar tendon allograft
- Outpatient ACL reconstruction feasible
- Postop continuous passive motion is longer standard of care
- Avoid open-chain quad extension exercises during rehab.

ANTERIOR KNEE PAIN

WILLIAM R. POST, MD
REVISED BY CHARLES NOFSINGER, MD

HISTORY

- Onset: insidious or activity-related
- Blunt trauma common
- Consider overuse: increased/unusual activity for individual
- Watch for some cause of weakness (systemic or local) preceding onset (creates relative overload)
- Question carefully: precipitating factor(s)
- Pain: typically peripatellar; often poorly localized
- Nature of pain: achy dull or sharp
- Giving way with knee flexion-quad weakness
- Pain worse with prolonged knee flexion and stair climbing
- Patient-drawn pain diagrams correlate with examination tenderness

PHYSICAL EXAM

- Standing alignment: varus/valgus/squinting patellae
- Have patient squat and stand to screen for severity
- Evaluate quadriceps atrophy and tone
- Peripatellar palpation: define tender soft structures
  - Quadriceps, vastus lateralis and patellar tendons
  - Retinaculum, medial and lateral
  - Previous scars for possible neuroma
- Evaluate for effusion
  - May cause reflex quad inhibition
  - Anterior knee pain may develop secondary to weakness
  - Consider other intra-articular cause of effusion (meniscal or chondral pathology)

- Compress patella into trochlea at various angles of flexion
  - Remember, the patella doesn't enter the trochlea until about 10–15°.
  - This localizes location of articular lesion.
- Leg length discrepancy
- Evaluate patellar mobility: ? patellar tilt
- Test iliotibial band flexibility (Ober's test)
- Check quadriceps flexibility (prone vs. supine knee flexion)
  - Heel should reach the buttock or at least be symmetric with other leg
  - >10° = quad contracture
- Evaluate hamstring, gastrocsoleus, and hip flexor flexibility
- Evaluate hip motion, flexibility, and irritability
- Straight leg raise to rule out lumbar radiculopathy

STUDIES
- Radiographs
  - AP, lateral, 45° patellar axial view with both patellae
    - Evaluate for arthrosis.
    - Evaluate for coexisting bone pathology.
  - Radiographic alignment
    - Is alignment symmetric with contralateral asymptomatic knee?
    - Is lateral border of patella tilted laterally (rotated posteriorly)?
    - Is patella translated laterally (subluxed laterally)?
- MRI scan
  - Indicated in workup of anterior knee pain if surgery contemplated
  - Can document depth of cartilage lesions
  - Helpful to document malalignment before realignment surgery
  - Images patellar alignment earlier in flexion than plain axial radiographs
  - More sensitive for soft tissue malalignment since less bony trochlear constraint in early flexion
- Bone scan
  - Helpful to document component of suspected articular overload
  - Unique compared to static tests above since it images biologic uptake

DIFFERENTIAL DIAGNOSIS
- Anterior knee pain is a symptom, not a diagnosis.

- Typical pathophysiology: Overload causes microinjury with possible inflammation
  - Pain secondary to above decreases activity
  - Stiffness/weakness result
  - Joint less able to absorb applied loads due to less elastic soft tissues
  - Less muscle strength to absorb eccentric loads
  - Result in further microinjury if loads applied exceed ability to absorb
  - Loss of biologic homeostasis
- Usual cause: loss of biologic homeostasis due to supraphysiologic loading
  - Repetitive
  - Acute blunt trauma
  - Combination of both
- Less common causes
  - Medial plica syndrome
  - Neuroma
  - Posterior cruciate ligament deficiency: 70% have anterior knee pain
  - Anterior cruciate ligament deficiency: 25% have anterior knee pain
  - Effusion of any source
  - Referred pain from hip in children (Perthes/slipped capital femoral epiphysis)
  - Sciatic, femoral, or saphenous nerve pathology
  - Neuroma

TREATMENT
- Surgery rarely necessary
- Avoid provocative activity
  - Patients must understand this and cooperate
  - Prescribed exercise must not provoke severe pain
  - Progress slowly
- Exercises to restore flexibility and strength
  - Quadriceps strengthening, especially vastus medialis obliquus
  - Many patients tolerate closed-chain strengthening better
  - Avoid isokinetic strengthening
  - Avoid open-chain quad strengthening
- Avoid painful arc of motion during early rehab
  - Gentle persistent stretching, especially prone quad stretch
- Physical methods that help with pain by control of alignment

- ➤ Patellar taping works well to decrease pain, likely by affecting soft tissue tension
- ➤ Knee sleeves with lateral patellar buttress
- ➤ Counterforce straps if pain localized to patellar or quad tendons
- ➤ Semirigid orthotics if excessive hindfoot pronation
- ■ Pain control: ice, analgesics, NSAIDs
- ■ Gradual return to desired activities
- ■ Surgery: depends on diagnosis
- ■ These principles are for pain, not patellar instability.
- ■ Surgical principles: resect localized synovial or chondral pathology, correct malalignment, and unload articular lesions
  - ➤ Arthroscopic debridement of plica (pathologic hypertrophic plica syndrome)
  - ➤ Chondroplasty: unstable chondral pathology without malalignment
  - ➤ Lateral release: excessive lateral patellar tilt
    - Contraindicated in hypermobile patients
    - Be cautious in patients with patellar instability
    - Caveat: medial patellar facet chondromalacia
  - ➤ Lateral release with anteromedialization (AMZ) of tibial tubercle
    - Lateral tilt with moderately advanced lateral patellar facet arthrosis
  - ➤ Chondral resurfacing not very successful in patellar or trochlear lesions

DISPOSITION
N/A

PROGNOSIS
- ■ Nonoperative treatment successful in >90%
  - ➤ Follow-up: 4–6 weeks
- ■ Return to activity depends on chronicity and severity of problem.
- ■ Use objective flexibility measures in follow-up.
- ■ Surgery results
  - ➤ Lateral release 90% good/excellent if minimal arthrosis and isolated tilt
  - ➤ Chondroplasty
  - ➤ Plica excision check
  - ➤ Lateral release/AMZ results consistent and durable.

CAVEATS AND PEARLS
- ■ Anterior knee pain is a symptom, not a specific pathology.

- Define specific pathology to treat successfully.
- History critical: uncover relevant factors
- Prescribe specific exercise program based on correcting flexibility deficits and using modalities over sites of greatest tenderness.
- Modify exercise/activities to reduce pain.
- Evaluate hip strength and flexibility; deficits common.
- Articular tenderness less common than soft tissue
- Always evaluate prone quad flexibility and hamstring flexibility.

ATHLETIC PUBALGIA

WILLIAM E. GARRETT, JR., MD, PhD

HISTORY
- Pain in groin with high-intensity exercise
- Onset usually insidious
- May follow an acute injury after many weeks
- Especially painful with powerful kicks, as in soccer
- Painful with sprinting, jumping, or hurdling
- Pain with powerful rotation of torso around hips
- Usually unilateral, may be bilateral
- Preponderance in men
- Usually in high-level athletes rather than recreational
- Often follows or accompanies adductor longus injury
- Common in soccer, hockey, football
- Diagnosis usually made primarily on history

PHYSICAL EXAM
- Tenderness just lateral to rectus abdominis insertion on pubis
- Tenderness at site of direct inguinal hernia
- Pain with sit-ups
- Pain with flexion and adduction of hip
- Pain above inguinal ligament
- No direct or indirect hernia
- Normal hip motion
- Not tender at adductor longus attachment unless coexistent with adductor strain
- May be tender over symphysis pubis
- Physical exam without characteristic history may not be convincing

STUDIES
- Radiographs of pelvis and hips usually normal
- Radiographs occasionally show reactive changes in symphysis
- MRI often negative in chronic cases
- MRI in acute injuries may show adductor longus or rectus abdominis strain
- MRI in acute injuries may show bone reaction in pubic symphysis or at attachment sites of involved muscles

DIFFERENTIAL DIAGNOSIS
- Adductor longus injury
  - Characteristic acute injury
  - Pain with abduction of hip and active adduction
  - Chronic conditions may have elements of athletic pubalgia and adductor strain
- Inguinal hernia
  - Palpation can reveal defect and bulge with Valsalva maneuver
  - General surgical consultation helpful
- Stress fracture of pubis
  - Tenderness over bone rather than soft tissue
  - Usually more frequent in women
  - Bone scan differentiates if there is question
- Rectus abdominis strain
  - Acute injury
  - Local tenderness at site of injury
- Osteitis pubis
  - Tender over symphysis pubis
  - Radiographs show widening, sclerosis, bone resorption
  - Often coexists with adductor or abdominal muscle injury

TREATMENT
- Acute
  - Rest from painful activity, especially in acute cases
  - Therapy to include:
    - Abdominal muscle and adductor stretching
    - Abdominal muscle strengthening, especially rectus abdominis and obliques
  - Nonsteroidal anti-inflammatory drugs
  - Return to activity as symptoms allow

- Chronic
  - ➤ Same therapy as for acute injuries
  - ➤ Extensive warm-up and stretch before athletic activity
- Surgery
  - ➤ Indications
    - Pain limits or prohibits performance
    - No improvement with conservative treatment
  - ➤ Procedure
    - Pelvic floor repair similar to Bassini-type herniorrhaphy for direct inguinal hernia
    - Usually performed by a general surgeon
    - Endoscopic procedures have been done successfully but documentation is lacking
    - May be done as an outpatient
    - May resume play in 2–3 months
    - Also need to address simultaneous pathology in adductor longus muscle and tenotomize if involved
    - Adductor problems often addressed by orthopedic surgeons

DISPOSITION
N/A

PROGNOSIS
- Conservative treatment most helpful in acute conditions but success rate unknown
- Operative treatment has high rate of success for isolated athletic pubalgia
- Patients can usually return in 3 months or less
- Complications infrequent

CAVEATS AND PEARLS
- Problem is more widespread than realized in soccer, hockey, and other sports.
- Diagnosis is difficult because of the relative lack of objective signs or tests.
- History is most characteristic element.
- Problem is often bilateral.
- There must be an (as yet not understood) relationship between adductor, abdominal, and pubic symphysis conditions.
- Rapport and involvement of a general surgeon are essential. A general surgeon colleague who understands this problem should be a part of the decision-making team.

AXILLARY VEIN THROMBOSIS

MARK BOWEN, MD

HISTORY
- Uncommon but >= arterial occlusions
- Mechanism
  - Primary – repetitive trauma of upper extremity – so-called effort thrombosis
  - Secondary – hypercoaguability, iatrogenic trauma from central venous catheter
- Primary – athletic, dominant extremity, males
- Compression at costoclavicular space most common
- Anatomic structures include subclavius muscle and first rib
- Direct trauma or stretch may injure vessel wall
- Thrombosis after clavicle fracture and figure-8 treatment also reported
- Minor symptoms = easy fatigability
- Major symptoms = pain, swelling
- Symptoms typically develop in first 24 hours

PHYSICAL EXAM
- Diffuse swelling, shoulder to hand
- Mottled, cyanotic discoloration with dependent rubor
- Palpation of axilla may reveal thrombosed cord
- Shoulder range of motion diminishes due to swelling
- Normal arterial exam

STUDIES
- Radiographs
  - Usually normal, unless associated with traumatic injury
  - Evaluate lower cervical, upper thoracic spine for anomalous ribs
- Venous Doppler exam
  - Noninvasive
  - Lab, operator dependent
- Venography
  - Gold standard
  - Documents size and location of thrombus
  - Small occlusion may progress in size
  - Documents recanalization

DIFFERENTIAL DIAGNOSIS
- Other trauma to athlete's arm
- Muscle strain, contusion
- Thoracic outlet syndrome
- Bone or soft tissue infection
- Cellulitis
- Systemic clotting abnormality
- Fracture – traumatic or pathologic
- Compartment syndrome

TREATMENT
- Immobilization, strict rest
- Elevation
- Nonsurgical
  - Anticoagulants prevent propagation, embolus
  - Thrombolytics (streptokinase, urokinase)
    - Some reports of increased risk of bleeding
- Surgical – acute
  - Appropriate when concern for chronic symptoms is high
  - Recommend first rib resection or scalene resection
  - Decompression area depends on pathology
  - Role for thrombectomy unknown
- Surgical – chronic
  - Recurrent symptoms

DISPOSITION
N/A

PROGNOSIS
- Good, but concern for swelling and return of function
- Competitive athlete – high risk of recurrence if underlying cause not corrected surgically
- Complications
  - Pulmonary embolism
  - Persistent swelling
  - Exertional fatigue and pain

CAVEATS AND PEARLS
- Unusual problem
- In athletes, look for repetitive overhead activity, fatigue, swelling
- Diagnostic test of choice: venogram for total information
- In competitive athletes, consider correcting underlying cause

BIPARTITE PATELLA

MATTHEW SHAPIRO, MD

HISTORY

- Result of congenital abnormality (failure of accessory ossification centers to fuse)
- Occurs in 2–5% of knees
- Usually exists as an asymptomatic fibrocartilaginous union (synchondrosis) of superolateral patellar ossification (75% of cases); also may occur inferiorly or at lateral margin
- Commonly an incidental finding on x-ray
- <15% are symptomatic
- Bilateral in 40%
- May be associated with traumatic knee injury
- Often becomes painful as a result of a direct blow to the patella (dashboard mechanism); fibrous union is injured and ossification becomes unstable and painful

PHYSICAL EXAM

- Tenderness present at (usually) superolateral portion of patella
- May be a sense of instability of ossification

STUDIES

- Visible as distinct ossification attached to main body of patella via pseudarthrosis
- Most typically exists at superolateral portion of patella
- Skyline view taken with patient squatting may reveal motion (Ishikawa view)
- Also visible on CT or MRI (again, usually incidental finding)

DIFFERENTIAL DIAGNOSIS

- Dashboard mechanism also associated with patella fracture, prepatellar bursitis, retropatellar traumatic chondromalacia, and posterior cruciate ligament rupture
- May be mistakenly referred as a patellar fracture
- May be confused with a lateral facet fracture; true fractures are usually longitudinal rather than oblique
- Must be differentiated from patellar stress fracture (rare)

TREATMENT

- Treat symptomatically.

- Often pain subsides with conservative treatment over several weeks.
- Consider corticosteroid injection if fragment remains painful.
- If conservative treatment fails, consider surgical excision.

DISPOSITION
N/A

PROGNOSIS
- Expect normal outcome with conservative or surgical treatment.

CAVEATS AND PEARLS
- After knee trauma, bipartite patella may be an incidental x-ray finding that is not connected to the injury; therefore, treatment should not be directed at the bipartite patella.

BOXER'S FRACTURE

JOHN FERNANDEZ, MD

HISTORY
- Symptoms
  - Pain at fracture site
  - Dorsal swelling
  - Deformity of hand/finger
- Mechanism
  - Direct impact injury metacarpal head/shaft
  - Common in football, basketball, boxing, wrestling, "hand combat" sports

PHYSICAL EXAM
- Assess for associated injuries
- Tendon ruptures/avulsions
- Metaphalangeal joint (MPJ) dislocations
- Carpal fractures/dislocations
- Dorsal swelling
- Tenderness to palpation
- Crepitance with palpation/motion
- Deformity
  - Malrotation of digit with flexion
  - Overlap of fingers
  - 5° of rotation = 1.5-cm overlap
- Dorsal prominence/angulation

- Loss of metacarpal height/shortening
- Loss in range of motion
- Extension loss at MPJ/proximal interphalangeal joint (PIPJ)
  - 2-mm shortening = 7° ext. loss
- Extrinsic tightness
  - Adhesions of extensor tendons
  - Less PIPJ flexion with MPJ flexion
- Intrinsic tightness
  - Contracture of intrinsic muscles
  - Less PIPJ flexion with MPJ extension
- Late findings
  - Deformity
  - Loss of motion
  - Loss of grip strength

STUDIES
- Radiographs
  - AP/lateral/oblique of hand
  - RF/SF: 30° supinated lateral
  - Points to assess
    - Shortening/loss of height
    - Angulation
    - Translation

DIFFERENTIAL DIAGNOSIS
- Contusion/soft tissue avulsion
- MPJ dislocation

TREATMENT
- Fracture considerations
  - Comminution
  - Proportional to energy of injury
  - Proportional to instability of fracture
  - Digits involved
  - Fracture "stabilized" by surrounding tissues
    - Intermetacarpal ligaments
    - Intrinsic muscles
  - Border metacarpals more likely to displace
    - Less soft tissue support
    - Index and small metacarpal
  - Ring/small fingers
    - Compensatory carpal metacarpal joint ROM
    - Increased deformity allowed

> Index/middle fingers
  - No compensatory carpal metacarpal ROM
  - Decreased deformity allowed
> Neck fracture
  - Allows for greater angular deformity
  - Compensation through MPJ ROM
> Assess for possible intra-articular involvement
- Acute
  > Splint in "intrinsic plus" position
  > Wrist 20° extension
  > MPJ 70° flexion
  > Interphalangeal joint full extension
  > Include adjacent uninjured digits
  > Strict elevation to limit swelling
  > Treatment-dependent factors
    - Stability of reduction
    - Residual alignment
- Criteria for acceptable alignment
  > Index/middle finger
    - Angulation: <10°
    - Shortening: <3 mm
    - Rotation: none
  > Ring/small finger
    - Angulation
      - SF: <40°
      - RF: <30°
    - Shortening: <3 mm
    - Rotation: none
- Nonoperative treatment
  > Reduction
    - Anesthetic block
      - Wrist level
      - Fracture level (hematoma block)
    - "Jahss" maneuver
      - Flex MPJ 90°
      - Flex PIPJ 90°
      - Support metacarpal shaft with fingers
      - Apply pressure to end of PIPJ with thumbs
    - Immobilize in "intrinsic plus" position
  > Cast or splint
    - Control rotation
    - "Buddy strap"

- Include adjacent uninjured digit
- Recheck reduction every week, 3 weeks
- After 3 weeks, recheck every 2–3 weeks
- After first 3 weeks, change splint/cast
- Consider placing in orthoplast splint
  - Allow interval ROM
  - Cut down splint
  - Allow PIPJ ROM
- Fracture requires 4–6 weeks to heal
- Radiographic healing may lag clinically
- Clinical healing occurs quickly
- If no pain to palpation/ROM
  - Allow ROM/early light use
- Allow normal use after radiographs healed
- Operative treatment
  - Indications
    - Unable to achieve acceptable reduction
    - Unable to maintain acceptable reduction
    - Unable to extend digit fully
    - "Pseudoclawing"
    - Significant swelling
    - Open injuries
    - Associated injuries
  - Several options depending on fracture type
    - Percutaneous pinning
    - Dorsal plating
    - Tension/cerclage wiring
    - Allows for early ROM
  - Percutaneous pinning
    - Intramedullary pin
    - Only if minimal comminution
    - 0.062/0.045 K-wire
    - Place through metacarpal head
    - Pull out proximal near wrist
    - Leave MPJ free to allow ROM
  - Cross-pinning
    - 0.045 K-wires
    - 1 pin proximal/2 pins distal to fracture
    - Pin to adjacent "intact" metacarpal
  - Dorsal plating
    - Comminuted fractures

- AO modular hand set
  - 2.7/2.5-mm plates
  - "Blade plate"
  - 2× longer than bone diameter
  - 2.7/2.0-mm screws
- ➤ Tension/cerclage wiring
  - 0.045/0.035 K-wires/24-gauge wire
- ➤ Postoperative management
  - Splint 1 week
  - Begin therapy in 1 week
  - Edema modalities
  - Scar massage
  - Protected ROM
  - Removable orthoplast splint
- Late
  - ➤ Malunion
    - Angular/rotational deformity
    - Osteotomy with ORIF
  - ➤ Nonunion
    - Revision ORIF with bone grafting
  - ➤ Loss of motion
    - MPJ release
    - Extensor tendon tenolysis

DISPOSITION
N/A

PROGNOSIS
- Nonoperative treatment
  - ➤ >90% good/excellent result, even with significant deformity
    - Return to play immediately
      - Padded splint/cast
    - Complications
      - Loss of MPJ ROM
      - Loss of extension
      - Malunion/nonunion
      - Deformity
- Operative treatment
  - ➤ Good results overall/25% complications
  - ➤ Risks
    - Outweighed by risk of malunion

- Infection
- Tendon adhesions
- Joint stiffness
➤ Return to play immediately
- Padded cast/splint
➤ Late repair/reconstruction
- Fair/poor result
- Complications
  - Residual deformity
  - MPJ/PIPJ stiffness

CAVEATS AND PEARLS
- Begin ROM as soon as possible.
- Refer to occupational therapist.
- Removable orthoplast splint
- Allow PIPJ ROM at very least.
- Try to use pins/screws when possible.
- Limit use of plates.
  ➤ More stripping necessary
  ➤ Increased adhesions/loss ROM
- Increase threshold for surgery if extensor lag in finger.
- Increase threshold for surgery if a lot of swelling.
- Always inform patient of residual deformity even with good retained function.
  ➤ Prominent dorsal bone
  ➤ Loss of metacarpal head profile with fist
  ➤ Mild rotational deformity

BRACHIAL NEUROPATHY (PARSONAGE-TURNER SYNDROME)

ELLIOTT HERSHMAN, MD

HISTORY
- Insidious onset of shoulder girdle pain
- Not associated with traumatic event
- Pain can be incapacitating, requiring narcotics
- Often described as "burning" pain
- Symptoms can develop during or following athletic activity
- Pain characteristically continues despite cessation of activity with shoulder

- May follow a viral illness or an immunization such as hepatitis B or influenza
- Symptoms usually unilateral

PHYSICAL EXAM
- Muscle weakness develops as acute pain subsides
- Proximal upper extremity muscles involved
- Rhomboid major and minor (dorsoscapular nerve), supraspinatus and infraspinatus (suprascapular nerve), deltoid (axillary nerve), and biceps nerve most commonly affected
- Scapular winging frequent
- Sensory deficit uncommon but can be present
- Multiple muscles affected, commonly due to diffuse plexus involvement
- Isolated or single nerve involvement has been clinically reported

STUDIES
- EMG
  - Most helpful test; confirms clinical impression
  - Diffuse plexus involvement present
  - Abnormalities present, 3 weeks after onset of paresis
  - Fibrillation potentials and positive waves consistent with denervation will appear
  - Distal nerve conductions normal (median/ulnar)
  - EMG abnormalities often present on contralateral, asymptomatic side, consistent with systemic condition
  - As strength recovers, giant polyphenic potentials appear on EMG needle exam, consistent with neural sprouting and recovery
- MRI
  - Weakened muscles may show high signal intensity on T2 imaging
  - Atrophy of involved muscles noted if weakness persists
  - Useful to rule out other conditions in cervical spine (disk herniation, spinal stenosis) and shoulder (rotator cuff tear)

DIFFERENTIAL DIAGNOSIS
- Cervical radiculopathy
  - Neck pain and restriction of motion present, unlike brachial neuropathy
  - EMG reveals root level distributions, not plexus involvement
  - MRI correlates root compression with clinical findings

- ➤ Weakness limited to myotomal distributions
- ➤ Sensory deficit (dermatomal) common
- ■ Rotator cuff tear
  - ➤ Weakness of supraspinatus and infraspinatus most common
  - ➤ Deltoid intact in rotator cuff tear, weak in brachial neuritis
  - ➤ MRI of shoulder will show rotator cuff tear; generally normal in brachial neuritis unless there is a previous history of shoulder problems
  - ➤ No sensory changes with rotator cuff tear
  - ➤ Scapular winging not present in rotator cuff tear

TREATMENT
- ■ Phase 1 (painful phase)
  - ➤ Support extremity
  - ➤ Analgesics
  - ➤ Rest
- ■ Phase 2 (rehabilitation, as pain resolves)
  - ➤ Most rehabilitate entire extremity due to subclinical involvement
  - ➤ Gentle range of motion to maintain mobility
  - ➤ Progressive strengthening and sports-specific training
- ■ Corticosteroids frequently prescribed but have not been proven to be of clinical benefit

DISPOSITION
N/A

PROGNOSIS
- ■ Variable recovery
- ■ Muscles may not regain normal strength in the long term
- ■ Scapular winging persists
- ■ Return to athletic participation individualized, based on level of recovery

CAVEATS AND PEARLS
- ■ Profound, intractable pain out of proportion to clinical picture is suggestive of neuritis
- ■ Let athletes know early on that recovery is variable and unpredictable
- ■ Known by many other names, including acute brachial radiculitis, acute neuropathy, neuralgic amyotrophy
- ■ Most likely etiology is immunologic

BRACHIAL PLEXUS INJURIES

JOHN D. KELLY, IV, MD
REVISED BY CHARLES NOFSINGER, MD

HISTORY
- Sports injury, especially football, rugby, wrestling, hockey (contact)
- Mechanism: traction (plexus), compression (root), or direct blow
- Traction
  - Head lateral-deviated with concomitant ipsilateral shoulder depression
  - Occurs in younger scholastic athletes
  - Brachial plexus "stretch" injury
  - Not associated with cervical or foraminal stenosis
- Compression
  - Cervical extension with or without concomitant ipsilateral lateral deviation
  - More common in collegiate/professional athletes
  - Cervical root compression injury
  - Associated with cervical or foraminal stenosis
- Direct blow
  - Shoulder pad or forearm to supraclavicular region
  - Direct blow to axillary nerve
- Initial complaints
  - Burning, tingling, pain emanating from neck/shoulder and radiating distally
  - Weakness immediately or delayed onset
- Chronic cases may present with prolonged weakness (months) or persistent paresthesias (rare)
- Dysesthetic pain follows no set dermatomal distribution

PHYSICAL EXAM
- Weakness may not be evident several hours or days after injury
- Deltoid, biceps, and spinati most frequently involved
- Detailed neurologic exam by nerve root and branch
- Neck range of motion often limited with compression (root) injury
- Spurling's test often positive for compression (root) injury
- Brachial plexus stretch test or Tinel's in supraclavicular fossa may be positive for traction (plexus) injuries

STUDIES
- Cervical radiographs, including lateral flexion/extension if neck pain or stiffness present
  - Loss of lordosis common
- MRI if prolonged or profound weakness; to rule out herniated disk or cord anomalies
- EMG not usually helpful
  - Reserve for weakness that persists beyond three weeks

DIFFERENTIAL DIAGNOSIS
- Cervical cord injury
  - Bilateral arm symptoms, burning hands, or concomitant ipsilateral upper and lower extremity symptoms
  - Burners always are evident as unilateral symptoms and never involve the lower extremities
- Cervical spine fracture or instability
  - Significant neck discomfort usually
  - Positive radiographs
- Herniated cervical disk
  - Rare in young athletes
  - Consider if compression burner with wide cervical canal (soft tissue vs. bony compression)
  - MRI diagnostic

TREATMENT
- Refrain from sports until symptoms resolve
- Return to play is based on clinical exam. Beware that EMG can be abnormal for 50 weeks in clinically asymptomatic patients.
- Full painless neck range of motion, resolution of paresthesias, negative provocative tests, and normal strength necessary for clearance
- "Chest out" position to open foramina
- Shoulder shrug and scapular retraction exercises helpful
- Apply axial compression of cervical spine and resisted hand pressure to head to elicit residual neck "soreness" before return to play
- Preventive measures
  - Year-round neck and trapezial strengthening
  - Cervical orthosis to limit extension and lateral deviation ("cowboy collar")
  - Correct errors in blocking and tackling

DISPOSITION
N/A

PROGNOSIS
- Generally favorable
- Protracted weakness or dysesthetic pain possible but rare

CAVEATS AND PEARLS
- Recurrent extension burner has high likelihood of cervical/foraminal stenosis
- EMG may take months to "normalize" and is not useful to determine return to play
- Cervical stenosis can be determined by lateral radiograph; Pavlov ratio <.80 considered stenotic
- "Shoulder tackling" has decreased incidence of cervical spine injury while likely increasing incidence of burners
- Compression (root) injuries occur at foramina
- Traction (plexus) injuries occur at division level of plexus
- Neck pain common in extension/compression (root) burners
- Neck pain rare in traction (plexus) injuries

CALCANEAL STRESS FRACTURES

MAYO A. NOERDLINGER, MD
BERNARD R. BACH, JR., MD

HISTORY
- Active involvement in sports, the military, or dancing
- Pain develops slowly over time
- Dull, nagging pain in the inferior heel with activity
- Pain and swelling on both sides of heel
- Pain relieved with rest

PHYSICAL EXAM
- Pain on direct side-side compression of calcaneal head

STUDIES
- Noted on oblique radiograph
  > From posterosuperior aspect of calcaneus to anteroinferior surface
- With negative radiographs, obtain bone scan

DIFFERENTIAL DIAGNOSIS
- Nerve entrapment
- Plantar fasciitis
- Heel spur
- Plantar fascia rupture

TREATMENT
- Reduce activity until athlete is asymptomatic
  - ➤ Clinically healed when bone is not tender to palpation
- Immobilization until radiographic evidence of bone healing
  - ➤ Short-leg cast
  - ➤ Cam walker

DISPOSITION
N/A

PROGNOSIS
- Complete healing may take 6-8 months

CAVEATS AND PEARLS
- This fracture is due to repetitive loads and traction of gastrocsoleus complex on the Achilles tendon.

CAPITELLAR FRACTURES

GEORGE A. PALETTA, JR., MD
STEVE BERNSTEIN, MD

HISTORY
- Traumatic event
- Mechanism: fall on outstretched arm w/ valgus moment across elbow
- Presentation: swelling & tenderness at lateral aspect of elbow

PHYSICAL EXAM
- Pain w/ elbow rotation
- Must R/O medial, posterior elbow instability
- Careful neurovascular exam

STUDIES
- Standard AP & lateral radiographs
- Radial head – capitellum view sometimes helpful

DIFFERENTIAL DIAGNOSIS
- Radial head fracture
- Lateral epicondyle fracture

TREATMENT
- Type I (complete noncomminuted fracture of capitellum in coronal plane)
  - Closed reduction
    - Patient supine
    - Traction w/ elbow at 90°, forearm supinated, & manual downward pressure applied to fragment
    - Immobilize in long-arm cast or posterior splint for 3–4 wks
  - ORIF
    - For failure of closed reduction
    - Through a lateral approach (extensor carpi ulnaris, anconeus)
- Type II (fracture involving a shell of anterior cartilage w/ a thin layer of subcondylar bone, "Kocher-Lorenz fracture")
  - Closed reduction
  - ORIF if fragment large enough & displaced
  - Excision if fragment too small
- Type III (comminuted)
  - ORIF vs. excision as in type II

DISPOSITION
N/A

PROGNOSIS
- Best w/ anatomic reduction & early mobilization
- Principal complication: loss of elbow ROM
- Results of excision are good in short term, unpredictable in long term

CAVEATS AND PEARLS
- Uncommon fracture
- Beware of associated medial or posterior elbow instability
- Radial head-capitellar radiograph view helpful
- Kocher-Lorenz Fracture (type II) may be difficult to pick up
- Anatomic reduction key for best result
- Most common complication is motion loss

CERVICAL DISK DISEASE

HOWARD S. AN, MD, PhD

HISTORY
- Differentiate between acute vs. chronic herniated nucleus pulposus (HNP)
- Acute
  - May recollect specific traumatic onset
    - Lifting
    - Movement of neck
    - Direct contact injury to head
  - Pain, usually severe
  - Acute HNP with myelopathy rare
  - Radiculopathy symptoms affected by neck position
  - Neck pain may precede radicular symptoms
- Chronic
  - May have slow insidious onset
  - Usually cannot recollect specific injury/time of onset
  - Pain may fluctuate
  - Radiculopathy may not be affected by neck position
  - May have numbness without pain
  - Cervical spine rotation may give vertebral artery occlusion symptoms
  - Anterior osteophytes may give visceral pressure symptoms (pharyngeal symptoms)
- Similar symptoms between acute and chronic
  - Painful stiff neck
  - Usually mid/upper neck
  - Radiation to suboccipital region
  - Referred pain to upper shoulders/trapezius region
  - Pain provoked by motion
  - May be precipitated by postural position during sleep
  - Suboccipital headache (upper cervical disease)
  - May have torticollis posturing
- Radicular pain
  - Depends on disk involved
  - Burning, radiating, electrical, knife-like description
  - Often related to neck position
    - Extension

- Ipsilateral side bending
- Contralateral side bending
- Rotation
- Flexion
➤ May note that hands seem clumsy

PHYSICAL EXAM
■ Assess cervical ROM
➤ Extension, flexion, side bending, rotation – correlate with pain, restriction, referred pain
➤ **Extension and rotation toward the painful side reproduces pain down the arm – positive Spurling's maneuver**
■ Palpation of cervical spine for tenderness
■ May have specific motor atrophy with chronic denervation
■ Motor testing upper and lower extremity
■ Assess for hyporeflexia, hyperreflexia
➤ Hyperreflexia may be sign of upper motor neuron, cord compression, myelopathy
■ Assess, sensation – light touch, vibratory, positional, temperature
■ Myelopathy findings

STUDIES
■ Radiographs
➤ AP – joints of Luschka, coronal alignment
➤ Lateral – loss of cervical lordosis, narrowing of intradiskal spaces, osteophytes, narrowing of AP canal
➤ Obliques – foraminal stenosis/spondylosis
➤ Open mouth – C1-2, dens assessment
➤ Instability
- Flexion/extension views
■ MRI
➤ Most sensitive for HNP
➤ Caveat: disk bulge is common
➤ Acute indication – weakness
➤ Usually defer 6 weeks; may be forced in athlete to obtain earlier
➤ Can rule out intrinsic cord process
■ EMG/nerve conduction study
➤ Helpful to assess for peripheral entrapment
■ MRI + gadolinium
➤ Helpful with previous surgery

- Myelography or CT myelography
  - ➤ Excellent assessment for neural compression due to osteophytes
- **Thin CT sections with 45-degree oblique sagittal reconstruction are helpful to assess foraminal stenosis.**

DIFFERENTIAL DIAGNOSIS
- Peripheral entrapment syndromes
  - ➤ Carpal tunnel (median nerve)
  - ➤ Guyon's canal entrapment (ulnar nerve)
  - ➤ Cubital tunnel syndrome (ulnar nerve)
  - ➤ Radial tunnel syndrome (radial nerve)
  - ➤ Pronator teres syndrome
  - ➤ Anterior interosseous syndrome (median nerve)
  - ➤ Posterior interosseous syndrome (radial nerve)
  - ➤ Suprascapular notch compression (suprascapular nerve)
  - ➤ Quadrilateral space syndrome (axillary nerve)
- Brachial plexus
  - ➤ Burner syndrome
  - ➤ Thoracic outlet compression
  - ➤ Parsonage-Turner syndrome
    - • Mononeuropathy
    - • Polyneuropathy
- Central CNS/cord considerations
  - ➤ Arnold-Chiari malformation
  - ➤ CNS/cord tumors (primary, metastatic)
  - ➤ Spinal cord atrioventricular malformations
  - ➤ Syringomyelia
  - ➤ Infections (e.g., spinal epidural abscess)
  - ➤ Meningitis
  - ➤ Guillain-Barré syndrome
  - ➤ Tabes dorsalis
  - ➤ Herpes zoster
  - ➤ Acute cerebellar ataxia
  - ➤ Multiple sclerosis
  - ➤ Amyotrophic lateral sclerosis
- Associated fracture + HNP

TREATMENT
- Acute without neurologic weakness
  - ➤ Radiographic and clinical evaluation

- ➤ Educate patient
- ➤ NSAIDs
- ➤ Ice/heat
- ➤ Short course of immobilization with cervical collar
- ➤ Short course of muscle relaxants
- ➤ Minimize/avoid narcotics
- ➤ Nonnarcotic analgesics
- ➤ Activity modification
- ➤ Physical therapy – strengthen muscles/traction
- ➤ Traction more helpful in younger patient with soft disk herniation
- ➤ Cervical epidural steroids
- ➤ Medrol Dosepak helpful for severe radicular symptoms
- ■ Acute with neurologic weakness
  - ➤ Consider earlier MRI evaluation
- ■ Acute with no improvement
  - ➤ MRI evaluation
- ■ Early surgical indications for HNP
  - ➤ Severe uncontrolled pain
  - ➤ Significant motor weakness
- ■ Surgical indications
  - ➤ Persistent radicular symptoms with HNP or foraminal stenosis
  - ➤ Failed conservative treatment
- ■ Conservative treatment
  - ➤ Neck pain secondary to degenerative joint disease without neurologic compression, radiculopathy, myelopathy
- ■ Surgical methods
  - ➤ Anterior diskectomy + fusion for neck and arm symptoms
  - ➤ Posterior surgical procedures: used for lateral disk HNP or foraminal stenosis in patients with primary radicular symptoms without significant neck pain

DISPOSITION
N/A

PROGNOSIS
- ■ Most patients with acute HNP will recover within 6 weeks.
- ■ Surgical treatment
  - ➤ Overall pain relief 80%
  - ➤ Full neurologic recovery 90%
  - ➤ Autograft vs. allograft for fusion controversial

➤ Anterior plating gaining popularity to enhance the fusion rates and avoid postoperative bracing for multiple-level cases

CAVEATS AND PEARLS
- Most patients recover within 6 weeks
- Consider extensive differential diagnosis with radicular symptoms
- Always rule out cord compression on physical exam
- Surgical treatment only with significant motor loss or failure of conservative treatment
- Hold out of play/practice with radicular symptoms
- Burner generally not associated with severe neck pain
- Some fracture/dislocations can have associated HNP
- Caveat: use of narcotics should be minimized

CERVICAL FRACTURES

HOWARD S. AN, MD, PhD

HISTORY
- Injury – direct or indirect
- Mechanism
  - ➤ Compressive flexion
  - ➤ Vertical compression
  - ➤ Distractive flexion
  - ➤ Distractive extension
  - ➤ Compressive extension
  - ➤ Lateral flexion
  - ➤ Rotation
  - ➤ Combination
- Traumatic
  - ➤ Fall
  - ➤ Axial load (e.g., spearing in tackle football)
  - ➤ Motor vehicle accident
  - ➤ Blow to side of head
- Pain
- Neurologic involvement
  - ➤ Classification of spinal cord injury
  - ➤ Muscle grading
  - ➤ Neurologic examination

PHYSICAL EXAM
- On field
  - ABCs of trauma evaluation/management
  - Stabilize spine
  - Establish neurologic examination
    - Fracture
    - Fracture with complete injury
    - Fracture with incomplete injury

STUDIES
- Radiographs
  - AP, shoot-through lateral, swimmer's view, obliques, open mouth
  - Hard cervical collar in place
- MRI
  - Helpful for silent noncontiguous fracture
  - With unilateral/bilateral facet may detect herniated nucleus pulposus
  - Helpful to assess associated soft tissue injury

DIFFERENTIAL DIAGNOSIS
- Burner
  - Not associated with neck pain
  - Usually C5 distribution
  - Return to play if no neck tenderness and full motor recovery
- Transient quadriplegia
  - Incidence 7/1,000 athletes
  - Varied mechanism – axial load, hyperextension
  - Sensory motor abnormalities last 10–15 minutes
  - Occasional abnormalities up to 48 hours
  - Associated with congenital spinal stenosis, congenital fusion, cervical instability, herniated nucleus pulposus

TREATMENT
- Initial treatment
  - As for spinal cord injury
- Hospital management
  - Depends on fracture type and subclassification
  - Depends on associated injuries if associated with multiple trauma
  - Depends on spinal cord injury complete/partial

- Upper cervical fracture
  - ➤ Occipital condyle fracture
    - Halo vest or cervical orthosis
    - Depends on subtype
  - ➤ Atlas fracture
    - Most treated nonsurgically
    - Type 1 may require acute surgical treatment
  - ➤ C1–2 subluxation
    - CT, cineradiography, MRI may be needed to evaluate
    - Usually nonsurgical treatment – cervical orthosis, halo, skeletal traction
    - Occasional surgery – posterior fusion + postop orthosis or halo
  - ➤ Odontoid fracture
    - May require closed reduction + halo
    - C1–2 posterior arthrodesis or anterior screw fixation of odontoid type II fracture
  - ➤ Axis fracture
    - Treatment depends on type
    - Type I – cervical orthosis
    - Type II – cervical orthosis
    - Type IIA – axial traction contraindicated, cervical extension + halo
    - Type III – surgical treatment
  - ➤ Subaxial cervical spine fracture
    - Compressive flexion injuries
      - Halo 8–12 wks for cases with mild angulation and intact neurologic status
      - More severe may require anterior corpectomy, fusion, stabilization
    - Vertical compression injuries
      - Anterior corpectomy, fusion, anterior plate stabilization for severe cases
    - Distractive flexion injuries
      - Immediate closed reduction
      - Secondary posterior fusion + stabilization
      - Caveat: Herniated nucleus pulposus; if so anterior diskectomy and fusion first
    - Compressive extension injuries
      - Posterior cervical stabilization

- Distraction extension injuries
  - Anterior cervical decompression + fusion
- Lateral flexion injuries
  - Treatment depends on degree of injury
  - Stage I – halo
  - Stage II – surgical stabilization

DISPOSITION
N/A

PROGNOSIS
- Depends on type of fracture and whether partial or complete

CAVEATS AND PEARLS
- Assume cervical fracture in head-injured patient until proven otherwise
- Do not remove athlete's helmet; remove face mask
- Controlled log roll if athlete prone
- Establish neurologic status carefully
- If associated spinal cord injury, use methylprednisolone protocol within 8 hours

---

CERVICAL SPRAINS OR STRAINS

HOWARD S. AN, MD, PhD

HISTORY
- Strain defined as muscle injury caused by contraction
- Sprain defined as ligamentous injury
- Injuries usually occur at myotendinous junction
- Flexion/extension or whiplash injuries
- Localized neck pain, or referred pain to shoulder and scapula without radiculopathy
- History of deceleration-type mechanism
- Soreness in paravertebral muscles
- Difficulty turning/moving neck
- Injury mechanism varied
  - Deceleration
  - Twisting
  - Bending

➤ Abnormal posturing
➤ Pushing
➤ Pulling

PHYSICAL EXAM
- Normal neurologic exam
- Reduced cervical spine motion
- Secondary muscle spasm
- Neck may "list" to one side

STUDIES
- May consider cervical spine radiographic series if no trauma
- Obtain if history of trauma
- Rule out significant instability with flexion/extension radiographs about 2–3 weeks later and herniated disk with MRI about 4–6 weeks after injury
- May note degenerative joint disease changes on x-rays
- Second-order imaging rarely indicated
- Caveat: significant night pain, immunosuppression, steroid use, history of cancer
- Lab studies: CBC/sed rate – infection/tumor consideration

DIFFERENTIAL DIAGNOSIS
- Consider if persistent symptoms >6 weeks
- Similar to lumbar sprain/strain considerations except intra-abdominal causes
- Degenerative joint disease
- Herniated nucleus pulposus
- Infection
- Fibromyalgia
- Tumor

TREATMENT
- Ice
- NSAIDs
- Brief course of muscle relaxants
- Nonnarcotic analgesics
- Avoid steroids
- Avoid epidural steroids
- With acute sprain/strain, avoid antidepressants
- Modify activities
- Modalities equivocal benefit

- Avoid traction
- Surgery not indicated for acute sprain/strains
- Chronic conditions may warrant pain clinic

DISPOSITION
N/A

PROGNOSIS
- Generally excellent
- Prognosis worsens with chronicity
- Consider secondary gains in chronic patient
  - Symptom magnification
  - Workers' compensation
  - Personal injury suit

CAVEATS AND PEARLS
- Reassure patient that prognosis is good
- Keep patient active
- Avoid prolonged muscle relaxants
- Avoid narcotics
- Caveat: secondary gains

CHILBLAINS

WILLIAM O. ROBERTS, MD

HISTORY
- Chronic vasculitis of dermis
  - Caused by chronic exposure to cold conditions above freezing
  - Affected areas
    - Dorsum hands and feet
    - Anterior tibia
    - Face

PHYSICAL EXAM
- Leathery, waterlogged skin
- Dusky, gray color

STUDIES
N/A

DIFFERENTIAL DIAGNOSIS
N/A

TREATMENT

Prevention
■ Keep feet dry and warm
■ Aluminum chlorhydrate solution to prevent sweating

DISPOSITION
N/A

PROGNOSIS
N/A

CAVEATS AND PEARLS
■ Moderate to severe cold injury best treated in the hospital
■ Severe cold injury and illness not common in athletes
  ➢ Occurs quickly in injured athlete in a cold outdoor setting
  ➢ Evacuation protocols are critical for remote activities
■ Risk increases if glucose and fluids are not replaced during activity
■ Wet environments increase risk of hypothermia at "warmer" temperatures
■ Preventing cold-related injuries and illness
  ➢ Behavioral adaptation ignored in competition
    • Safety of competitive arena is left to event administration
  ➢ Physiologic adaptation to cold stress is limited
  ➢ Define environmental conditions that pose a threat to safety
    • Nordic skiing limits race starts to −20° C (−4° F) and above
    • Wind chill cooling, duration of exposure, and wet environments increase risk
  ➢ Stop, postpone, or modify activities in high-risk settings
  ➢ Buddy system to watch for behavior changes and tissue freezing
  ➢ Athlete and coach education for risks, hydration, and proper clothing
  ➢ Equipment and clothing
    • Layer clothing
    • Avoid cotton materials
    • Limit exposed skin
    • Shield high-risk area with vapor-barrier clothing
    • Remove metal jewelry, especially circumferential and pierced

CHRONIC EXERTIONAL COMPARTMENT SYNDROME

JEFFREY GUY, MD

HISTORY

- **Definition:** ache, sharp pain, or pressure in the lower leg experienced during sporting activity, usually relieved at rest
- Most commonly anterior compartment but may occur in all
- Usually nontender on exam
- No history of trauma
- Common in runners or any athletes with high demands placed on their lower extremities
- 75–95% have symptoms bilaterally
- Etiology unclear

Pathogenesis

- Pressure elevation due to muscle hypertrophy or noncompliant fascia causing pain by direct mechanical deformation of pain fibers
- Muscle injury: edema/hemorrhage – increased pressure in enclosed space – ischemia – further soft tissue damage

PHYSICAL EXAM

- Often have negative exams in the office
- Possible tenderness or increased tension over involved compartment after exercise
- Passive stretching of involved compartment may induce pain after exercise
- Reduced sensation over first dorsal web space with involvement of deep peroneal nerve
- Weakness or paresthesias may also occur with chronic cases

STUDIES

- Compartment pressure measurement
  - ➤ Direct measurement of involved compartments using needle catheter such as Stryker STIC catheter, WICK catheter, or transducer from arterial line
  - ➤ Operative treatment: fasciotomy recommended with a measured pressure > 15 mmHg at rest, > 30 mmHg after 1 min exercise or 20 mmHg after 5 minutes after exercise

DIFFERENTIAL DIAGNOSIS

- Stress fracture
- Periostitis
- Tendinitis
- Nerve entrapment
- Infection
- Neoplasm
- Venous stasis
- Excessive pronation

TREATMENT

- Nonoperative
  - Activity modification
  - Orthotics
  - Generally unsuccessful
  - Compartment measurements if clinically suspicious
- Operative
  - Anterior compartment is usually the only decompression necessary.
  - Anterior compartment release: 2- to 3-cm incision off the tibial crest
  - Careful of superficial peroneal nerve as it exits the fascia approximately 10 cm above fibula
  - Additional compartment release as clinically necessary

DISPOSITION

N/A

PROGNOSIS

- Good if recognized and treated early
- Persistent weakness or nerve damage can occur in chronic untreated cases.

CAVEATS AND PEARLS

- Early recognition is the key to successful treatment.
- Always consider exertional compartment syndrome in cases of vague lower extremity pain in athletes.

CLAVICLE FRACTURES

JOEL SHAPIRO, MD
FRANCES CUOMO, MD

HISTORY

- Mechanism: fall on outstretched arm or on point of shoulder
- Commonly associated with contact and high-speed sports: rugby, bicycling, skiing, etc.
- Epidemiology: M > F
- Patient reports pain over clavicle/fracture site
- Symptoms may be acute with injury, or chronic with malunion or nonunion
- Also commonly seen in newborns with "pseudoparalysis" of arm after delivery

PHYSICAL EXAM

- Deformity over fracture site
- Edema and ecchymosis, may extend down arm
- Subcutaneous bone: requires careful exam for open fracture
- Evaluate surrounding structures: neurovascular exam, pneumothorax (associated injury in 3% of fractures)
- Attempts at motion of the arm will elicit pain and crepitus at fracture site and should be limited

STUDIES

- Radiographs
  - Include AP of clavicle, AP view with 45° cephalic tilt, PA chest and shoulder trauma series, if indicated by exam
  - Zanca view (AP clavicle with 15° cephalic tilt) if fracture at lateral third
  - Serendipity view (AP sternum with 45° cephalic tilt) or CT scan to evaluate injury to medial third, or sternoclavicular joint
- Special studies
  - Arteriogram and vascular surgical consultation if vascular injury suspected

DIFFERENTIAL DIAGNOSIS

- Diagnosis usually straightforward, confirmed with x-ray

- Other anatomic disruptions may be confused with fracture: subluxation/dislocation of acromioclavicular, sternoclavicular, or glenohumeral joints; acromial or coracoid fracture
- Consider other injury with high-energy mechanism: floating shoulder, scapulothoracic dissociation, high rib fracture
- Look for associated head/cervical spine injuries

TREATMENT
- Based on location of fracture
- Include middle (85%), lateral (10%), and medial (5%) third fractures
- Acute fractures
  - Middle-third fracture treated with sling/swath and/or figure-of-eight brace for 6–8 weeks in adults, 4–9 weeks in children
  - Medial-third fracture treated with sling/swath and/or figure-of-eight brace for 6–8 weeks in adults, 4–6 weeks in children
  - Distal-third fracture may require surgery
  - No reduction maneuver required
  - May consider reduction in case of severe skin tenting/impending open injury; risk of injury to nearby neurovascular structures (consider performing in OR)
  - Newborns may be treated by safety-pinning sleeve to shirt-front for 2 weeks for most fractures
- Indications for ORIF for middle- and medial-third fractures
  - Open injury (or impending open injury with severe skin tenting), associated neurovascular injury, floating shoulder, nonunion or malunion
  - Greater than 1.5 cm fragment displacement is relative indication (associated with increased incidence of delayed/nonunion)
  - ORIF carries nonunion rate of approx. 10%
  - Usual implant is 3.5 reconstruction plate; requires contouring
- Nonunion/malunion treatment
  - Goals are solid union with re-established length to prevent dysfunction (may need intercalary bone graft, usually tricortical iliac crest)

DISPOSITION
N/A

PROGNOSIS
- Generally a benign injury with good outcomes and minimal disability
- Nonoperative treatment has >96% union rate for middle-third fractures

- 25% of nonunions that do occur are asymptomatic
- Malunions with shortening up to 1.5 cm are well tolerated with minimal functional deficit
- Regular follow-up at 2- to 4-week intervals needed to assess clinical and radiographic healing
- Return to sports 12–16 weeks, contingent on radiographic evidence of union
- Complications of nonoperative treatment include nonunion, malunion, neurovascular impingement from callus, and cosmetic deformity
- ORIF carries approx. 10% nonunion rate (significantly worse than closed treatment)

CAVEATS AND PEARLS
- Warn patients about final cosmetic outcome regardless of treatment (bump vs. scar)
- If ORIF done, may need future hardware removal
- Avoid nonheaded IM devices for fixation
- Complications due to pin migration

CONCUSSIONS

BERNARD R. BACH, JR., MD

HISTORY
- Definition
  - ➤ Latin derivation; "to shake violently"
  - ➤ Injury resulting in temporary disturbance of brain function caused by neuronal, chemical, or neuroelectrical changes without structural changes
  - ➤ Lack of universal definition
- Sports associated with concussions
  - ➤ Auto racing
  - ➤ Boxing
  - ➤ Cheerleading
  - ➤ Cycling
  - ➤ Diving
  - ➤ Equestrian sports
  - ➤ Football
  - ➤ Gymnastics
  - ➤ Hang gliding

- Ice hockey
- Lacrosse
- Martial arts
- Motorcycling
- Parachute
- Rugby
- Skating/Rollerblading
- Skiing
- Skydiving
- Soccer (goalie)
- Track (pole vaulting)
- Trampolining
- Wrestling
- Symptoms
  - Feeling of being stunned
  - Brief loss of consciousness (LOC), variable amnesia
  - Lightheadedness
  - Vertigo
  - Loss of balance
  - Headaches
  - Blurred vision
  - Cognitive and memory dysfunction
  - Difficulty concentrating
  - Lethargy
  - Fatigue
  - Personality changes
  - Inability to perform ADLs
  - Sleep disturbances

PHYSICAL EXAM
- On-field evaluation
  - ABCs
  - Is patient conscious?
  - Did athlete lose consciousness?
  - Is athlete amnestic?
  - Level of orientation
  - Neck pain?
  - Glasgow Coma Scale
- Sideline evaluation
  - Cranial nerve check (I-IV)
  - Pupillary assessment

> Battle's sign (posterior auricular hematoma)
> Otorrhea
> Rhinorrhea
> Raccoon eyes
■ Coordination: special tests
> Romberg
> Single-leg Romberg
> Tandem (heel-toe) Romberg
> Finger-to-nose test

STUDIES
■ Radiographs generally not obtained

DIFFERENTIAL DIAGNOSIS
■ Acute subdural hematoma
> Head trauma results in venous bleeding
> Low pressure
> Slow clot formation
> Delayed symptoms (hrs/days/wks)
> Treatment: surgical decompression
■ Epidural hematoma
> Head trauma results in bleeding from middle meningeal artery
> Severe head trauma mechanism
> Skull fracture, temporoparietal region
> Rapid neurologic changes within 10–20 minutes
> Treatment: immediate surgery
■ Intracerebral hematoma
> Trauma causes intracerebral bleeding
> LOC
> Possible partial paralysis
> Possible pupillary dilation
> Progressive edema may affect noninjured brain tissue
> Treatment: nonsurgical; eventual recovery
■ Second impact syndrome
> Recurrent concussion prior to recovery from initial concussion
> Second injury may be minor
> Athlete collapses
> Rapidly dilating pupils; semicomatose
> Loss of eye movement
> Respiratory failure
> Incidence unknown

➤ Mortality 50%
➤ Morbidity 100%
➤ Athlete must be asymptomatic for at least 1 week postconcussion
➤ Caveat: athlete who does not report symptoms for fear of not playing
➤ Pathophysiology
- Loss of autoregulation of brain's blood supply
- Vascular engorgement
- Marked increase in intracranial pressure
- Herniation of uncus of temporal lobe below tentorium of cerebellar tonsils through foramen magnum
- Demise more rapid than epidural hematoma
- Time interval from injury to brain stem herniation 2–5 minutes
- Brain stem herniation and compromise followed by ocular involvement and respiratory failure

TREATMENT
■ Establish diagnosis
■ Rule out catastrophic head injury
■ If LOC, assess for associated cervical spine injury
■ Determine grade of concussion
➤ LOC
- None, any, 1, <2–3, <5 minutes
➤ Amnesia
- Time intervals vary (1, 15, 30 minutes, 24 hours)
■ Guidelines/grading systems multiple and varied
■ Criteria for return to play controversial

DISPOSITION
N/A

PROGNOSIS
■ Postconcussion symptoms
➤ Headache (+/− exertion)
➤ Dizziness
➤ Fatigue
➤ Irritability
➤ Impaired memory
➤ Impaired concentration

- Postconcussion syndrome
  - ➤ Incidence unknown
  - ➤ Altered neurotransmitter function
  - ➤ Correlates with duration of amnesia
  - ➤ Workup with CT scan & neuropsychiatric tests
  - ➤ Return to sport: resolution of symptoms and studies normal
- Neuropsychological tests

CAVEATS AND PEARLS
- In athlete who is evaluated on field with LOC, assume concomitant cervical spine injury until proven otherwise
- Guidelines are guidelines; treat each athlete individually

CONGENITAL CERVICAL SPINE STENOSIS

JOHN D. KELLY, IV, MD

HISTORY
- Recurrent "burners" or "stingers"
- Episode of cord neuropraxia
- Associated with hyperflexion, hyperextension, and/or axial loading cervical spine
- No lasting deficits usually seen in chronic cases

PHYSICAL EXAM
- Acute
  - ➤ Check for spinous process tenderness
  - ➤ Comprehensive neurologic exam, especially upper extremities
  - ➤ Spurling's test for recurrent burners
  - ➤ Axial load head and elicit resisted hand pressure to head to rule out occult ligamentous injury
- Chronic
  - ➤ Check for spinous process tenderness
  - ➤ Comprehensive neurologic exam, especially upper extremities

STUDIES
- Lateral cervical spine radiograph
  - ➤ Pavlov or Torg ratio <.80 suggests stenosis
    - Ratio of canal size/vertical body sagittal diameter
    - Independent of x-ray magnification

- Sensitive in predicting stenosis but low positive predictive value
➤ Sagittal cervical canal diameter (corrected for magnification), 13 mm
  - Accurately represents midline dimensions of canal
  - Obtain if Torg ratio abnormal
- Plain CT
  ➤ Excellent for quantitative assessment of bony cervical canal
  ➤ May miss soft tissue impingement
  ➤ Addition of myelography enhances resolution
- MRI
  ➤ Best image of soft tissue encroachment on canal (herniated nucleus pulposus)
  ➤ Obtain if lateral radiograph abnormal to determine size of spinal cord and assess "functional reserve" of canal
- Cross-sectional area of cervical spinal canal (per CT) most frequently abnormal parameter in patients with congenital spinal stenosis

DIFFERENTIAL DIAGNOSIS
- Both recurrent burners and cord neuropraxia may mimic cervical spine instability, disk disease, and fracture

TREATMENT
- Acute
  ➤ Rule out serious cervical spine injury
  ➤ Spine injury precautions if significant neck pain or tenderness
- Chronic
  ➤ Advise patient of risk of recurrent burners and cord neuropraxia
  ➤ Diminished functional reserve of cord and nerve roots predisposes to recurrent injury
  ➤ Neck, trapezial strengthening
  ➤ "Cowboy collar," neck rolls to avoid hyperextension
  ➤ "Chest out" posture to open foramen
  ➤ Attention to blocking, tackling technique

DISPOSITION
N/A

PROGNOSIS
- Neurologic sequelae of recurrent burner and cord neuropraxia self-limiting

- Return to play if full, painless neck range of motion, normal strength, no pain with provocative maneuvers, and no symptoms
- Contraindications to play
  - Recurrent burners with residual symptoms or deficit
  - Cord neuropraxia with
    - One or more recurrences
    - Associated instability, disk disease, significant degenerative changes
    - Neurologic symptoms >36 hours
    - MRI evidence of cord injury

CAVEATS AND PEARLS
- "Spear tackler spine"
  - Subset of football players at risk for cord neuropraxia who demonstrate
    - Congenital stenosis
    - Loss of cervical lordosis
    - "Spearing" tackling techniques
  - Athletes with above best advised to avoid collision sports
- Diminished functional reserve of cord suggests heightened risk of neural injury (nonsports literature supports this)
  - MRI evidence of cord compression or edema is a red flag and supports cessation of contact sports
  - Canal can also be encroached by degenerative changes, soft tissue (disk), or instability

CORACOID FRACTURES

JOEL SHAPIRO, MD
FRANCES CUOMO, MD

HISTORY
- Mechanism: fall on point of shoulder, direct blow to coracoid, acromioclavicular (AC) separation, violent contraction of the biceps/coracobrachialis
- Commonly associated with contact and high-speed sports: rugby, bicycling, skiing, etc.
- Alternate mechanism is fatigue fracture from trapshooting or medial migration with rotator cuff arthropathy

PHYSICAL EXAM
- No deformity usually seen
- Edema and ecchymosis, may extend down arm
- Evaluate surrounding structures: neurovascular exam
- Pain with active shoulder elevation or elbow flexion

STUDIES
- Radiographs include axillary view, AP with 60° cephalic tilt, Stryker notch view
- CT scan if plain x-rays not sufficient

DIFFERENTIAL DIAGNOSIS
- Diagnosis sometimes difficult, confirmed with radiographs
- Other anatomic disruptions may obscure fracture: subluxation/dislocation of AC, sternoclavicular, or glenohumeral joints; acromial fracture
- Consider other injury with high-energy mechanism: floating shoulder, scapulothoracic dissociation, high rib fracture

TREATMENT
- Classification: types I–V
  - Type I: tip fracture (tip avulsion most common)
  - Type II: fracture extends to 50% of coracoid body
  - Type III: fracture extends to 75% of coracoid body
  - Type IV: fracture extends to 100% of coracoid body
  - Type V: fracture at base of coracoid (type IV) with extension into glenoid (intra-articular)
- Treatment
  - Type I–III: nonoperative
  - Types IV–V: nonoperative if nondisplaced; ORIF if displaced
  - ORIF technique: cannulated screw
- Other indications for ORIF
  - Associated AC separation
  - Associated clavicle fracture
  - Suprascapular nerve compression (by displaced fragment)
  - Athlete or heavy laborer (relative indication)

DISPOSITION
N/A

PROGNOSIS
- Good results for most fractures with nonoperative management

- Results worse when associated with AC separation (loss of suspensory mechanism of upper extremity)
- Uncommon nature of the injury and scant literature make treatment recommendations difficult

CAVEATS AND PEARLS
- Injury often discovered late
- Routine axillary views for shoulder trauma should help avoid missed diagnosis

---

CUBITAL TUNNEL SYNDROME

CHAMP BAKER, MD
DAVID D. NEDEFF, MD

HISTORY
- Ulnar neuropathy at the elbow
- Most common form of ulnar nerve entrapment
- Second most common compressive neuropathy in the upper extremity (carpal tunnel syndrome most common)
- Symptoms may include numbness or paresthesias in ring and little finger, medial elbow pain, or hand weakness
- Chronic cases are more likely to present with marked intrinsic hand muscle weakness
- Five potential sites of compression: arcade of Struthers, medial intermuscular septum, epicondylar groove, between two heads of flexor carpi ulnaris, and exit from flexor carpi ulnaris

PHYSICAL EXAM
- Clinical history may be the most important diagnostic tool
- Physical exam should start at cervical spine
- Detailed exam of the elbow
  - Carrying angle
  - Range of motion
  - Crepitus and/or tenderness
  - Ligamentous stability
  - Ulnar nerve subluxation with flexion
- Elbow flexion test is most reliable (elbow flexion and wrist extension for 1 minute; positive if numbness and/or paresthesias occur in ulnar distribution)

- Elbow flexion test is more sensitive than specific (false positives in up to 10% of normal individuals)
- Detailed sensory exam (vibratory perception, monofilaments, two-point discrimination)
- Wartenberg's sign (inability to adduct little finger)
- Intrinsic motor weakness indicates chronic compression (weakness of thumb pinch; positive Froment's sign)

STUDIES
- Plain radiographs
  - AP, lateral, and tunnel or axial view
  - Look for loose bodies, osteophytes, angular deformity, or malunion
- MRI generally not necessary for diagnosis
- Electrodiagnostic studies (EMG, nerve conduction velocity) not essential when diagnosis is obvious on history and physical exam
- Nerve conduction studies should be done with elbow flexed and are better for diagnosis of earlier compressions

DIFFERENTIAL DIAGNOSIS
- Cervical disk disease
- Ulnar compression at wrist
- Brachial plexopathy
- Spinal tumors
- Syringomyelia
- Thoracic outlet syndrome
- Pancoast tumor
- Metabolic disorders (diabetes, hypothyroidism, alcoholism, vitamin deficiencies)

TREATMENT
- Initial treatment includes avoidance of prolonged elbow flexion with activity modification or splinting
- NSAIDs
- Avoid local steroid injections around nerve
- Surgical indications
  - Persistent numbness, paresthesia after conservative management
  - Progressive muscle weakness
  - Persistent mild weakness for 3–4 months
  - Chronic neuropathy with weakness
- Several surgical options

➤ Simple decompression
  • Incise cubital tunnel retinaculum
  • Technically easy and immediate mobilization
  • More proximal or distal sites of compression not addressed
➤ Anterior transpositions
  • Subcutaneous, intramuscular or submuscular
  • All procedures move nerve to more protected position
  • 2 to 3 cm of length is gained, which decreases nerve tension
  • All five sites of potential compression are addressed
  • Disadvantages include extensive manipulation of nerve and disruption of neural blood supply
➤ Medial epicondylectomy
  • Seldom used
  • Eliminates medial epicondyle as source of compression
  • Contraindicated in throwing athletes
  • Risk of ulnar-sided elbow instability if too much bone removed
  • Risk of persistent symptoms if too little bone removed (more common)

DISPOSITION
N/A

PROGNOSIS
▪ Nonsurgical treatment successful in about 50% of patients
▪ Surgical results best in mild and moderate cases
▪ No significant differences between various types of anterior transposition
▪ Anterior transposition: 82–95% good or excellent results
▪ Simple decompression: good results for mild cases with isolated compression in cubital tunnel
▪ Short period (7 days) of immobilization in semiflexed position followed by gradual active extension
▪ Some authors favor immediate range of motion
▪ Complications are often technique-related
  ➤ Most common: persistent, severe dysesthesias
  ➤ Medial epicondylectomy may produce elbow instability
  ➤ Simple decompression may cause ulnar nerve instability
  ➤ Submuscular anterior transposition has been associated with elbow flexion contractures (may be negated with early range of motion)

➤ Neuroma (most commonly medial antebrachial cutaneous nerve)

■ Treatment of failed cubital tunnel surgery extremely difficult

➤ Poor prognostic factors include age >50 years, EMG evidence of denervation, and previous submuscular transposition

CAVEATS AND PEARLS

■ Listen to the patient; history may be the best diagnostic tool

■ Elbow flexion test is more sensitive than specific

■ Best results in mild and moderate cases

■ Anterior transposition is preferred for most cases

DIGITAL DISLOCATIONS

GERARD T. GABEL, MD

HISTORY

■ Sports > work injury

■ Mechanism: Hyperextension > torsional or deviation force

■ Proximal interphalangeal joint (PIP) more often than distal interphalangeal (DIP) or metaphalangeal (MP) joints

■ PIP/DIP may spontaneously reduce or be reduced by bystander or patient

■ MP joint usually irreducible

■ Prompt swelling, limitation of motion

■ Common sports: football, basketball, volleyball

■ May have associated tendon or structural ligamentous injuries

PHYSICAL EXAM

■ Acute: Swelling, deformity

■ May be open injury

■ PIP/DIP – Extensor tendon injury in volar dislocations

■ MP

➤ Dimpling palmarly (indicates complex dislocation)

➤ Parallelism – proximal phalanx and metacarpal lie parallel – complex dislocation

➤ Hyperextension – proximal phalanx lies extended relative to metacarpal – simple dislocation

STUDIES

■ Plain x-rays: True AP/lateral

➣ DIP – dorsal > volar, with or without articular surface fracture
➣ PIP – dorsal > volar, size of articular surface fracture generally dictates postreduction stability; may be rotational or deviational dislocation
➣ MP – dorsal – if parallel, irreducible; if extended, reducible; may have chip or avulsion fracture or incarcerated sesamoid
■ MRI, arthrogram not used

DIFFERENTIAL DIAGNOSIS
■ Clinically may appear as displaced fracture
■ Radiographs diagnostic

TREATMENT
■ DIP joint
➣ Closed reduction/digital nerve block
➣ Axial distraction/slight hyperextension
➣ Splint at neutral/active range of motion at a few days
➣ Sports with protective splint
■ PIP joint
➣ Dorsal
• Digital block
• Axial distraction/slight hyperextension
• Check active range of motion stability (usually stable unless structural fracture)
• Early active and passive range of motion
• Extension block splinting if unstable
• Splint short of unstable angle
• Decrease flexion block over 3 weeks
• If large fracture fragment, instability a problem; may need open reduction and internal fixation or volar plate arthroplasty
➣ Volar – central slip avulsion – extension splinting as boutonniere or surgical repair
■ MCP joint
➣ Simple
• Hyperextension subluxation – no distraction (may convert to complex injury)
• Wrist block – reduction maneuver of simply pushing on the base of the proximal phalanx to rotate the digit into flexion
➣ Complex
• Closed reduction rarely possible

- Operative reduction via dorsal approach
- Push volar plate out of interposed position (with or without splitting the plate)
- Immediate active range of motion with extension block for 1–2 weeks

DISPOSITION

N/A

PROGNOSIS

- Usually excellent range of motion and stability if early range of motion possible
- Associated fractures: more unstable injury, poorer prognosis
- Buddy tape digit for earlier but protected return to sport

CAVEATS AND PEARLS

- Don't convert simple to complex MP dislocation by inappropriate reduction maneuver.
- Don't overlook central slip avulsion in PIP dislocations (test PIP extension strength with or without digital block).

DISCOID MENISCUS

ANSWORTH A. ALLEN, MD
MARK C. DRAKOS, MD

HISTORY

Definition

- Abnormal-shaped meniscus
- Oval or disc-shaped with variable coverage of tibial plateau
- Medial or lateral discoid meniscus, usually in lateral compartment; medial discoid meniscus is rare
- Types (refers to coverage of tibial plateau): incomplete, complete
- Wrisberg type – No posterior meniscotibial attachments

Symptoms

- Children
  - ➢ Frequently no history of trauma
  - ➢ Symptoms may be variable, vague, or inconclusive
  - ➢ Snapping knee syndrome in children
  - ➢ Pain in affected compartment
  - ➢ Audible clunking with ROM knee is common

- Adults
  - ➤ Incidental finding at arthroscopy
  - ➤ Symptoms of meniscal tear
  - ➤ Occasionally have long history of clunk in knee

PHYSICAL EXAM
- Mild effusion – Variable
- Joint line tenderness
- Audible or palpable clunk as knee is brought into extension
- Flexion contracture
- Provocative maneuver for meniscal pathology
- McMurray's positive – Clunk
- Pain with forced hyperextension

STUDIES
- **Radiographs**
  - ➤ Usually normal
  - ➤ AP, lateral, Tunnel, infrapatellar (Merchant) (four views)
  - ➤ Cupping of lateral tibial plateau
  - ➤ Widened tibiofemoral joint space
  - ➤ Hypoplasia of lateral tibial spine
  - ➤ High-riding fibular head
  - ➤ Squaring of lateral femoral condyle
- **MRI**
  - ➤ Usually diagnostic
  - ➤ Specific criteria for diagnosis
  - ➤ Meniscal tear/degeneration
- **Arthroscopy**
  - ➤ Incidental finding

DIFFERENTIAL DIAGNOSIS
- Meniscal tears
- Meniscal cysts
- Osteochondritis dissecans
- Chondromalacia patellae
- Instability of tibiofibular joint
- Snapping of tendons around knee
- Iliotibial band syndrome

TREATMENT
- Only in symptomatic knee
- Establish diagnosis

- Consider MRI
- Arthroscopic evaluation
- Treatment considerations
  - ➤ Incomplete/complete discoid
    - No tear – Observe; do not remove or reshape if no tear
    - If torn – Reshape to contoured stable rim
  - ➤ Wrisberg discoid meniscus
    - Arthroscopic or open meniscus repair
    - Consider fibrin clot

DISPOSITION
N/A

PROGNOSIS
- Nonsurgical treatment
  - ➤ Asymptomatic patients with discoid meniscus do well without surgery
- Surgical treatment
  - ➤ Arthroscopic resection to contoured stable rim – 80% good to excellent
  - ➤ Meniscal excision (Wrisberg type) – Avoid if possible
  - ➤ Repair – Better long-term results
- Return to play
  - ➤ 8 weeks with partial meniscectomy
  - ➤ 6 months after repair
- Complications of surgical treatment
  - ➤ Re-tear meniscus
  - ➤ Deep vein thrombosis/pulmonary emboli (<1%)
  - ➤ Osteoarthritis (long-term) if total meniscectomy

CAVEATS AND PEARLS
- Suspect discoid meniscus in children with clunking/snapping knee.
- Diagnosis can be confirmed with MRI in most cases.
- Asymptomatic patients with incidental findings of discoid meniscus are not surgical candidates.
- Preserve as much of meniscus as possible during surgery.
- Wrisberg type: repair with fibrin clot; avoid excision if possible.
- Repair has better long-term results.
- Discoid medial meniscus relatively rare

DISTAL BICEPS TENDON RUPTURES

CRAIG M. BALL, MD, FRACS
KEN YAMAGUCHI, MD
REVISED BY CHARLES NOFSINGER, MD

HISTORY

- Males 40–60 years of age
- Sporting or work injury
- Dominant arm
- Single traumatic event with unexpected forceful extension applied to an actively flexed elbow
- Most common symptom: sudden, sharp tearing sensation in antecubital fossa
- Pop or snap may be heard
- Initial intense pain subsides to dull ache
- Subjective weakness in flexion and supination is a variable complaint, especially in chronic cases

PHYSICAL EXAM

- Ecchymosis and swelling in antecubital fossa and medial aspect of arm
- Tenderness in antecubital fossa
- Palpable defect in antecubital fossa with a complete rupture
- Bicipital aponeurosis (lacertus fibrosis) may still be intact, in which case the deformity is not as pronounced
- The medially located lacertus fibrosis should not be mistaken for the biceps tendon, which is felt more laterally in the antecubital fossa
- Active elbow flexion in supination accentuates the defect in the antecubital fossa by causing proximal retraction of the muscle belly
- Acutely, weakness may be accentuated because of pain
- Flexion strength may be mildly reduced but supination power is often decreased by 30%
- Chronically, supination power and endurance may remain permanently compromised
- Neurovascular examination should be performed

STUDIES

- AP and lateral radiographs are usually normal but rarely show a small fleck of bone from radial tuberosity or irregularity and enlargement of tuberosity

- MRI not usually necessary in the diagnosis of a complete tendon rupture but may be useful in equivocal cases or if suspect tendinosis or a partial tear
- Ultrasound quite accurate

DIFFERENTIAL DIAGNOSIS
- Biceps tendinosis – tendon degeneration without rupture, presents with pain in antecubital fossa but usually more chronic, may exist with partial tears, MRI diagnosis
- Partial rupture – increasingly being reported, women also affected, similar mechanism, tendon still palpable, fatigue pain common, MRI diagnosis
- Musculotendinous junction rupture – rare, usually diagnosed at surgery or on MRI
- Cubital bursitis – inflammation of bursa between biceps tendon and anterior aspect of tuberosity, may occur in isolation (tendon intact) or associated with biceps tendon pathology
- Entrapment of lateral antebrachial cutaneous nerve – rare, tenderness localized to lateral elbow flexion crease, tendon remains intact

TREATMENT
- **Acute**
  - Early immediate repair to radial tuberosity recommended
  - Nonoperative management only for elderly sedentary patients
  - Repair within 6 and preferably 2 weeks to ease reattachment
  - Exposure can be achieved by either a two-incision or a one-incision technique; good results reported for both
  - Risk of synostosis using two-incision technique minimized by not exposing ulna
  - Fixation achieved by various methods, with bone tunnels and suture anchors the most common
- **Chronic**
  - Need to repair chronic ruptures is questionable as gains in strength are modest
  - Significant disability associated with rupture may justify an attempt
  - For tears >6 weeks old, tendon may be retracted and scarred
  - Tenodesis to brachialis can be considered for activity-related pain
  - Anatomic repair to tuberosity may help improve strength and endurance, especially in supination

➤ Inadequate tendon length should be anticipated
➤ Autologous tendon or fascia lata grafts may be required to lengthen the tendon

■ **Partial ruptures**
➤ Surgery recommended following failure of nonoperative management
➤ Completion of tear with reinsertion at tuberosity recommended

■ **Rehabilitation**
➤ Posterior splint at 90° for 7–10 days
➤ Need for continued splinting with extension block determined by tension of repair
➤ Ideally, gradual stretching and use of the extremity allowed from 2 weeks
➤ Progressive strengthening begun at 6 weeks
➤ Rehabilitation following delayed repair is similar, although a splint with an extension block is usually used for the first 4–6 weeks

DISPOSITION
N/A

PROGNOSIS
■ **Nonsurgical treatment**
➤ Results can be acceptable, especially in the elderly, low-demand patient
➤ Activity-related pain can occur
➤ Decreased strength and endurance in flexion and especially supination

■ **Surgical treatment**
➤ Predictably good results regardless of whether bicipital aponeurosis intact or not
➤ Return of normal or near-normal strength and function possible
➤ High patient satisfaction
➤ Results of repair of chronic ruptures less predictable

■ **Return to play**
➤ Full activity allowed in 4–6 months

■ **Complications**
➤ Injury to radial or anterior interosseous nerves with one-incision approach
➤ Proximal radioulnar synostosis with two-incision approach (rare with muscle-splitting technique)

➤ Minor flexion contracture
➤ Rerupture, although possible, is uncommon

CAVEATS AND PEARLS
- History and examination usually sufficient for diagnosis
- Hallmark is a palpable defect accentuated by attempted elbow flexion
- If in doubt, an MRI or ultrasound scan can be useful to confirm
- Rupture probably occurs in a tendon weakened by intrasubstance degeneration or external mechanical impingement
- Symptomatic partial ruptures are rare
- Results of one- and two-incision techniques are similar
- Use of suture anchors may simplify the procedure
- Results of late repair are unpredictable for return of strength, but activity-related pain is diminished
- Protect repair against lifting force for first 6 weeks

DISTAL QUADRICEPS TENDINITIS

CHARLES A. BUSH-JOSEPH, MD

HISTORY
- Anterior knee pain, typically after period of overuse
- Gradual onset, no clear injury
- Associated with running or jumping sports
- Seen in ages 30–60
- Males more common than females
- May be recurrent based on activity
- Complaints of swelling or instability uncommon

PHYSICAL EXAM
- Tender proximal pole of patella, quad tendon
- Rarely involves joint swelling (presence of joint effusion leads to other diagnosis)
- Pain with resisted knee extension or single leg squat
- Quadriceps and hamstring tightness common
- No instability or loss of motion

STUDIES
- Radiographs

➤ Usually normal
➤ May show traction osteophyte at proximal pole of patella
■ MRI
  ➤ Not necessary, clinical diagnosis
  ➤ May use to rule out intra-articular injury
  ➤ Typical finding is tendon degeneration at proximal pole of patella

DIFFERENTIAL DIAGNOSIS
■ Patella tendonitis – Tenderness inferior pole of patella
■ Quadriceps rupture – Traumatic knee injury, loss of active knee extension
■ Degenerative arthritis – Diffuse joint pain and swelling, radiographic arthrosis
■ Inflammatory knee synovitis – Noted by joint swelling and synovial thickening
■ Prepatella bursitis – Extra-articular fluid collection

TREATMENT
■ Acute onset – Relative rest (avoid high-impact activities), ice, oral anti-inflammatories/analgesics
■ Quadriceps stretching
■ Chronic recurrent – Quadriceps/hamstring strengthening and stretching, knee sleeve, consider physical therapy, avoid open-chain exercises
■ No indication for cortisone injections (risk of rupture)
■ Arthroscopic or surgical debridement in rare refractory cases

DISPOSITION
N/A

PROGNOSIS
■ Generally excellent; minor recurrences typical
■ No improvement (over 4–6 weeks) warrants further investigation for alternative diagnosis.

CAVEATS AND PEARLS
N/A

ELBOW DISLOCATION

CRAIG M. BALL, MD, FRACS
KEN YAMAGUCHI, MD

HISTORY
- Common; second in frequency only to shoulder dislocation
- Usual mechanism a fall on outstretched hand, typically during sports
- Median age 30 years
- Diagnosis often straightforward
- Presents with painful soft tissue swelling and deformity about elbow
- Recurrent instability probably more common than previously thought
- Chronic dislocation rare in developed countries

PHYSICAL EXAM
- Deformity usually obvious
- Posterior dislocations most common (90%); anterior dislocations rare
- Detailed neurovascular examination required before and after reduction
- Concomitant upper extremity injury in up to 15%
- Extensive swelling can occur

STUDIES
- AP and lateral radiographs to determine direction of dislocation and presence of associated fractures
- Oblique views may also be helpful
- Associated fractures common (complex dislocation) – radial head and neck (5–10%), epicondyle avulsions (up to 12%), coronoid process (10%)
- High incidence of osteochondral injuries not seen on radiographs
- Radiographs must be repeated following reduction (AP and true lateral)
- Any distraction of joint should raise suspicion of interposed soft tissue or bony fragment
- Additional studies not usually required

DIFFERENTIAL DIAGNOSIS
- Displaced periarticular fractures
- Chronic unreduced elbow dislocation

■ Nontraumatic elbow dislocation (rheumatoid arthritis, neuropathic joint)

TREATMENT
■ **Acute – Nonoperative**
➤ Treatment in absence of associated fracture is immediate closed reduction
➤ If seen before significant swelling and spasm has occurred, reduction may be possible without sedation; otherwise, complete relaxation is preferred
➤ Posterior dislocations reduced by first supinating the forearm to clear the coronoid past the trochlea
➤ After reduction, assess range of motion and stability with forearm in pronation
➤ Tendency for redislocation in extension is most important
➤ Most simple dislocations are stable following reduction
➤ Recurrence is uncommon (<1–2% for simple dislocations)
➤ **Rehabilitation**
  • Elbow splinted in full pronation at 90° of flexion for 3–5 days, then active motion is started
  • If elbow feels unstable in terminal extension (<45°), a range-of-motion brace with an extension block can be used
  • Frequent follow-up radiographs required to document maintenance of reduction
  • 3–6 weeks of protected motion is adequate
■ **Acute – Operative**
➤ Only rarely is surgical treatment indicated
➤ Two situations when surgery may be required:
  • When elbow requires flexion beyond 50–60° to maintain reduction
    • High incidence of interposed soft tissue or bony fragments
    • Medial and/or lateral ligaments require repair and/or reconstruction
  • When elbow dislocation is associated with unstable fractures about the joint
    • Best approached by early surgery
    • Treatment goals: mobility and stability
    • Lateral support restored by reconstruction or replacement of radial head
    • Anterior buttress restored by fixation of type II and III coronoid fractures

- Ulnohumeral articulation restored by fixation of olecranon fractures
- Reassess stability following fracture fixation
- Ligament repair usually required
➤ **Rehabilitation:** early protected motion if elbow stable
■ **Chronic**
➤ Open reduction may be required after 5–10 days
➤ Longstanding cases with minimal pain and a functional range of motion may not require treatment
➤ Joint should be freed of scar tissue and bony articulation reconstructed
➤ Ligament reconstruction should be performed
➤ Hinged fixator may be required
➤ Active and passive range of motion started immediately

DISPOSITION
N/A

PROGNOSIS
■ Motion should be commenced early
■ Stiffness directly related to length of immobilization (>3 weeks associated with significant stiffness)
■ Majority of patients (>80%) regain excellent function and strength
■ Minor flexion contracture not uncommon
■ Improvement possible for at least 6–12 months
■ Results for fracture-dislocations less predictable, but early clinical results following aggressive treatment are promising
■ Role of hinged external fixators is evolving
■ **Complications**
➤ Stiffness
  - Typically affects terminal 10–20° of extension
  - Related to length of immobilization
➤ Neurovascular injury
  - Both arterial and nerve injury uncommon
  - Ulnar nerve most frequently injured (stretch)
➤ Heterotopic ossification
  - Soft tissue calcification common but rarely limits motion
  - True heterotopic ossification rare
➤ Recurrent instability
  - Not commonly reported
  - Deficiency of ulnar part of lateral collateral ligament most common cause

➤ Distal or radial ulnar joint (DRUJ) injury – important to consider in fracture-dislocations

CAVEATS AND PEARLS
- Primary stabilizers – ulnohumeral articulation, anterior medial collateral ligament, ulnar lateral collateral ligament
- Secondary stabilizers – radial head, anterior capsule, dynamic from muscles
- Dislocation the final of three sequential stages of instability, with soft tissue disruption progressing from lateral to medial
- The body internally rotates on the pronated hand, producing an external rotation and valgus moment on the elbow
- Associated injuries common
- Treatment dictated by stability of elbow after reduction and stabilization of associated fractures
- Vast majority of dislocations stable after closed reduction
- Patients do well if started on early rehab program
- Careful follow-up to prevent redislocation during treatment is essential
- Recurrent instability uncommon but important to recognize and treat early
- Patients should be aware that some loss of motion is typical

---

EPIPHYSEAL FRACTURES MEDIAL CLAVICLE

BERNARD R. BACH, JR., MD
REVISED BY CHARLES NOFSINGER, MD

HISTORY
- Direct or indirect injury mechanism
  - ➤ Direct blows – usually posterior displaced fracture
  - ➤ Indirect – injury to shoulder
    - Anterior shoulder compression – anterior displacement
    - Posterior shoulder compression – posterior displacement
- Sports – football, rugby
- Presenting symptoms similar to sternoclavicular (SC) joint injuries in adult
- Anatomic considerations with posterior displacement
  - ➤ Structures at risk – potentially life-threatening
    - Innominate artery/vein
    - Trachea

- Esophagus
- Brachial plexus

PHYSICAL EXAM
- Swelling locally
- Crepitance over fracture
- Local pain
- Deformity – more apparent with anterior displacement
- Late presentation – mass secondary to fracture callus
- Dyspnea
- Dysphagia
- Venous congestion
- Reduced pulses

STUDIES
- Radiographic views
  - Standard shoulder series inadequate
  - Difficulties viewing SC joint with osseous overlap
  - Serendipity view
    - Tangential radiograph (40° cephalic) – bilateral
      - Relationship to opposite clavicle indicates direction of displacement
      - Anterior displacement – superior position
      - Posterior displacement – inferior position
- Tomograms
  - Helpful but replaced by CT or MRI
- CT scan
  - Allows excellent differentiation of medial clavicle

DIFFERENTIAL DIAGNOSIS
- Medial clavicle fracture – nonepiphyseal
- SC joint dislocation
  - Anterior vs. posterior

TREATMENT
- Diagnosis and treatment depend on understanding of anatomy
  - Medial epiphyseal fracture unusual (1%)
  - Clavicle fracture – 6% of all fractures
  - Medial clavicle epiphyses are last long bone to appear
  - Ossifies late (18–20 years)
  - Fusion may not occur until early 20s
  - Clavicular motion greatest at SC joint
  - Physis lies outside joint capsule

> Stability dependent on
  • Intra-articular disk
  • Capsular ligaments (anterior/posterior)
  • Interclavicular and costoclavicular ligaments
> Medial clavicle contributes 80% longitudinal growth
  • Excellent ability to remodel
■ Classification
  > Categorized using Salter-Harris classification
    • I – Through growth plate
    • II – Includes portion of metaphysis
    • III – Fracture through portion of physis
    • IV – Fracture through metaphysis and physis
    • Most fractures – Salter-Harris I or II
  > Classify based on direction of shaft displacement anterior vs. posterior
■ Nondisplaced fracture
  > Sling 2–4 weeks
■ Displaced fracture – anterior
  > Marked displacement – closed reduction
  > Sling 2–4 weeks
  > Avoid ORIF
  > Never use pins (can migrate)
  > Most treated without reduction secondary to remodelling ability
■ Displaced fracture – posterior
  > Emergency treatment if mediastinal compression
    • Reduce in OR
    • Vascular consultant available
    • Towel clip reduction technique
■ Unrecognized late fractures
  > Leave alone

DISPOSITION
N/A

PROGNOSIS
■ Majority of medial epiphyseal fractures treated without reduction
■ Shoulder motion not impaired
■ Long-term sequelae not well documented
■ Return to play
  > Assess for tenderness
  > Usually 4–6 weeks

Complications

■ Pinning never recommended secondary to hardware breakage/migration
■ Pins may migrate to lung, pleura, heart, spinal cord, great vessels
■ Nonunions rare
■ Prominence related to fracture callus is not a complication

CAVEATS AND PEARLS

■ Medial clavicular epiphyseal fractures may be underrecognized and usually interpreted as SC joint dislocation
■ Ossifies late teens, fuses early 20s
■ Injuries extremely uncommon
■ Direct or indirect injury mechanisms
■ Excellent healing and remodelling potential
■ Posterior injuries can compress mediastinal structures
■ Avoid fixation with hardware

EXERCISE-ASSOCIATED MUSCLE CRAMPING (HEAT CRAMPS)

WILLIAM O. ROBERTS, MD

HISTORY

■ Involuntary muscle spasms after or during exercise
■ Mechanism of onset related to triad of muscle fatigue, dehydration, and salt loss
■ Possible neural etiology
■ More frequent in hot, humid environments
■ Heat not true cause
■ Can occur with hyponatremia and exercise exhaustion
■ More frequent with no acclimatization or salty sweat

PHYSICAL EXAM

■ Painful, palpable muscle spasm
■ Usually muscles involved in activity

STUDIES

■ Normal serum sodium level

DIFFERENTIAL DIAGNOSIS

■ Exertional hyponatremia

- Exercise exhaustion
- Exertional heat stroke

TREATMENT
- Oral fluid, glucose, and salt replacement rather than water alone
  - Gatorade (21 mEq/L) with additional 1 tsp salt added per liter
  - Chicken bouillon/broth
  - Pedialyte (Ross) with 45 mEq Na/L
  - Rehydralyte (Ross) with 75 mEq Na/L
  - Pickle juice
  - Alka-Seltzer 2 tabs in water
- Neuroinhibition techniques with prolonged stretch and deep pressure
- Assisted walking
- If IV fluids needed, use normal saline or D5%NS
- Medications
  - IV D50%W, 50 mL
  - Diazepam 1–5 mg IV push (off label)
  - Mg++ sulfate 1–5 g IV (off label)
  - Dantrolene 1–7 mg/kg IV/PO (off label)

DISPOSITION
- Discharge when spasm controlled; longer observation if medications used

PROGNOSIS
N/A

CAVEATS AND PEARLS
N/A

EXERCISE EXHAUSTION (HEAT EXHAUSTION)

WILLIAM O. ROBERTS, MD
REVISED BY CHARLES NOFSINGER, MD

HISTORY
- Inability to continue exercise
- Most common form of "heat illness"
- Related to exercise volume or intensity more than "heat"
  - Combined cellular energy, salt, and water deficiency

➤ Possible neural fatigue
➤ More frequent in hot conditions
  • Energy demands of temperature regulation
■ Symptoms of water depletion associated with low fluid intake
  ➤ Intense thirst
  ➤ Fatigue
  ➤ Weakness
  ➤ Flushing
  ➤ Chills
  ➤ Dizziness
■ Symptoms of salt depletion associated with profuse sweating replaced by water
  ➤ Weakness
  ➤ Giddiness
  ➤ Frontal headache
  ➤ Anorexia
  ➤ Nausea
  ➤ Muscle cramps
■ Athletes usually have combined salt and water deficiency with energy deficit

PHYSICAL EXAM
■ Always rule out heat stroke first with core temperature
■ Water-depletion exercise exhaustion
  ➤ Impaired judgment
  ➤ Hyperventilation
  ➤ Normal rectal temperature up to 39°C
  ➤ Irritability
  ➤ Lethargy
  ➤ Muscular incoordination
  ➤ Oliguria
■ Salt-depletion exercise exhaustion
  ➤ Giddiness
  ➤ Vomiting
  ➤ Diarrhea
  ➤ Muscle cramps
  ➤ No weight loss
  ➤ Normal to low-normal rectal temperature

STUDIES
■ Serum Na+

DIFFERENTIAL DIAGNOSIS
- Exertional heat stroke
- Exertional hyperthermia
- Hyponatremia
- Exercise-associated muscle cramping

TREATMENT
- Oral water and salt replacement
- Intravenous rehydration
  - D5% 1/2NS or D5% NS for <4 hours duration
    - 1/2NS or NS for >1 liter IV fluid
  - D5% NS for first liter for >4 hours duration
    - NS for >1 liter IV fluid
- Control muscle contractions
  - Neuromuscular inhibition techniques
  - Salt replacement
  - Pharmacologic treatment
    - Diazepam IV
    - Magnesium sulfate IV

DISPOSITION
- Return to activity after rehydration and resolution of fatigue

PROGNOSIS
N/A

CAVEATS AND PEARLS
N/A

EXERTIONAL HEAT STROKE

WILLIAM O. ROBERTS, MD

HISTORY
- Collapse with high body temperature and CNS changes during or after exercise
  - Greatest risk in fast-paced and/or high-intensity activities
  - Associated with dehydration in long-duration activities
- Body heat removal during exercise impaired by high humidity
- If hypothalamus overheats, increased morbidity and mortality
- Severe complications if not promptly treated
  - Death

- ➤ Seizure
- ➤ Rhabdomyolysis
- ➤ Renal failure
- ➤ Lactic acidosis
- ➤ Disseminated intravascular coagulation
- ➤ Adult respiratory distress syndrome
- ➤ Cardiac muscle damage
- ➤ Immune system suppression
- Occasional isolated mortality during hot, humid road races and July/August football practices
- Long-term heat tolerance not altered in 80% of athletes with exertional heat stroke
- Measurement of environmental heat stress
  - ➤ Ambient temperature – relative humidity risk chart
    - Recommend Kulka and Kenney, Phys Sportsmed 30(7):37, 2002
  - ➤ WBGT (wet bulb globe temperature) chart
- Dehydration decreases effective blood volume available
  - ➤ Heat transfer to the shell
  - ➤ Sweating response
- Risk factors
  - ➤ Continuous heat exposure (not cooling at night)
  - ➤ Cumulative and acute dehydration
  - ➤ Child athletes have increased ratio of surface area to mass
    - Greater heat gain from environment
    - More metabolic heat for surface area
    - Less sweating capacity for cooling
  - ➤ Older athletes have decreased cardiac output for heat transfer
  - ➤ Sleep deprivation
  - ➤ Malnutrition
  - ➤ Supplements and medications
  - ➤ Family or personal history of malignant hyperthermia
  - ➤ Football uniform inhibits heat transfer
- Symptoms
  - ➤ Fatigue
  - ➤ Dizziness
  - ➤ Weakness
  - ➤ Feel hot
  - ➤ Flushing
  - ➤ Chills
  - ➤ Profuse sweating

PHYSICAL EXAM

- Rectal (core) temperature >40°C
  - ➤ Oral, tympanic, and axillary temps not accurate
- Pulse 100–120 bpm
- Low blood pressure
- Hyperventilation
- CNS dysfunction most important marker
  - ➤ Impaired judgment
  - ➤ Bizarre behavior
  - ➤ Amnesia from time of body temperature elevation
    - Contact sports, mistaken for head injury
  - ➤ Loss of lower limb function and unable to ambulate
  - ➤ Collapse to ground
  - ➤ Delirium
  - ➤ Stupor
  - ➤ Coma
- Ashen skin color due to circulatory collapse
- Sweaty, cool skin
  - ➤ Heat loss system functioning
    - Unable to remove metabolic heat
  - ➤ Dry, hot skin typical finding in classic heat stroke
  - ➤ Screen for dry, hot skin = missed exertional heat stroke
- Seizure can occur
  - ➤ Athletic setting, also think of cardiac arrest or hyponatremia

STUDIES

- Check Na+ for hyponatremia
- Potassium often decreased
- Glucose for hypoglycemia
- CK (CPK) and K+ increased with exertional rhabdomyolysis
- Elevated SGOT >1,000: increased morbidity and mortality

DIFFERENTIAL DIAGNOSIS

- Exertional heat stroke
- Exertional hyperthermia
- Exercise (heat) exhaustion
- Exertional hyponatremia
- Head injury

TREATMENT

- Field treatment is immediate cooling

- ■ Ice water "tub" immersion method of choice
  - ➤ Cooling rates of 15–24°F/hr
- ■ Ice packs or ice water-soaked towels to neck, axilla, and groin
  - ➤ Cooling rate half of immersion
  - ➤ Add fans to improve cooling rate
- ■ Cooled IV fluids may decrease core temp
- ■ Monitor temperature every 5–10 minutes during and after therapy
- ■ Cooling endpoint is 102°F to prevent overcooling
- ■ Careful fluid replacement until core is cooled
  - ➤ For IV fluid use D5% NS, D5% 1/2NS, NS, or 1/2NS
- ■ Medications to relieve muscle cramping or treat seizure
  - ➤ Diazepam 1–5 mg IV push (off label)
  - ➤ Magnesium sulfate 5 g IV push (off label)
- ■ Dopamine for blood pressure support (hospital)
- ■ Miscellaneous hospital-based cooling techniques
  - ➤ Iced gastric, peritoneal, or rectal lavage
  - ➤ Extracorporeal circulation with bypass blood pump or dialysis
  - ➤ Warm air mist sprays or wet gauze (or sheets) and fans
    - • Cool at 7°F/hr in heat stroke victim

DISPOSITION
- ■ Release from medical area when clinically stable and normothermic
  - ➤ Instruct in fluid and energy replacement
  - ➤ Re-evaluate if change in status
  - ➤ Recommend follow-up exam for severe casualties
- ■ Transfer to emergency facility
  - ➤ Not responding to on-site treatment
  - ➤ Any sign of single- or multi-organ failure
  - ➤ Moderate to severe dehydration

PROGNOSIS
- ■ Good if recognized and treated immediately
  - ➤ In "golden" hour
- ■ Poor if not recognized and treatment is delayed
  - ➤ Organ damage a function of area under temperature and time curve elevated above 106°F

CAVEATS AND PEARLS
- ■ Treat first, then transfer
- ■ The football uniform traps heat and increases risk of heat stroke
- ■ Dehydration negates the effects of acclimatization to heat

- Football players in full uniform for 2-hr practice
  - Can lose 25 lbs of fluid
  - Can lose 10 gr of salt
- Acclimatization is essential for heat tolerance
  - For football consider: no pads day 1, helmet only days 2–3, helmet and shoulder pads days 4–5, and full pads from day 6 on if ambient temp and relative humidity in "safe" zone
  - Helmets and pads off for conditioning drills and rest breaks
  - Replace fluid losses
  - Supplement with extra salt in fluids and at meals

EXERTIONAL HYPERTHERMIA

WILLIAM O. ROBERTS, MD

HISTORY
- Elevated core temperature during or after exercise without CNS changes
- Presentation with exercise exhaustion
  - Hyperthermic exercise-associated collapse

PHYSICAL EXAM
- Rectal (core) temperature $>40°C$
- No CNS dysfunction
- Check for signs of dehydration

STUDIES
- Serum Na+

DIFFERENTIAL DIAGNOSIS
- Exertional heat stroke
- Hyponatremia
- Exercise exhaustion

TREATMENT
- Observe
- Oral hydration with salted fluids

DISPOSITION
- Release when normothermic

PROGNOSIS
N/A

CAVEATS AND PEARLS
N/A

EXERTIONAL HYPONATREMIA

WILLIAM O. ROBERTS, MD

HISTORY
- Collapse associated w/ serum sodium <130 mmol/L
  - Range from 110–130 mmol/L
- Events >4.5 hours long
- "Common" in Ironman-length events
- Increasing in marathon races with slow runners
- More frequent in hot, humid conditions
- Female > male (9:1)
  - Current recommendations may overhydrate smaller body sizes
  - Individualize fluid intake based on needs for pace and conditions
- May present with muscle cramping
- Can be minimally symptomatic for several hours
- Rapid deterioration, progressing to seizure, respiratory distress, and coma
  - Due to pulmonary and cerebral edema
- Two mechanisms of onset
  - Water intake greater than sweat rate without normal renal water clearance
    - Overhydration
  - Large salt losses in sweat replaced with water
    - Often associated with dehydration
    - Decreased urine production during exercise
- Presenting history and symptoms of water intoxication
  - High fluid intake of 1–2 full glasses of water at every aid station
  - Lightheaded
  - Dizzy
  - Nausea
  - Progressively severe pounding headache
  - Feeling of impending doom or feeling scared
  - Feeling puffy, with tight skin and clothing
  - Sleepy

- Presenting history and symptoms of salty sweaters
  - Sweat burns eyes and tastes salty
  - Salt precipitate on skin, hair, and clothing
  - Water as primary replacement fluid
  - Signs of dehydration

PHYSICAL EXAM
- Ashen skin color, including lips
- Overhydration
  - Minimal weight loss or weight gain
  - "Puffy"
    - Rings, watches, and shoes tight
    - Face swollen
    - Hand and foot edemal
    - BP, pulse, and respiratory rate usually normal
- Salt depletion
  - Minimal to severe weight loss
  - Sunken eyes
  - Orthostatic BP and pulse changes
- Vomiting
- Mental status intact until late in course
- Confusion
- Muscle cramps
- Clonus
- Dyspnea
- Prolonged seizure
- Obtundation

STUDIES
- Serum Na+ <130 mmol/L
  - Mean Na+ in obtunded patients 121 ± 3 mmol/L
  - Range 111–127 mmol/L
- O2 sat may be decreased (<90%) with pulmonary edema
- Hematocrit
  - Decreased in overhydration
  - Increased in dehydration

DIFFERENTIAL DIAGNOSIS
- Cardiac arrest
- Exertional heat stroke
- Exercise-associated muscle cramps

TREATMENT
- Initial evaluation
  - ➤ Check pulse and breathing
  - ➤ Check rectal temperature
  - ➤ Check for medical alert tag
- IV start for medication access
  - ➤ Diazepam and/or Mg^{++} sulfate on standby for clonus or seizure
- Serum sodium 125–130 mmol/L and clinical signs of dehydration
  - ➤ Rehydration with normal saline in medical tent
  - ➤ Check electrolyte levels after each liter of IV fluid
- Initial sodium level <130 mmol/L and fluid overload
  - ➤ If asymptomatic, allow natural diuresis
  - ➤ Close observation
  - ➤ Hypertonic saline or NS in hospital

DISPOSITION
- Medical teams may choose to treat on site if safer for athlete
- Transfer to emergency facility if no labs onsite
  - ➤ Initial sodium <125 mmol/L
  - ➤ Initial sodium level <130 mmol/L and obvious fluid overload
  - ➤ Unresponsive to initial therapy
  - ➤ Worsening sodium levels
  - ➤ No diuresis
  - ➤ Seizure
  - ➤ Obtunded
- Alert emergency room of transfer and expected complications
- Prevention
  - ➤ Match fluid intake to sweat losses
  - ➤ Salted fluids during and after activity

PROGNOSIS
N/A

CAVEATS AND PEARLS

Acute heat disorders
- Suspect as a cause of collapse in exercise settings
- Early recognition is critical to outcome
  - ➤ Athletes die from unrecognized exertional heat stroke or hyponatremia
- Increasing wet bulb global temperature (WBGT) correlates with slower distance running performances

■ Heat causes accelerated cell metabolism and destruction
  ➤ Prompt cooling critical for optimal outcome

Behavioral adaptations to heat stress
■ Normal to stop activity when heat stress perceived during activity
■ Athletes in competition will ignore normal behavioral responses
■ Safety of the competitive arena is left to event administration
■ Predetermined guidelines will protect the athletes

Physiologic adaptation to heat stress is acclimatization
■ Physiologic effects of adaptation to a hot environment
  ➤ Decreased heart rate
  ➤ Increased plasma volume
  ➤ Increased sweating
  ➤ Earlier sweating
  ➤ Decreased skin blood flow
  ➤ Decreased $Na+$ losses
■ Body system response to adaptation
  ➤ Decreased core body temperature
  ➤ Increased exercise tolerance time
  ➤ Decreased perceived exertion
■ Time course for acclimatization
  ➤ Usual onset in 10–14 days
  ➤ Greatest improvement occurs at 8–12 weeks
  ➤ More rapid induction with
    • Harder training in heat
    • Higher cardiorespiratory fitness level
    • Greater VO_{2max}
  ➤ Induced in cool environments by training in heavy clothing
■ Maintaining acclimatization
  ➤ Daily exposure of half-hour
  ➤ Protection lost in few days to weeks
■ Salt intake <3 g/d for first 3–5 days
  ➤ Increased risk of heat illness
  ➤ Blunts acclimatization response
  ➤ Salt supplementation improves acclimatization

Preventing heat-related "emergencies" during athletic competition
■ Recommendations for athletes training and competing in the heat
  ➤ Get fit in cool environment
  ➤ Use the cool part of the day for intense workouts
  ➤ Monitor hydration
  ➤ Extra salt early in heat exposure or for muscle cramping

- ➤ Monitor rectal temperature and keep below 39°C
- ➤ Schedule daily heat exposure for adaptation maintenance
- ◼ Salted fluids
  - ➤ 0.1% saline solution freely available during hot work
- ◼ Acclimatization to heat for 8–10 days
- ◼ Fluid replacement matched to actual losses
- ◼ Plan and schedule events for safest thermal environment
- ◼ Define hazardous heat and humidity conditions that pose a threat to safety
  - ➤ Risk increases above 65°F and 50% relative humidity
  - ➤ Modify the event or practice to increase safety margin
    - Add quarter breaks and allow free access to fluids
    - Shorten games or allow unlimited substitution
    - Alternate schedule to move midday games to cooler hours
    - Cancel all nongame activities
    - Move to air-conditioned environments when not playing
    - Shortening a road race may increase pace and heat stroke risk
  - ➤ Postpone the event until cooler conditions prevail
  - ➤ Consider cancellation above 82°F and 100% relative humidity
    - Especially in high-sun conditions
- ◼ Announce the current heat risk prior to competition or practice
- ◼ Runner education and preparation
  - ➤ Acclimatization to heat
  - ➤ Hydration instructions and overhydration risks
  - ➤ Proper clothing
  - ➤ Heat illness symptoms

Body temperature measurement
- ◼ Temperature differences between body core and shell in heat
  - ➤ Temperature measurements at natural openings are influenced by shell temperature
  - ➤ Greatest difference during evaporation of sweat
  - ➤ Exertional heat stroke may differ by 5°C
- ◼ Rectal temperature provides good core estimate in the field
  - ➤ Diagnostic and treatment criteria based on rectal temperature
  - ➤ Infrared temperature scanner measures shell temperature accurately
    - Does not estimate core temperature in sweating athletes
  - ➤ Oral temperature cooled by rapid respiratory rates and cool saliva
  - ➤ Axillary temperature cooled by evaporating sweat

FEMORAL NECK STRESS FRACTURES

EDWARD YIAN, MD
EDWARD M. WOJTYS, MD

HISTORY

- Clinical history
- Groin pain
  - Inguinal pain
  - Deep aching within hip
  - Pain in thigh
  - Referred pain to knee or back
  - Pain worsens with activities
  - Usually no specific injury or trauma
  - History of altered activities
    - Change in intensity of training/frequency/distance
  - Seek menstrual history (oligomenorrhea/amenorrhea)
  - Evaluate for eating disorders/nutritional issues
- Athletes at risk
  - Long-distance runners
  - Ballet dancers
  - Soccer players
  - Military recruits
- Incidence variable
  - Japan – 3% all hip fractures
  - Israeli military recruits – 5%
  - Royal Marine recruits – 3%
- Mechanism
  - Trabecular microfractures through normal bone
  - Time-dependent
  - Spontaneous healing occurs with reduced bone loading
  - Related to repetitive subthreshold forces/mechanical loads
- "Insufficiency fractures" – variant of stress fracture
  - Elderly patients
  - Fatigue strength diminished
  - Lower loads result in osseous failure
  - Associated diseases
    - Hyperparathyroidism
    - Diabetes
    - Osteoporosis
    - Osteomalacia

- Rheumatoid arthritis
- Irradiation
- Classification systems
  - Devas
    - Compression
      - Mechanically stable
      - Callus formation – Inferior neck region
      - No cortical break noted radiographically
    - Tension
      - Superior surface femoral neck origin
      - Fracture perpendicular to axis of force
      - Increased risk of displacement
  - Blickenstaff
    - 1 – Periosteal reaction/callus along inferior neck region, no visible fracture line
    - 2 – Visible nondisplaced fracture
    - 3 – Completely displaced fracture
  - Fullerton
    - Tension type
      - Superolateral neck origin
      - Increased risk of displacement
      - Callus forms on tension side
      - Elderly at risk
    - Compression type
      - Internal inferior neck callus formation
    - Displaced type
      - Separation of fracture fragments

PHYSICAL EXAM

- Antalgic gait
- Pain at extremes of hip motion
- Tenderness over groin/inguinal region
- Evidence of "hip irritation" with rotation
- Difficulties performing straight-leg raise
- Groin pain on heel percussion
- Groin pain with single-leg hops

STUDIES

- Radiographic
  - AP pelvis, AP & lateral affected hip
    - Usually normal in early phase

- Assess for osteopenia
- Injury changes – Sclerosis, cortical disruption along superior/inferior neck

■ Bone scan
  - ➤ Early detector/reliable
  - ➤ False-positive tests occur in sickle cell, infection
  - ➤ May detect 10 days from initial injury
■ MRI
  - ➤ Positive study may be detected within 24 hours
  - ➤ Studies suggest more sensitive and specific than bone scan
  - ➤ Decreased signal intensity T1 images
  - ➤ Increased signal changes T2 images
■ Quantitative ultrasound bone density screening
  - ➤ Predictive of future stress fracture

DIFFERENTIAL DIAGNOSIS

■ Groin strain
■ Infection
■ Tumor
■ Lumbar referred pathology
■ Intra-abdominal referred pathology
■ Hernia
■ Osteitis pubis
■ Synovitis
■ Slipped capital femoral epiphysis in teenager

TREATMENT

■ Type-dependent
■ Compression type
  - ➤ Stable fracture pattern
    - Nondisplaced
      - Nonoperative treatment
      - Nonweight-bearing until pain-free at rest
      - Progress to protected weight-bearing
      - Serial radiographs to assess healing
    - Displaced
      - ORIF
        - Cannulated screws
        - Knowles pins
        - Compression hip screw
      - Open reduction usually not needed

- Cortical break mandates surgical treatment
- Consider curetting/reaming fracture to stimulate healing

DISPOSITION
N/A

PROGNOSIS
- Prognosis is good with early detection and appropriate treatment if fracture remains nondisplaced.
- Once displacement occurs, anatomic reduction is needed with rigid internal fixation.
- Recurrence is dependent on correction of predisposing factors such as training errors, diet.
- Complications
  - Delayed union
  - Nonunion
  - Malunion
  - Refracture
  - Avascular necrosis
    - Related to time interval if displacement
    - Related to type of fracture
- Return to play
  - Nonimpact conditioning – Begin when athlete pain-free (bicycling, swimming, etc.)
  - Symptoms recur – Conditioning must stop
  - If athlete is symptom-free for 6 weeks, light resistance training implemented (e.g., single-leg leg press with 25–30% body weight)
  - If athlete symptom-free for 12 weeks – Impact loading can be reintroduced provided patient did well with nonimpact conditioning and has performed 6 weeks of resistance training
  - Training errors, nutritional and endocrine issues should be addressed prior to resumption of running.

CAVEATS AND PEARLS
- Suspect stress fracture in athlete with groin pain.
- Suspect stress fracture in athlete with changes in training activities.
- Seek menstrual dysfunction in female athlete with stress fracture.
- If cortical involvement, recommend surgical fixation.
- Compression fracture (inferior neck) can be treated nonoperatively.
- Although often normal, obtain radiographs to rule out other pathology.
- Place athlete on crutches during work-up to avoid catastrophe.

FIBULA STRESS FRACTURES

JEFFREY GUY, MD
REVISED BY CHARLES NOFSINGER, MD

HISTORY
- *Most common*: Overuse injuries usually related to sporting activities requiring repetitive and/or high-impact activity such as long-distance runners, gymnasts, and dancers
- *Less common*: Overuse or normal physical activity in athletes with poor-quality bone
- Disruption of bone equilibrium: Bone destruction or breakdown exceeds bone formation and repair
- *Risk factors*: High-impact activities, tight muscles and tendons, flat feet, high arches, leg length discrepancy, poor nutrition/eating disorders, menstrual irregularities
- Most common in distal fibula 2–3 inches above lateral malleolus
- Symptoms usually have a gradual onset; however, may also develop with a sudden increase in duration, frequency, or intensity of training
- Pain especially intense with activity, usually relieved with rest
- May progress to complete fracture if not recognized and treated

PHYSICAL EXAM
- May be normal as the patient may be asymptomatic during periods of inactivity
- When symptomatic, pain can described as dull or sharp depending on the progression of fracture.
- Pain localized over the distal fibula; may be sensitive to percussion or tapping proximal or distal to involved area

STUDIES
- Plain radiographs
  - ➤ May appear normal acutely
  - ➤ Radiodense lines are a sign of attempted healing.
- Bone scan
  - ➤ More effective than plain films at identifying an area of increased bone activity
- MRI
  - ➤ Also effective at identifying stress fractures but more useful when diagnosis is in question

➤ May demonstrate bone edema and fracture lines associated with a stress fracture but also will identify pathologic lesions and soft tissue masses
■ CT scan
➤ Best test to further characterize bony detail of area involved
➤ Helpful in surgical planning

DIFFERENTIAL DIAGNOSIS
■ Chronic ankle instability
■ Chronic compartment syndrome
■ High ankle sprain
■ Peroneal tendon subluxations
■ Bone tumor

TREATMENT
■ Acute
➤ Immediate cessation of activity and employ rest, ice, compression, and elevation regimen
➤ Modified weight-bearing until painless ambulation achieved
➤ Six weeks of modified activity (varies with extent of symptoms)
➤ Anti-inflammatory medication as needed
➤ Identify and modify training regimen or other etiology thought to contribute to the stress fracture
➤ Encourage nonweight-bearing cardiovascular activity such as swimming and stationary bike
➤ Physical therapy emphasizing stretching regimen
➤ Progressive and controlled return to activity
■ Chronic nonoperative
➤ Permanent cessation of involved sport
➤ Fosamax
➤ Bone stimulator
■ Chronic operative
➤ Internal fixation with plate and bone graft

Treatment considerations
■ Age
■ Training regimen
■ Nutrition
■ Chronicity

DISPOSITION
N/A

PROGNOSIS
- Good if etiology identified and modified

CAVEATS AND PEARLS
- Beware of pathologic bone! Stress fractures can result from normal physical activity in patients with poor bone quality such as osteomalacia.
- Stress fracture can be initial presentation of eating disorder in young women.
- Close follow-up essential to safe return to sport

FLEXOR PROFUNDUS AVULSION (JERSEY FINGER)

JOHN FERNANDEZ, MD

HISTORY
- Often not initially recognized/misdiagnosed
- Not reported immediately
- Lack of significant complaints
- Diagnosis requires high index of suspicion and accurate exam
- Symptoms
  - Usually mild/short-lived
  - Swelling of finger
  - Loss of motion/strength
  - Pain in finger/palm
- Mechanism
  - Forced finger extension against active flexion
  - Finger usually caught in clothing ("jersey finger") during grasping
  - Ring finger most commonly affected
  - Anatomically longest with metacarpophalangeal joint/proximal interphalangeal joint (PIPJ) flexion
- Common in football, basketball, wrestling
- Three main types of avulsions identified

PHYSICAL EXAM
- Swelling/ecchymosis
- Tenderness to palpation
- Note site of tenderness, finger or palm

- Loss of active flexion at distal interphalangeal joint (DIPJ)
- "Make a fist," note fingertip cannot flex to palm
- Hand on table palm up, block middle phalanx while trying to flex finger, note loss of DIPJ flexion
- Loss of passive flexion "tenodesis effect"
- Hyperextend wrist passively, should have some DIPJ flexion
- Loss of normal "flexion cascade" of fingers at rest
- Late findings: hyperextension instability of DIPJ

STUDIES
- Radiographs
  - AP/lateral/oblique or hand/finger
  - Usually normal appearance
  - Look for fracture fragment from proximal/volar part of distal phalanx
- MRI
  - Sagittal cuts can reveal site of distal tendon retraction A4 pulley, PIPJ, or palm

DIFFERENTIAL DIAGNOSIS
- DIPJ/PIPJ dislocation
  - Instability/tenderness at joint
  - Active DIPJ flexion intact
- Phalangeal fracture
  - Tender at fracture
  - Active DIPJ flexion intact
- Nerve palsy
  - Active DIPJ flexion intact
  - Passive DIPJ flexion (tenodesis) is lost
  - Multiple digits involved

TREATMENT
- Leddy/Packer classification
  - Type I
    - Tendon retracted to palm/A1 pulley
    - Tender mass in palm
    - Reinsert within 2 weeks
    - Least common
  - Type II
    - Tendon retracted to PIPJ level

- Reinsert within 3 months
- Most common
➤ Type III
  - Tendon retracted to DIPJ level/A4 pulley
  - Associated bone fragment
  - Reinsert/repair bone with 2 weeks
  - Type IIIa: tendon avulsed from bone fragment
■ Acute
  ➤ Rapid, accurate diagnosis critical
  ➤ Establish type of avulsion
  ➤ Repair as quickly as possible depending on type
  ➤ Repaired directly to phalanx with pull-out suture button over nail
  ➤ Midlateral/zigzag approach
  ➤ Bunnell criss-cross suture in tendon end (3-0 monofilament)
  ➤ Decorticate palmar bone distal to DIPJ
  ➤ Drill two free Keith needles through insertion site and through nailplate dorsally
  ➤ Pull sutures through with Keith needles
  ➤ Tie suture over nylon button/felt pad over nailplate
  ➤ Reinforce repair site with 4-0 figure-eight sutures
■ Postoperative supervised occupational therapy
  ➤ Dorsal block splint
  ➤ Dynamic traction
  ➤ Protected mobilization
  ➤ Follow-up every 2 to 3 weeks
■ Late
  ➤ If no DIPJ instability, no special need for DIPJ flexion
■ No treatment
  ➤ If DIPJ unstable/weak pinch
  ➤ Fusion/tenodesis of DIPJ
  ➤ Free flexor tendon graft
  ➤ Young, motivated, and compliant patient
  ➤ Only if there is specific need for DIPJ flexion
  ➤ Technician/musician
  ➤ Risk of worsening finger function
  ➤ Loss of PIPJ motion/contracture

DISPOSITION
N/A

PROGNOSIS
- Early recognition and proper repair
  - Very good result
  - Return to play 6–8 weeks
  - Complications
    - May lose some DIPJ extension
  - Grip strength almost normal
- No repair
  - Fair/good result
  - Function of "superficialis finger" is very good
  - Return to play immediately
  - Complications
    - Loss of DIPJ flexion
    - Diminished grip strength
    - Hyperextension instability
- Tenodesis/fusion DIPJ
  - Good result
  - Return to play immediately with splint
  - Complications
    - Loss of DIPJ flexion
    - Diminished grip strength
- Late repair/tendon graft
  - Fair/poor result
  - Return to play 6–8 weeks
  - Complications
    - Make finger worse
    - Adhesions/scarring
    - Loss of PIPJ motion
    - Contracture

CAVEATS AND PEARLS
- Always examine for profundus function in any finger injury/complaint.
- Repair as quickly as possible.
- Tendon contracture worsens rapidly.
- Begin therapy within 2–3 days.
- Ensure therapist is qualified; perform 3 times weekly.
- Leave button in place at least 6 weeks.
- Consider leaving late injury alone, depending on type of avulsion; risk worsening existing function.

FROSTBITE

WILLIAM O. ROBERTS, MD

HISTORY
- Frostbite is freezing of tissue, including intracellular contents
- Occurs with exposure to ambient temperatures <28–31°F
  - Eutectic point of saline solution
- Risk greatest in appendages and watershed areas
- Risk factors for athletes
  - Outdoor activity in ambient temperatures <31°F
  - Previous frostbite increases risk twofold
  - Altered mental status
    - Hypothermia
    - Exercise exhaustion
  - Tobacco use
  - Black race
  - Petroleum product spill
    - Cooled below tissue freezing level
    - Evaporative heat loss accelerates tissue freeze

PHYSICAL EXAM
- Clinical picture
  - White, cold, firm or hard tissue
  - Vascular changes and inflammation with rewarming
    - Free radical oxidative stress tissue damage
- Classification based on initial exam
  - Superficial
    - Mobile subcutaneous tissue
  - Deep
    - Deep tissue hard
    - Cool and insensitive post-thawing
- Severity rating determined after several days
  - First-degree
    - Numbness
    - Erythema
    - Edema
  - Second-degree
    - Clear, fluid-filled blisters
    - Erythema

- Edema
➤ Third-degree
  - Hemorrhagic blisters
➤ Fourth-degree
  - Injury to bone and muscle
  - Tissue mottled and lifeless

STUDIES
N/A

DIFFERENTIAL DIAGNOSIS
■ Self-evident from exam

TREATMENT
■ Protect and insulate frozen tissue until rewarmed
■ Do not rewarm frozen tissue until there is no chance of refreezing
■ Rapid rewarming in a water bath at 40–42°C (104–108°F)
■ Pharmacologic interventions
  ➤ Topical aloe vera (70% aqueous extract)
    - Dermaide™ aloe cream
  ➤ Oral ibuprofen, 400 mg bid
  ➤ Prophylactic antibiotic use controversial
■ Observe for demarcation of viable tissue before surgical debridement or amputation

Prevention
■ Avoid practice and competition in high-risk settings
■ Safety and prevention education of athletes and coaches
■ Equipment and clothing
  ➤ Layer clothing
  ➤ Limit exposed skin
  ➤ Shield high-risk area with vapor-barrier clothing
■ Remove metal jewelry, especially circumferential and pierced
■ Buddy system to watch for tissue freezing

DISPOSITION
N/A

PROGNOSIS
N/A

CAVEATS AND PEARLS
N/A

GAMEKEEPER'S THUMB (AKA SKIER'S THUMB)

GERARD GABEL, MD

HISTORY
- Sports > Work injury
- Mechanism: forceful radial deviation of thumb, usually a fall on outstretched arm/abducted thumb
- May feel "pop" – tear of ulnar collateral ligament (UCL)
- Immediate pain
- Dysfunction due to pain and instability
- Weakness of pinch, grasp
- Swelling along ulnar aspect of metacarpophalangeal (MCP) joint
- Chronic cases complain of weak pinch, pain with use
- Common sports: skiing, football, basketball
- May be acute superimposed on chronic
- May have dorsal capsular or volar plate injury (but UCL injury primary issue)

PHYSICAL EXAM
- Swelling, tenderness to palpation along ulnar > radial aspect of metaphalangeal (MP) joint
- May have palpable Stener's lesion (6- to 8-mm nodule along ulnar metacarpal neck)
- Stener's lesion
  - Eversion of UCL from its anatomic course by adductor aponeurosis
  - Held in displaced position by adductor aponeurosis margin
  - UCL cannot heal if everted in this manner
- Occasional mild interphalangeal or carpometacarpal level tenderness
- Obtain plain x-rays prior to stress testing (if nondisplaced avulsion fracture, don't do stress exam)
- Radial deviation stress exam of UCL
  - Usually requires Xylocaine block – 5 cc 2% Xylocaine, inject along ulnar metacarpal neck
  - Hold MP joint in neutral deviation, 30° of flexion (to relax volar plate)
  - Radially deviate MP joint
  - Check for degrees of laxity as well as firm end point

➤ Check in full extension to assess involvement of volar plate
➤ Check opposite thumb stress exam
➤ >25–30° of increased laxity indicative of complete UCL avulsion – probability of Stener's lesion 35–90%
➤ <25° of asymmetry, incomplete lesion
- Chronic cases (>6 weeks postinjury)
  ➤ Less tenderness, but similar laxity findings
  ➤ May have firm end point
  ➤ Stener's lesion smaller on physical exam (3–5 mm)
  ➤ Thumb rests in abducted position, ulnar metacarpal head prominent

STUDIES
- Plain radiographs
  ➤ True AP/lateral of thumb centered at MP joint
  ➤ Findings: avulsion fracture (displaced or nondisplaced), volar subluxation, radial deviation of MP joint
  ➤ Specific tests – stress AP x-rays (postblock)
    • To quantify/document degrees of angulation, to rule out Salter I or II growth plate fracture
    • Obtain on all patients except those with nondisplaced avulsion fractures (due to risk of conversion to Stener's lesion)
- Arthrogram may show leak along UCL, may outline UCL – rarely used
- MRI: excellent visualization in acute cases (>95% accuracy), less so in chronic cases (<50% accuracy)
- Ultrasound inconsistent, not recommended

DIFFERENTIAL DIAGNOSIS
- Salter fractures – Salter I fractures, if nondisplaced, may mimic UCL injury on exam and nonstress x-ray
  ➤ Must do stress x-ray on all patients with open growth and negative initial x-ray
- Volar plate injuries – hyperextension injury, tender to extension stress, negative radial deviation stress exam
- MCP dislocation – hyperextension injury, plain film diagnosis; no stress exam

TREATMENT
- Incomplete injuries
  ➤ Stable

- Splint protection
- Immediate active and passive range of motion
- No varus/valgus
- Resume sports as tolerated
➤ Unstable
  - Splint or cast immobilization 3 weeks, followed by active and passive range of motion
  - No varus/valgus
  - Return to sports as tolerated with or without thumb-based MP protective splint
■ Complete injuries: operative
➤ 2.0-cm incision along ulnar MP joint
➤ Split adductor, reduce/pin MP in 15° of flexion/slight ulnar deviation
➤ Minisuture anchor repair of UCL to proximal phalanx margin (anatomic)
➤ Cast, start protected range of motion at 3 weeks
➤ Arthroscopic – technically possible to "invert" Stener's lesion, arthroscopic assisted repair of UCL, results ? in comparison to open
➤ Chronic cases – ligament reconstruction using palmaris longus (or partial strip of radial wrist extensor or flexor)
  - Same exposure as in acute cases
  - Split remaining UCL longitudinally
  - Identify/prepare anatomic origin and insertion, pin joint
  - Harvest palmaris longus graft
  - Minisuture anchors at origin and insertion double-strand graft reconstruction

DISPOSITION
N/A

PROGNOSIS
■ >90% good and excellent results (stable with good range of motion)
■ Mild to moderate loss of motion common (10–30°) – minimize with early/protected range of motion
■ Prognosis dependent on MP stability
■ Return to play
➤ Nonabduction-requiring sports or positions (e.g., volleyball, offensive lineman) – may tape thumb to hand and return quite early once pin removed

➤ Abduction-requiring positions (e.g., basketball, receiver, quarterback)
  • Incomplete injuries – as permitted by pain (may follow tip pinch to monitor recovery)
  • Complete injuries – minimum of 2 months postoperatively; monitor tip pinch

CAVEATS AND PEARLS
■ Don't misdiagnose Salter injury
■ Palpable Stener lesion most diagnostic finding; if present, operative
■ During rehabilitation have patient "skin a cat differently"
  ➤ Tip pinch along radial rather than ulnar tip
  ➤ Tape thumb securely to palm to play
  ➤ Allow earlier return without compromise

GROIN MUSCLE STRAIN

EDWARD YIAN, MD
E. M. WOJTYS, MD
REVISED BY CHARLES NOFSINGER, MD

HISTORY
■ Common injury in athletes
■ Mechanisms of injury
  ➤ Hip hyperabduction
  ➤ Abdominal wall hyperextension
  ➤ Rapid deceleration or eccentric contraction
  ➤ Lateral movements, kicking, twisting
  ➤ Directional changes
■ **Sports at risk**
  ➤ Football
  ➤ Soccer
  ➤ Figure skating
  ➤ Hockey
  ➤ Track and field
■ Risk factors
  ➤ Poor conditioning
  ➤ Fatigue
  ➤ Cold environment, inadequate muscle warm-up
  ➤ Inadequate rehabilitation of previous injury
■ Hip adductor muscles most commonly involved

- Symptoms dependent upon severity of strain
  - Grade I
    - Gradual tightening of muscle after injury
    - Pain with stretching
  - Grade II
    - Pop or tearing sensation
    - Muscle spasm
    - Inability to continue play
  - Grade III
    - Dramatic, painful injuries
    - Pop or tearing sensation
    - Soft tissue swelling, spasm, edema

PHYSICAL EXAM

- Assess hip ROM – Abductor/adductor, flexion/extension, internal/external rotation
- Identify area of local tenderness, or gapping in muscle-tendon unit
- Assess active resistance to hip flexion, extension – Abductor/adductor, internal/external rotation

STUDIES

- Radiographic
  - AP pelvis; AP, lateral of hip
  - Usually normal, rule out bone avulsion
    - Iliac crest and sartorius, tensor fasciae latae origin
    - ASIS and rectus femoris origin
    - Lesser trochanter and psoas
    - Ischial tuberosity – hamstrings
- MRI
  - May help define percent of disruption in muscle-tendon-bone unit
  - Can determine hematoma formation
- Ultrasound
  - Helps determine muscle integrity
  - Localize hematomas

DIFFERENTIAL DIAGNOSIS

Strains

- Muscles inserting onto pelvis and symphysis
  - External oblique
  - Internal oblique
  - Transversus abdominis

➤ Inferior pelvic muscles
  • Adductors
  • Pectineus
  • Gracilis
  • Obturator internus
  • Quadratus femoris
  • Gluteus
  • Hip flexor strain
➤ Sports hernia
➤ Orthopedic entities
  • Slipped capital femoral epiphysis
  • Stress fracture femoral neck or pelvis
  • Obturator nerve entrapment
  • Osteitis pubis
  • Inguinal hernia
  • Snapping hip – psoas
  • Labral tears
  • Osteitis pubis (pubalgia)
  • Unusual causes of hip pain
▪ Septic hip
▪ Pelvic inflammatory disease
▪ Inflammatory bowel disease
▪ Prostatitis
▪ Referred pain herniated lumbar disk
▪ Rectal/testicular cancer
▪ Avascular necrosis femoral head

TREATMENT
▪ Dependent on grade of muscle-tendon injury (I, II, III)
  ➤ Rest, ice, compression, initially
  ➤ Protected weight-bearing until injury extent determined
▪ Consider operative treatment if tendon detached from bone with displacement and loss of strength, failure of conservative treatment
▪ Must re-establish strength, flexibility
▪ Isometric strengthening as pain subsides
▪ Start with concentric exercises and proceed to eccentric for fastest return
▪ Progress to isotonic exercises and functional activities as strength improves

DISPOSITION
- Return to play criteria: normal hip ROM, flexibility and strength, functional rehabilitation with plyometrics

PROGNOSIS
- Results dependent on accuracy and completeness of diagnosis and appropriate treatment
- All grades of injury must regain full, pain-free range of hip motion to avoid repeat injury
- Strength must be satisfactory for size and activity level of patient
- Functional training and plyometrics training crucial for full recovery
- Complications
  - Recurrent strain, usually due to under-appreciation of the degree of injury
  - More common when athlete returns to play without full rehabilitation

CAVEATS AND PEARLS
- Correct diagnosis critical for effective treatment
- Radiographs rule out more significant pathology
- Flexibility and strengthening are crucial following injury
- Cannot rush athlete back to play; allow soft tissue healing and maturation

---

GROIN PAIN

EDWARD YIAN, MD
E. M. WOJTYS, MD

HISTORY
- Common disabling problem in athletes
- Sports requiring side-to-side movements, kicking, twisting
- Majority of groin pain in athletes secondary to adductor strains
- Multiple etiologies – Considerations in patient with complaint of groin pain
  - Muscular
  - Articular

➤ Periarticular
➤ Intra-abdominal
  • Urologic
  • Gynecologic
  • GI
■ Muscular-anatomic considerations
  ➤ Muscles inserting onto pelvis and symphysis
    • External oblique
    • Internal oblique
    • Transversus abdominis
  ➤ Inferior pelvic muscles
    • Adductors
    • Pectineus
    • Gracilis
    • Obturator internus
    • Quadratus femoris
    • Gluteus
■ Mechanism of injury – hip hyperabduction/abdominal hyper-extension
  ➤ Forceful muscle contraction
  ➤ May recollect a misstep
  ➤ Usually related to rapid deceleration or eccentric contraction
  ➤ Symptoms dependent on severity of strain
■ **Severity of injury**
  ➤ Grade I
    • May note gradual tightening of muscle
    • Pain with stretching
  ➤ Grade II
    • Single step/movement
    • May feel pop or tearing sensation
    • Muscle spasm
    • Inability to continue play
  ➤ Grade III
    • Dramatic, abrupt injuries
    • Pop or tearing sensation
    • Soft tissue swelling
    • Initial burst of pain
    • Diffuse pain later – secondary to spasm/edema
    • Muscle spasm
    • Occasional palpable gap in muscle

- Location may affect severity of strain
  - Grades I/II – Usually more distal in muscle level
  - Grade III – Usually to the muscle attachment at pelvis
- May present with localized soft tissue pain
- Ecchymoses can be significant
- Risk factors
  - Poor conditioning
  - Fatigue
  - Cold environment
  - Inadequate rehabilitation of previous injury
- **Presentation**
  - Common in sports with quick directional changes
    - Football
    - Soccer
  - Propulsion
    - Figure skating
    - Hockey
    - Track and field

PHYSICAL EXAM
- Assess hip ROM – flexion/extension, abductor/adductor, internal/external rotation
- Identify area of maximal tenderness
  - Tendon
  - Muscle

STUDIES
- Radiographic
  - AP pelvis; AP, lateral of hip
    - Usually normal
    - May identify avulsion of muscle-tendon units
      - Iliac crest – Sartorius, tensor fasciae latae origin
      - ASIS – Rectus femoris origin
      - Lesser trochanter – Psoas
      - Ischial tuberosity – Hamstring
- MRI
  - May reveal extent of grade II injuries (10% vs. 90%)
  - Location of grade III injuries

DIFFERENTIAL DIAGNOSIS
- Orthopedic entities
  - Hip flexor strains

- ➤ Slipped capital femoral epiphysis (SCFE)
- ➤ Degenerative joint disease (DJD)
- ➤ Stress fracture
- ➤ Psoas bursitis
- ➤ Obturator nerve entrapment
- ➤ Osteitis pubis
- ➤ Inguinal hernia
- ■ Differentiating features
  - ➤ SCFE
    - Young athlete (9–15 yr)
    - Athlete at risk: obese, sedentary, African-American
    - Medial thigh referred pain common
    - Referred knee pain possible
    - Trendelenberg gait
    - Pain with weight-bearing
    - Pain with hip motion
    - Presentation can be acute or gradual over months
    - Exam demonstrates loss of hip internal rotation
    - Hip flexion results in hip abduction and external rotation
    - Can be associated with endocrine disorders
    - Bilaterality in 40%
    - Contralateral presentation within 18 months
    - Radiographs
      - Widening of epiphyseal line
      - Loss of sphericity as head slips
  - ➤ DJD
    - Gradual onset over time
    - Morning stiffness
    - DJD – early loss of internal external rotation before flexion, abduction
    - Pain can be referred to thigh and/or knee
    - Radiographic diagnosis
      - Loss of joint space
      - Marginal osteophyte formation
      - Subchondral sclerosis/cyst formation
    - Bone scan may detect early DJD
  - ➤ Obturator nerve entrapment
    - Anterior division ventral rami L2-4
    - Two branches within obturator canal
    - Compression by trauma, hematomas, fractures in athletes
    - Medial thigh and groin pain

- Activity-related pain
- Resolution of pain with rest
- Pain produced by stretching pectineal
  - Passive external rotation and hip abduction while standing
- Radiographs: normal
- MRI: possible atrophy of innervated muscles
- Bone scan: equivocal for origin of adductor muscles
- EMG: chronic changes
- Local anesthetic diagnostic
➢ Hernia
  - Diagnosis by clinical exam
  - Groin swelling or bulge
  - Dragging sensation
  - Symptoms may be referred to scrotum
  - Complaint of aching, discomfort
  - Direct hernias less symptomatic
  - Direct hernias less likely to incarcerate
  - Femoral hernias more common in females and more likely to incarcerate
  - Differentiate from hydrocele, lymphadenopathy, groin abscess, undescended testes
➢ Intra-articular etiology
  - Groin, thigh pain associated with
    - Popping, clicking, catching, locking
    - "Giving way" sensation
  - Radiographs may demonstrate loose body, fracture
  - May require CT scan to establish diagnosis
  - MRI arthrogram: labral tear, synovitis, hypertrophic ligamentum teres
  - Hip arthroscopy may be needed to establish diagnosis
➢ Snapping hip
➢ Hip flexor strain
➢ Stress fracture
➢ Labral tears
➢ Osteitis pubis (pubalgia)
➢ Pelvic stress fracture
➢ Unusual causes of groin pain
  - Septic hip
  - Pelvic inflammatory disease
  - Inflammatory bowel disease
  - Prostatitis

- Referred pain herniated lumbar disk
- Rectal/testicular cancer
- Avascular necrosis femoral head

TREATMENT
- Establish correct diagnosis – critical
- Rest, ice, compression
- Re-establish strength, flexibility
- Isometric strengthening as pain subsides
- Progress to isotonic exercises and functional activities
- Return to play criteria
- Role of neoprene compression sleeves

DISPOSITION
N/A

PROGNOSIS
N/A

CAVEATS AND PEARLS
- Correct diagnosis critical for effective treatment
- Imaging to rule out more significant pathology
- Flexibility and strength are keys to recovery
- **Allow adequate recovery time – soft tissue healing often takes 6 weeks – soft tissue maturation will take months**

HAMSTRING STRAIN

DAVID C. NEUSCHWANDER, MD
REVISED BY CHARLES NOFSINGER, MD

HISTORY
- Most common thigh muscle injury
- Among most frequent injuries in athletes involved in running, jumping, and kicking sports (sprinting, basketball, football, soccer)
- Ischial tuberosity avulsion injuries from severe hip flexion while knee maintained in full extension (waterskiing, dancing, weightlifting, ice skating)
- Can occur in early or late stages of athletic participation
- Often associated with inadequate warm-up or fatigue
- Majority occur in acute setting with sudden onset of posterior thigh pain during strenuous exercise.

- May have audible pop heard by athlete and/or competitors that limits ability to participate
- Can also occur in more chronic setting
- Feel tightness or "pull" limiting subsequent participation

PHYSICAL EXAM
- Acutely, athlete may be on ground grabbing at posterior thigh.
- May have palpable defect in severe cases, but in most cases, it is important to palpate muscle from origin to insertion, which is best done with athlete lying prone and knee flexed 90°.
- Attempts may be made to determine severity by testing the position for maximal tenderness with the straight-leg raise test.
- Another guideline for severity is a determination of the amount of restriction of passive knee extension with the hip flexed 90°.
- Ecchymosis usually present, but does not tend to be correlated with severity of injury.
- With time, localized discomfort with palpation becomes more diffuse and less defined.

STUDIES
- Plain x-rays are not helpful in diagnosis or determining the extent of muscle strains, except in cases of ischial tuberosity avulsion.
- Ultrasound, bone scan, and CT scan have been used to evaluate hamstring injuries.
- MRI scans can clearly delineate high signal intensity on T2 images, but are not thought to be cost-effective and do not alter treatment.

DIFFERENTIAL DIAGNOSIS
- More important determination is that of musculotendinous injury vs. avulsion injury from ischial tuberosity.

TREATMENT
- RICE (rest, ice, compression, elevation)
- Rest can simply be cessation of sports, with the most severe cases needing bed rest.
- Bagged crushed ice conforming to the thigh is used and crutches are useful just after the injury.
- Compression reduces hemorrhage and helps control edema.
- Want to control hemorrhage, edema, and pain in the first 3–5 days with the RICE regimen
- Gradual increasing ROM and strengthening exercises are followed by gradual resumption of activities.

- Prior to resumption of activity, it is important to restore hamstring strength, flexibility, and muscle balance.
- An attempt is done to classify strains by clinical means into grade I, II, and III.
  - Grade I has little hemorrhage and no structural damage and resolves rapidly with little loss of time.
  - Grade II – Partial tear of musculotendinous unit. Patient gives a more accurate history and functional loss is usually immediate with swelling.
  - Grade III – Complete muscular tear or avulsion injury
- Operation is recommended for proximal injuries with ischial tuberosity avulsions displaced >2 cm.
- Distal avulsion injuries are usually associated with lateral knee injuries and should be operatively treated.
- Therapeutic exercises help restore strength and flexibility (isometrics initially, then isotonic in concentric mode, and finally high-speed low-resistance isokinetic exercise program or progressive eccentric program).
- NSAIDs are also helpful.

DISPOSITION
N/A

PROGNOSIS
- Return to play based on athlete's progress in functional activities and isokinetic testing.
- Isokinetic testing within 10% of normal at slow and fast speeds and a hamstring quadriceps ratio of 0.5 to 0.6 is recommended.
- Restoration of flexibility and endurance also important
- Attempt to reproduce sporting activity; if can be done pain-free, then resume activities.

CAVEATS AND PEARLS
- Associated factors can be inadequate warm-up, inadequate stretching, poor endurance, poor technique, poor posture, leg length inequality, muscle strength imbalances.
- Identification of these factors may allow rehabilitation program to deal with correction of problems prior to injury.
- High incidence of recurrent hamstring strains due to inadequate treatment and premature return to play
- Surgery rarely necessary except in cases of proximal avulsion

- May be some correlation of hamstring strain to sacroiliac joint dysfunction and one report of sacroiliac joint mobilization helping in the treatment of hamstring strains

---

HIP DISLOCATIONS

JOHN W. NOBLE, JR., MD

HISTORY
- Mechanism
  - Uncommon in the athlete
  - Usually the result of contact sports
  - Occurs with force applied to flexed knee
- Symptoms
  - Extreme pain
  - Immediate disability
- Direction
  - Majority of dislocations are posterior
  - Up to 10% may be anterior

PHYSICAL EXAM
- Neurovascular status must be assessed prereduction
  - Limb held in flexion, adduction and internal rotation with a posterior dislocation
  - Limb typically held in external rotation with an anterior dislocation
  - Knee must be carefully examined because of associated ligamentous injuries

STUDIES
- Plain radiographs generally suffice at time of injury
- CT scan recommended postreduction to rule out incarcerated fragments
- Radiographic follow-up recommended for up to 2 years postdislocation
- MRI useful for the detection of post-dislocation avascular necrosis

DIFFERENTIAL DIAGNOSIS
- Acetabular fracture-dislocation
- Femoral head fracture with or without dislocation

- Femoral neck fracture
- Proximal femur fracture

TREATMENT
- Closed reduction
  - Closed reductions must be carried out emergently
  - Reduction carried out under general anesthetic or IV sedation
  - Bigelow, Allis, or Stimson maneuvers typically used
- Surgical treatment
  - Required for irreducible dislocation
  - Required for incarcerated osteochondral fragmentation
  - May be required for associated acetabular fracture
  - Arthroscopy may be considered for removal of osteochondral fragmentation

DISPOSITION
   N/A

PROGNOSIS
- Best without associated fracture
- Risk of avascular necrosis lowered with prompt reduction
- Late instability rare

CAVEATS AND PEARLS
- True orthopedic emergency
- Must evaluate neurovascular status before and after reduction
- Prompt reduction lowers risk of avascular necrosis
- Must check for congruent reduction
- Rule out incarcerated fragments

HIP FLEXOR (RECTUS) STRAINS

BERNARD R. BACH, JR., MD

HISTORY
- Definition – injury to muscle-tendon unit
  - May be partial or complete
- Anatomy
  - Rectus femoris originates from superior/inferior iliac spine

- Mechanism
  - Variable onset
    - Insidious – overuse
    - Specific event – forceful hip flexion or eccentric contraction on extended hip
  - May feel tearing or "pull" sensation
  - Pain
  - Acutely may have swelling, anterior hip discomfort
  - Painful active hip flexion

PHYSICAL EXAM
- Tenderness over proximal origin of rectus
- Tenderness over ASIS/AIIS
- Pain with active hip flexion
- Pain with passive hip extension
- Pain with resistance against hip flexion
- Resistance against adduction nonpainful
- Limp
- Passive hip motion normal
- Neurovascular exam normal
- Pain with attempts to perform abdominal "situps"

STUDIES
- Radiographs to rule out ASIS avulsion fracture
- Radiographs to rule out hip joint pathology
  - Slipped capital femoral epiphysis (SCFE) in adolescent
  - Degenerative joint disease in adult
- MRI rarely indicated

DIFFERENTIAL DIAGNOSIS
- Contusion
  - Direct contact mechanism rather than indirect forceful contraction
- Adductor strain
  - Pain more medial, groin region
  - Pain with resistance against adduction
  - Pain with passive abduction
- Psoas strain
- Sartorius strain
- SCFE
  - Often insidious

- ➤ Hip flexion with compensatory external rotation
- ➤ Radiographic confirmation
- ➤ Bilaterality 40%
- Legg-Perthes
  - ➤ Groin/hip pain in child 5–10 yr
  - ➤ Radiographic diagnosis
- Toxic synovitis
  - ➤ Differential with Legg-Perthes
- Quad strain
  - ➤ Similar mechanism
  - ➤ Distal location within muscle
- External oblique strain
  - ➤ Tenderness along iliac crest
- Avulsion fracture ASIS
  - ➤ Radiographic diagnosis
- Avulsion fracture AIIS
  - ➤ Radiographic diagnosis
- Chronic overuse "apophysitis"
- Snapping hip
- Osteitis pubis
- Hip pointer

TREATMENT
- Establish correct diagnosis
- Dependent on grade/severity
- Phase 1
  - ➤ Goals – Reduce pain, swelling, inflammation, bleeding
  - ➤ Treatment – RICE; crutches may be needed; NSAIDs
  - ➤ Time frame – 48–72 hrs
- Phase 2
  - ➤ Goals – Motion recovery
  - ➤ Treatment – Protected ROM, ice, heat, ultrasound, EMS; ± NSAIDs
  - ➤ Time frame – 72 hrs-7 days
- Phase 3
  - ➤ Goals – Increased strength, flexibility, endurance
  - ➤ Treatment – Isometrics, well leg bicycling
  - ➤ Time frame – 1–3 weeks
- Phase 4
  - ➤ Goals – Increase strength

➤ Treatment – Isotonic, ± isokinetic, proprioception, core strengthening

DISPOSITION
N/A

PROGNOSIS
- Usually good
- Recurrences possible
- Consider use of compression shorts
- Warm-up/cool-down important
- Heterotopic bone may form in soft tissues

CAVEATS AND PEARLS
- Chronic "hip flexor strain" – rule out pelvic/hip joint pathology

---

HIP POINTERS

WILLIAM E. GARRETT, JR., MD, PhD
REVISED BY CHARLES NOFSINGER, MD

HISTORY
- Painful injury at or below iliac crest
- Follows a direct injury
- May involve hematoma
- Common in contact sports or following a fall

PHYSICAL EXAM
- Tender over iliac crest, anterior superior iliac spine, gluteal muscles, or greater trochanter
- Swelling or hematoma may be present
- Activation of abdominal muscles painful

STUDIES
- Usually unnecessary
- Radiographs to rule out fracture if needed

DIFFERENTIAL DIAGNOSIS
- Iliac crest avulsion fracture, usually no contact
- Stress fracture of iliac apophysis
  ➤ More insidious onset

- Acute fracture of ilium
  - Higher-energy trauma
  - Pain more severe
  - Deformity or crepitus sometime present

TREATMENT
- Rest as needed
- Ice, analgesics, anti-inflammatory medications
- Compressive dressing early
- Rarely aspiration
- Early motion, stretching
- Increasing mobility/strengthening as tolerated
- Appropriate hip pads
- Injection of local anesthetic into hematoma for temporary relief

DISPOSITION
  N/A

PROGNOSIS
- Excellent
- May miss a few days to several weeks
- Faster return if recurrence avoided

CAVEATS AND PEARLS
- Easier to prevent than to treat
- Insist on use of hip pads when possible

HOOK OF HAMATE FRACTURES

ARTHUR RETTIG, MD
RON NOY, MD

HISTORY
- Mechanism of injury
  - Racquet, stick, and bat sports
    - Golf, baseball, softball, tennis, racquetball, squash
  - Stress fracture most often
  - Insidious onset of pain
  - Repetitive stress caused by torque
  - Acute direct palmar trauma
  - Acute trauma during bad swing (duff, etc.)

- Complaints
  - Ulnar wrist pain
  - Pain causing difficulty gripping and swinging club racquet, bat, etc.
  - Decreased performance, compensatory technique changes

PHYSICAL EXAM
- Tenderness over hook of hamate (1-2 cm distal and radial to pisiform)
- Tenderness over dorsal ulnar hand
- Pain with resisted DIP flexion of ring/small fingers with palmar-flexed/ulnar-deviated wrist
- Decreased grip strength

STUDIES
- Radiographs
  - Routine views often do not show the fracture
  - Carpal tunnel view
  - 20° supinated oblique view
- CT: gold standard
- Bone scan invasive but accurate
- MRI less accurate than CT but shows other soft tissue structures as well

DIFFERENTIAL DIAGNOSIS
- Wrist sprain
- Triangular fibrocartilage complex (TFCC) tear
- Ulnar nerve neuritis
- Ganglion cyst
- Carpal instability dissociative (CID): instability between bones in same carpal row
  - Carpal instability nondissociative (CIND): instability between carpal rows
- Hypothenar hammer syndrome

TREATMENT
- Acute traumatic fracture
  - Nonoperative
    - Cast
    - Indications
      - Out-of-season athlete
      - Nonswinging athlete

- High rate of nonunion – 50% healing time 12 weeks
- Higher union rate with acute trauma vs. stress fracture
➤ Operative
  - Indications
    - In-season athlete
    - Decreased performance secondary to pain
    - Failure of nonoperative treatment
    - Persistent pain
    - Painful nonunion
➤ Techniques
  - Excision
    - Gold standard
    - Splint for 1 week, then removable splint for 2–3 weeks
    - Return to sport at 6–10 weeks
    - Earlier return in playing cast
  - ORIF
    - Screw fixation
    - Difficult
    - High nonunion
    - Better with acute fracture than chronic stress fracture
    - Approach: volar curved incision, protect ulnar nerve and artery
■ Chronic stress fracture
  ➤ Nonoperative
    - Cast
    - High failure rate
    - Indication: medically unable to undergo surgery
  ➤ Operative
    - Indications
      - In-season athlete
      - Failure of nonoperative treatment
      - Pain
  ➤ Techniques
    - Excision
      - Gold standard
      - Splint for 1 week, then removable splint for 2–3 weeks
      - Return to sports at 6–10 weeks
      - Earlier return with playing cast
    - ORIF
      - Screw fixation
      - Difficult
      - High nonunion rates

DISPOSITION
   N/A

PROGNOSIS
- Nonsurgical treatment: better with acute trauma
- Surgical treatment: excision – best prognosis
- Follow-up routine
  ➤ Persistent pain – evaluate for nonunion
  ➤ CT scan
- Return to play: earliest return with excision
- Complications
  ➤ Nonunion
  ➤ Pain
  ➤ Ulnar nerve neuropathy
  ➤ Rupture flexor digitorum profundus – small finger

CAVEATS AND PEARLS
- High index of suspicion
- Golf, baseball, racquetball, tennis
- CT scan diagnostic
- Nonoperative treatment – higher union rate for acute trauma
- High nonunion rate with nonoperative treatment
- Excision is gold standard

HYPOTHERMIA

WILLIAM O. ROBERTS, MD

HISTORY
- Core body temperature <36.5°C (97°F)
- Classification scheme
  ➤ Mild: 34–36°C (93–97°F)
  ➤ Moderate: 30–34°C (86–93°F)
  ➤ Severe: <30°C (<86°F)
- Environmental conditions that increase risk
  ➤ Air temperature <18°C (64°F)
  ➤ Wind speed and wind chill factor cooling
  ➤ Wet conditions from sweat, rain, or sleet
  ➤ Cold water immersion
    • Water thermal conductivity 32 times > air

- Other risk factors in athletes
  - Older age, decreased metabolic rate
  - Younger age; larger ratio of body surface to mass speeds body heat loss
  - Hypoglycemia
    - Diabetes mellitus
    - Depleted glycogen store
  - Medical conditions
    - Head injury causing CNS dysfunction
    - Loss of shivering thermogenesis
- Cardiac effects of decreased core temperature
  - Heart rate slows to <3 bpm at 10°C core temp
  - Cardiac contractility normal to very low core temp
  - Atrial fibrillation <30°C
  - Ventricular fibrillation <28°C
  - Asystole <20°C
  - Treatment response poor <30°C

PHYSICAL EXAM
- Rectal temperature is diagnostic in field conditions – <30° (<70°F)
- Impaired judgment
- Confusion and apathy
- "Paradoxical undressing"
- Shivering response decreases <33°C
- Muscle stiffness
- Decreased level of consciousness
- Decreased pulse and respiratory rate
- Coma and loss of consciousness

STUDIES
- Blood glucose low
- EKG for rhythm and asystole
  - J-wave (extra deflection at QRS-ST junction) in 80%
- Chemistry changes
  - Elevated enzyme markers of cell injury
- Blood gases
  - Combined respiratory and metabolic acidosis

DIFFERENTIAL DIAGNOSIS
- Cardiac arrest
- Drug stupor
- Stroke or intracranial hemorrhage
- Head trauma

TREATMENT

- Immediate core rewarming
- Passive core rewarming methods with endogenous heat production
  - 1°C per hour at basal rate
  - 2°C per hour if shivering
  - Exercise for rewarming only for temperature >35°C
- Active external (surface) rewarming methods
  - Plumbed garments field method of choice
    - Bare Hugger™
  - Heating blankets
    - 0.5–3°C per hour
    - Burn risk
  - Warm (40–45°C) water immersion
    - Warming rate 5+°C per hour
    - Extremities out of water
    - Difficult to do CPR
    - Evaporative heat loss when taken from tub
  - Heated objects or containers (IV bags) in axilla, neck, and groin
  - Radiant heat sources
  - Other "animal" bodies (field technique)
- Active internal core rewarming methods
  - Extracorporeal cardiopulmonary bypass
    - Up to 10°C per hour
    - Method of choice in cardiac arrest
  - Continuous thoracostomy (pleural) lavage
    - Two chest tube method
    - Up to 8°C/hour
  - Peritoneal irrigation (dialysis)
    - 4–6°C per hour
    - Two bladder catheters for fluid exchange
    - Ringer's lactate or saline at 10–12 L/h at 40°C warmed in blood warmer
  - Augment field and hospital therapy
    - Warmed and humidified air inhalation
    - Warmed IV fluids at 43°C
- Field treatment and initial first aid
  - Remove from cold environment
  - Remove wet clothing
  - Dry skin
  - Insulate with blankets to stop core temperature drop
    - Prewarm with clothes dryer or microwave

➢ Warm packs in neck, axilla, and groin for mild to moderate hypothermia
- Hot-water bottles
- Warmed IV bags

➢ Blanket with circulation tubes for warmed air or fluid
- Bare Hugger™

➢ Breathe warmed, humidified air at 42–46°C
- Use O2 if available

➢ Mild to moderate hypothermia and conscious
- Oral fluid and glucose
- Consider IV dextrose 50% in water
- Walk to generate intrinsic heat

■ Field disposition

➢ Mild casualties can be released if normothermic and stable

➢ Transfer severe and most moderate casualties to hospital
- Evaluation
- Core rewarming

➢ EKG monitoring if available at maximum amplification
- Electrodes may not stick, so puncture skin with needle through electrode pad

➢ CPR for pulseless and apneic
- Start for asystole, not bradycardia
- Do not start CPR if unable to continue to treatment site

■ Hospital treatment

➢ Rapid internal extracorporeal rewarming for severe hypothermia
- Method of choice
- Alternatives are peritoneal dialysis or two chest tube irrigation
- Augmentation methods

➢ Monitor temp at 5- to 10-min intervals

➢ Endpoint for active rewarming
- Stop rewarming at 32–34°C
- Avoid hyperthermia and increased cell metabolism

➢ Cardiac arrhythmia prophylaxis with bretylium (5 mg/kg) for temp <28°C

➢ Defibrillation trial up to 3 shocks for temp <30°C

➢ Support hypovolemia with fluid resuscitation D5% NS or NS
- No lactated Ringer's, as cold liver cannot metabolize lactate

➢ Glucose monitoring and replacement

➢ Electrolyte, renal, and hepatic lab monitoring

➢ Antibiotics for pneumonia prophylaxis (controversial)

- Rewarming pitfalls
  - Peripheral rewarming reduces vasoconstriction, causing shock
  - Increased O_2 demand in warmed tissues
  - Afterdrop in core temperature occurs as warming begins
    - Heat exchange cools blood circulating through cold peripheral tissues
    - Up to 3°C adults and 5°C children

DISPOSITION
N/A

PROGNOSIS
- Rapid onset and rapid correction has better outcome
  - Decreased cell metabolism with lower cell temperature
  - Cold promotes cell preservation until cell contents frozen
- Mild hypothermia has general recovery with endogenous heat
- Moderate hypothermia has general recovery with active rewarming
- Severe hypothermia has 30-80% mortality
  - Pulse present at initial exam, better survival
  - Longer duration of hypothermia, increased morbidity
- Complications
  - Pneumonia
  - Pulmonary edema
  - Cardiac arrhythmia
  - Myoglobinuria
  - Disseminated intravascular coagulation
  - Seizures
  - Compartment syndromes

CAVEATS AND PEARLS
N/A

ILIOTIBIAL BAND SYNDROME

ANSWORTH A. ALLEN, MD
MARK C. DRAKOS, MD

HISTORY

Definition
- Iliotibial band (ITB) syndrome is an overuse injury.

■ Result of excessive friction between distal ITB and the lateral epicondylar eminence

Symptoms
■ Lateral knee pain that radiates proximally or distally
■ Usually associated with running 20–40 miles/week for >1 year
■ Also frequently seen in cyclists
■ Pain frequently develops after long run
■ Chronic cases have pain while running
■ Pain exacerbated by running on hills/banked surfaces
■ Increased pain with downhill running

PHYSICAL EXAM
■ Point tenderness at lateral epicondyle
■ Soft tissue swelling/crepitation
■ Pain with compression test thumb pressure over condyle and active knee flexion and extension – Pain at 30° of flexion
■ Prominent lateral epicondyle
■ Tight ITB
■ Excessive foot pronation, genu varum and internal tibial torsion may be present

STUDIES
■ **Routine knee series**
  ➤ Normal
  ➤ Take to rule out other causes for symptoms
■ **MRI/ultrasound**
  ➤ Soft tissue inflammation/edema ITB
  ➤ Fluid collection in bursa
  ➤ Signal abnormality in posterior fibers ITB

DIFFERENTIAL DIAGNOSIS
■ Lateral meniscal tear
■ Patellofemoral chondromalacia
■ Fabella syndrome
■ Proximal tibiofibular joint instability
■ Popliteus tendinitis

TREATMENT
■ Treatment options
  ➤ **Nonsurgical**
    • Rest/activity modification (reduce distance running/cycling)

- Alter training techniques
- Orthotics
- Anti-inflammatory medications
- Corticosteroid injection

➤ **Surgical**
- Chronic cases refractory to nonoperative management >1 year
- Document lesion on MRI/ultrasound
- Bursectomy and excision portion of ITB
- Debridement of lateral epicondylar eminence

DISPOSITION
N/A

PROGNOSIS
■ **Nonoperative treatment**
➤ High likelihood of improvement with nonoperative management
➤ Most patients do well
■ **Surgical treatment**
➤ Rarely indicated
➤ Overwhelming majority will not need surgery
➤ High patient satisfaction
Return to play
■ Nonoperative
➤ Usually 6–8 weeks
➤ Most return to pain-free running/cycling
■ Surgery
➤ Usually 3–4 months
➤ Criteria: pain-free running/activities

CAVEATS AND PEARLS
■ Suspect ITB syndrome in runners/cyclists with lateral knee pain.
■ Beware of anatomic predisposition.
■ Injection can be used for diagnostic and therapeutic purposes.
■ MRI can be used to rule out other causes of lateral knee pain.
■ Activity modification/NSAIDs/physical therapy and shoe modification are extremely effective.
■ Most patients do not need surgery.

INTERSECTION SYNDROME

CHRISTOPHER D. HAMILTON, MD

HISTORY
- Mechanism of injury
  - Repetitive trauma involving grasping, gripping
    - Bat or racquet sports
    - Industrial causation
  - Insidious onset
- Initial complaints and symptoms
  - Pain in wrist, dorsal forearm
  - Swelling
  - Pain with grasping
  - Crepitance in wrist extensors
  - Redness (uncommon)
- Chronic complaints
  - Continued initial complaints
  - Pain
  - Swelling
  - Crepitance
  - Loss of grip strength
  - "Clicking" with wrist extension

PHYSICAL EXAM
- Acute
  - Tenderness over second dorsal wrist compartment
    - Extensor carpi radialis longus and extensor carpi radialis brevis compartment
  - Swelling proximal to region of abductor pollicis longus and extensor pollicis brevis
  - Redness and erythema rarely seen
    - Area can be normally prominent
    - Compare to contralateral side
- Acute and chronic
  - Tenderness in dorsal wrist
  - Crepitance in second dorsal compartment
  - Pain with resisted wrist extension
  - Crepitance with wrist extension
  - Weak grip due to pain

STUDIES
- Radiographs
  - Generally a clinical diagnosis
  - Use to rule out other abnormalities
- Laboratory studies
  - Usually normal
  - No definitive laboratory findings
- MRI
  - Order for unusual cases, increased swelling
  - May find tendon abnormalities, ruptures, anomalies
  - Rule out unusual tumors
- Bone scan: rare stress fractures
- Ultrasound generally not helpful

DIFFERENTIAL DIAGNOSIS
- Overuse syndromes
- DeQuervain's syndrome generally more proximally located
- Tendinitis
- Stress fracture of radius
- Tendon ruptures: careful clinical exam of all wrist extensors
- Extensor retinaculum tears

TREATMENT
- Nonoperative
  - Relative rest
    - Modification of wrist activities to reduce stress
    - NSAIDs may decrease pain and swelling
  - Splinting: wrist splint molded in 15° of extension
  - Corticosteroid injection
    - Into second dorsal compartment
    - Just proximal to intersection point
    - Continued splinting after injection
- Operative treatment
  - Should be needed infrequently as conservative care is the main-stay of treatment
  - Release of second dorsal compartment
    - Longitudinal incision from wrist to proximal to affected area
    - Release of deep fascia and extensor compartment
  - Synovectomy
    - Acute and chronic inflammation encountered
    - Leave compartment open

> Closure of skin only
> Postoperative splint in 15° of extension
- Postoperative management
  > Splinting for 10 days to 2 weeks
  > Resume motion
  > Resume activities as tolerated
  > Return to sports over 4–6 weeks

DISPOSITION
N/A

PROGNOSIS
- Most should resolve with conservative treatment, often in 6–8 weeks
- Surgery indicated rarely
- Return to sports over 4–6 weeks as symptoms resolve

CAVEATS AND PEARLS
- Diagnosis primarily clinical
- Pathophysiology is a stenosing tenosynovitis of the second dorsal compartment
- Pain is more dorsal and proximal than DeQuervain's syndrome
- Injection of steroids can be very helpful early on

KNEE ARTHRITIS

KENT E. YINGER, MD
BERT R. MANDELBAUM, MD

HISTORY
- Primary degenerative osteoarthritis
  > Idiopathic
  > Enzymatic changes result in loss of cartilage proteoglycans
  > Rare before age 40
  > Common in obese people over 50
  > Often involves multiple joints (e.g., hips, hand distal interphalangeal joints)
- Secondary osteoarthritis
  > Injury to articular cartilage from trauma, instability, infection, or hemophilia

- Osteoarthritis (both types)
  - Morning pain and stiffness, better with activity
  - More pain and swelling with weight-bearing activities
  - May be associated with deformity – varus most common
  - No mechanical symptoms (e.g., locking, catching) unless associated with degenerative meniscus tear
- Inflammatory arthritis
  - Many types, such as rheumatoid, lupus, psoriatic, infectious (Lyme disease)
  - Autoimmune destruction of articular cartilage
  - Proliferation of synovium
  - May begin early in life (e.g., juvenile rheumatoid arthritis)
  - Often involves multiple joint (e.g., hips, feet, shoulders, hand metacarpophalangeal and proximal interphalangeal joints)
  - Cyclical flare-ups of pain and swelling

PHYSICAL EXAM
- Osteoarthritis
  - Effusion
  - Joint line tenderness
  - Often palpable spurs
  - Usually varus alignment
  - Loss of full extension
- Inflammatory arthritis
  - Effusion
  - Warm if flare-up
  - Joint line tenderness
  - Boggy synovium
  - Valgus or varus alignment
- May have instability due to autoimmune ligament destruction
- Eye exam

STUDIES
- Radiographs
  - Standing bilateral AP, Tunnel views, lateral, and sunrise views
  - Narrowing of joint space
  - Subchondral sclerosis and cysts, spurring in osteoarthritis
  - Varus or valgus alignment
- MRI
  - Can detect associated meniscal pathology

- Lab work
  - Rheumatoid factor
  - Antinuclear antibody (lupus)
  - Synovial fluid analysis with:
    - 50,000–70,000 WBCs, and poor viscosity (string test) in inflammatory flare
- Renal function tests

DIFFERENTIAL DIAGNOSIS
- Acute intra-articular infection
  - Rule out via aspiration
  - Infection with 80,000–100,000 WBCs and positive Gram stain/culture
- Villonodular synovitis
  - Unique MRI appearance and diagnostic synovial histopathology

TREATMENT
- Osteoarthritis – conservative
  - Physical therapy for strengthening
  - Oral nutraceutical (chondroitan sulfate, glucosamine)
  - NSAIDs
  - Intra-articular corticosteroid injection
  - Hyaluronate injection
  - Cane or crutch on least symptomatic side
- Inflammatory – conservative
  - Medication – NSAIDs, steroids, methotrexate
- Usually managed by rheumatologist
- Cane or crutch
- Surgical – osteoarthritis
  - Arthroscopy with debridement of meniscal tears and cartilage lesions gives temporary relief of symptoms
  - Osteotomy or unicompartmental arthroplasty for unicompartmental disease
  - Total knee arthroplasty
- Surgical – inflammatory arthritis
  - Arthroscopy with synovectomy for short-term relief
  - Total knee arthroplasty (TKA)

DISPOSITION
N/A

PROGNOSIS

- Osteoarthritis
  - ➤ After osteotomy, 85% good to excellent results after 5 years, then increasing failure rates
  - ➤ After unicompartmental or TKA, 90% survivability at 15 years
- Inflammatory arthritis – If patient has positive rheumatoid factor:
  - ➤ 75% will have progressive radiologic destruction of hands, feet, hips, and knees
  - ➤ After TKA, prosthetic survivability similar to osteoarthritis

CAVEATS AND PEARLS

- Osteoarthritis: Younger patient may be candidate for newer cartilage transplant technologies.
- Inflammatory arthritis: Early and aggressive rheumatologic workup and medical treatment can slow disease progress.

KNEE DISLOCATIONS AND COMBINED KNEE LIGAMENT INJURIES

PETER T. SIMONIAN, MD

HISTORY

- Generally high-energy trauma injury mechanism
  - ➤ Motor vehicle accident, motorcycle, pedestrian vs. motor vehicle, fall
- May occur with low-energy mechanism
  - ➤ Athletics (e.g., football, soccer, skiing, basketball, rugby)
  - ➤ Obese patient (e.g., slip or fall, misstep – minor trauma)
- Dislocation may be open or closed soft tissue injury
  - ➤ 30% of high-energy injuries
- Vascular injuries
  - ➤ Variable
    - Dependent on high vs. low energy
    - Dependent on direction of dislocation
    - Anterior and posterior have increased incidence
  - ➤ Generally 30% incidence (range 5–64%)
  - ➤ Involves popliteal artery
  - ➤ Artery tethered at Hunter's canal and soleus

➢ Intimal tears may present late (1 wk)
  • Arteriogram can assess intimal injury
■ Neurologic injuries
  ➢ Variable incidence
    • Peroneal nerve most commonly affected
      • Variable recovery
      • 30–40% incidence
    • Tibial nerve can be injured
■ Associated fractures
  ➢ Ipsilateral lower extremity fracture: 30–40% incidence
■ Amputations
  ➢ Secondary to vascular injury
  ➢ Incidence varies
    • Low energy, <5%
    • Ischemic time >8 hours, 85%
■ General priorities
  ➢ Limb salvage/viability
  ➢ Stabilization of ipsilateral fracture
  ➢ Address ligamentous stability
■ Definition
  ➢ Disruption of tibia-femoral articulation
■ Classification
  ➢ Energy type: high vs. low
  ➢ Direction of tibia relative to femur
    • Anterior
      • Most common (30%)
      • Mechanism – Hyperextension
    • Posterior
      • Incidence approaches 25%
      • Mechanism – Posteriorly applied force to flexed knee
    • Lateral
      • Incidence approaches 10–15%
      • Mechanism – Varus force
    • Medial
      • Incidence, 5%
      • Mechanism – Valgus force
    • Rotary
      • Combination rotation with applied force (e.g., posterolateral)
        • Possibly irreducible
        • Buttonhole of femoral condyle through capsule

PHYSICAL EXAM

- ABCs of trauma management
  - A – Airway
  - B – Breathing
  - C – Circulation
- Vascular status
  - Pulses
    - Dorsalis pedis
    - Posterior tibialis
    - Popliteal
  - Knee dislocated – Emergency
    - Pulse present – Reduce dislocation
      - Obtain arteriogram
      - Vascular consult
      - Pulse obliterated postreduction, schedule OR
    - No pulse – Reduce dislocation
    - Postreduction, no pulse
      - OR
      - Vascular consult
      - Shoot-through A-gram in OR
    - Postreduction, pulse present
      - Obtain arteriogram
      - Vascular consult
      - Consider MR angiogram
      - Some trauma centers monitor pulse & ankle/brachial ratio
- Neurologic
  - Must carefully document status
    - Normal, absent, diminished
  - Caveat – Compartment syndromes may occur postdislocation
    - May occur when vessel injured and surgically revascularized
      - Pain out of proportion
      - Pain on passive stretch of respective compartments
  - Peroneal nerve function (motor)
    - Ankle dorsiflexion
    - Great toe extension
    - Ankle eversion
    - Ankle inversion
  - Peroneal nerve function (sensation)
    - Dorsum of foot – Superficial peroneal nerve
    - Dorsal 1st web space – Deep peroneal nerve

➤ Tibial nerve function (motor)
  • Ankle plantarflexion
➤ Tibial nerve function (sensation)
  • Lateral foot – Sural
  • Plantar foot – Tibial nerve
■ Extremity screening
  ➤ Palpate thigh/lower leg/ankle/foot in trauma patient to uncover possible fracture
  ➤ Hip fracture can occur in high-energy – Assess hip ROM
■ Knee ligamentous exam
  ➤ Is joint "open" injury?
  ➤ Status of extensor mechanism
  ➤ Soft tissue swelling
  ➤ Thorough exam may be precluded by pain and swelling
  ➤ Anterior cruciate ligament (ACL)
    • Lachman test – Most sensitive
    • Anterior drawer – Least sensitive
    • Pivot shift – Pathognomonic, difficult to perform in acute setting
  ➤ Posterior cruciate ligament (PCL)
    • Posterior drawer – Most sensitive
    • Quad active test
    • Posterior sag
    • Recurvatum test
    • Reverse pivot shift test
  ➤ Medial collateral ligament (MCL)
    • Valgus at 30° – Most sensitive for MCL
    • Valgus at 0° – Implies associated secondary restraints injury
  ➤ LCL and posterolateral corner (PLC)
    • Varus at 30° – Most sensitive for lateral collateral ligament (LCL)
    • Varus at 0° – Implies associated secondary restraints injury
    • Posterolateral spin
      • 30°>90° knee flexion – PLC
      • 90°>30° flexion – PCL
    • Dial test/external tibial rotation – Asymmetry implies PLC injury

STUDIES
■ Radiographs
  ➤ AP, lateral, obliques

➤ Oblique helpful for tibial plateau fracture
➤ Findings
  • Second fracture – Lateral marginal capsular avulsion fracture
    • Almost always associated ACL injury
  • PCL avulsion fracture
    • Noted on lateral x-ray
  • Tibial eminence avulsion fracture
    • ACL avulsion
  • Tibial plateau fracture
  • Patellar fracture – Best noted on lateral x-ray
  • Fibular head fracture/avulsion – Best noted on AP
■ Angiogram
  ➤ See algorithm in "History"
  ➤ Obtain in all knee dislocations
  ➤ Assesses for intimal injury
■ MR angiogram
  ➤ Preferred by some centers instead of A-gram
■ MRI
  ➤ Generally obtained
    • Ligamentous injuries
    • Meniscal pathology
    • Bone bruise extent
    • Occult fracture
  ➤ Aids in surgical planning
■ Compartment pressure measurements
  ➤ High index of suspicion
  ➤ Measure all four compartments
  ➤ Normal compartments <10 mm
  ➤ Irreversible changes occur within 8 hours

DIFFERENTIAL DIAGNOSIS
■ Supracondylar femoral fracture with severe displacement
■ Tibial plateau fracture with severe displacement
■ Displaced patellar dislocation
■ Two- or three-ligament injured knee
  ➤ ACL, PCL ± PLC
  ➤ ACL, MCL
  ➤ ACL, LCL ± PLC
  ➤ PCL, MCL
  ➤ PCL, LCL ± PLC
■ Patellar tendon rupture

- Quadriceps tendon rupture
- Patellar fracture with displacement

TREATMENT
- Vascular status/limb salvage takes priority.
- Caveat – Assume reduced knee dislocation in multiligament-injured knee
- Generally acute immediate ligament reconstruction/repair not performed
- At time of vascular repair, some surgeons perform limited repairs.
- Reduced dislocation must be maintained
  - Splint
  - Drop lock postoperative knee orthosis
  - External fixator
  - If surgery deferred confirm that reduction maintained per x-ray.
- Studies support nonsurgical and surgical treatment methods.
- More contemporary approaches recommend surgical treatment
  - Function generally better
- Nonsurgical treatment acceptable in nonathletic, medically ill, obese situations.
- Surgical principles
  - Treat involved pathology.
  - PCL is central pivot – Single most important structure to reconstruct
    - Acutely may avulse and can be repaired
  - ACL and PCL can be repaired arthroscopically.
  - Tension ACL in extension.
  - Tension PCL at 70–90° knee flexion.
  - Tension PLC repair at 30° pre-ACL tensioning.
  - Allograft tissues helpful in multiligamentous/knee dislocation situations
  - Employ early motion in postop rehab protocol.
  - Watch for arthrofibrosis postop.

DISPOSITION
N/A

PROGNOSIS
- Postreconstructive complications
  - Stiffness
  - Heterotopic bone
  - Posttraumatic arthritis

➤ Motion loss
➤ Ligament laxity ± failure
➤ Deep venous thrombosis ± pulmonary embolus
➤ Compartment syndrome

CAVEATS AND PEARLS

■ Suspect reduced knee dislocation in multiligament-injured knee.
■ Radiographs necessary to exclude fracture
■ Always obtain arteriogram in knee dislocation.
■ If pulse absent postreduction, surgical exploration indicated
■ Rule of thirds – Incidence approaches 33%
　➤ Vascular, neurologic, ipsilateral fracture, amputation
■ Immediate ligament repairs/reconstruction not necessary
■ Compartment syndromes can occur
■ Intimal vessel injuries may present up to 1 week postdislocation.
■ PCL repair/reconstruction key structure
■ Severity of injury must be addressed with patient, family, coaches.
■ Return to play after surgical treatment of knee dislocation guarded

---

LABRAL TEARS OF THE HIP

JON SEKIYA, MD
E. M. WOJTYS, MD
REVISED BY CHARLES NOFSINGER, MD

HISTORY

■ Forced, excessive hip motion a common cause, especially flexion and extension
■ Impact injuries from falls, dismounts, jumps
■ Groin and/or inguinal pain
■ Audible and/or palpable click
■ Unable to exercise "hard"
■ Nonimpact exercises usually tolerated

PHYSICAL EXAM

■ Pain at extremes of hip motion
■ Pain with hip flexion, internal rotation and adduction; some clinicians compare pain with compression vs. distraction
■ Audible and palpable clunk or click with rotation
■ Resistance to hip motion can decrease because of pain.

STUDIES
- CT arthrogram
- MRI with or without contrast – contrast may help delineate tears
- AP and lateral x-rays – rule out loose bodies in hip joint

DIFFERENTIAL DIAGNOSIS
- Intra-articular loose body – most common are chondral
- Groin muscle strain
- Hernia
- Degenerative joint disease
- Snapping iliopsoas tendon

TREATMENT
- If asymptomatic other than popping sensation, nonoperative treatment advised
- If symptomatic, dysfunctional and imaging studies suggestive of tear, recommend hip arthroscopy

DISPOSITION
N/A

PROGNOSIS
- Results of operative treatment good if tear can be identified and hip joint degeneration is not significant
- If hip joint architecture is not normal (pediatric subluxation, slipped capital femoral epiphysis) or if a significant flexion contracture exists, prognosis is guarded
- Return to play: consider return when ROM, flexibility, and strength return to normal
- Complications of hip arthroscopy
  - Neurovascular injuries
  - Traction injury to pudendal or sciatic nerve
  - Iatrogenic intra-articular damage
  - Infection

CAVEATS AND PEARLS
- Many irregularities of hip labrum seen on MRI are not labral tears
- Operations indicated for significant pain and dysfunction
- Many loose intra-articular fragments not seen unless contrast used on imaging studies

LATERAL ANKLE SPRAINS

CAROL FREY, MD

HISTORY

- Mechanism of injury: plantarflexion and inversion
- Initial complaints
  - Pain over injured ligaments
  - Swelling
  - Loss of function
- Chronic cases
  - History of previous sprain
  - History of previous "giving way"
  - Chronic instability usually not painful between "giving way" episodes
  - Chronic pain is usually a misdiagnosis
- Patients who report a "pop" followed by immediate swelling are more likely to have suffered a severe sprain.

PHYSICAL EXAM

- Acute
  - Ecchymosis
  - Swelling
  - Tender to palpation over injured ligaments
    - Anterior talofibular
    - Calcaneal fibular
    - Posterior talofibular
  - Location of tenderness to determine what injured
  - Palpate lateral & medial malleolus & base of fifth metatarsal to crepitation or tenderness to rule out fracture
  - "Squeeze test"
    - Positive if injured syndesmosis
    - Compress tibia & fibula at midcalf
    - Reproduces pain at syndesmosis if "positive"
  - External rotation test
    - External rotation of foot
    - Ankle in dorsiflexion
    - Identifies injury to syndesmosis
    - Positive if creates pain in syndesmosis
- Chronic
  - As above for acute

➤ Varus stress test
➤ Anterior drawer test
➤ Always check subtalar motion.

STUDIES
■ Basic tests
  ➤ AP, mortise, and lateral x-rays
    • Go through the differential and rule out other conditions
    • Measure the syndesmosis 1 cm from the joint line on AP & mortise; should not measure >5 mm
    • Medial clear space should not be >5 mm
■ Specialized tests
  ➤ Stress tests
    • Varus stress
      • Neutral position
      • Compare to opposite side
      • >6° difference abnormal
    • Anterior drawer
      • Plantarflexion
      • Tibia stabilized
      • Anterior subluxation measured
      • >4 mm subluxation abnormal
    • Results differ depending on
      • Load
      • Relaxation
      • Machine or manual
      • Duration of load
      • Anesthesia/local anesthetic
      • Measurement methods differ
      • Foot position
    • Used only in evaluation of chronic instability
  ➤ MRI
    • Not recommended in acute cases
    • Used in workup of chronic pain
    • Periarticular hemorrhage
    • Irregular wavy contour to torn ligament
    • Discontinuity
  ➤ Arthrography
    • Must be done soon (3–7 days) after injury
    • Anterior talofibular – leaks anterior to lateral malleolus
    • Calcaneal fibular – peroneal tendonography leaks into lateral joint

DIFFERENTIAL DIAGNOSIS

- Peroneal tendon tear
- Peroneal tendon subluxation
- Osteochondral lesion
- Traction injury to nerves
- Fracture anterior process of calcaneus
- Fracture of the fifth metatarsal
- Fracture of the lateral process of talus
- Subtalar injury
- Syndesmosis injury
- Cuboid subluxation
- Tarsal coalition

TREATMENT

- Goal
  - Prevent chronic instability
  - Protect
  - Rehabilitation
- Phase 1
  - Protection – Commercially available splints
  - Ice, compression, elevation
- Phase 2
  - Peroneal and dorsiflexion strengthening
  - Achilles tendon stretching
- Phase 3
  - Functional conditioning
    - Brisk walking
    - Running
    - Figure 8 running
    - Hopping
    - Jumping
    - Cutting
  - Proprioception
    - Coordination exercises
  - Agility
  - Endurance
- Grade I and II injuries progress rapidly
- During phase 2 & 3, grade 2 and 3 protected with tape or brace
- Surgery
  - No study proves better than nonsurgical treatment
  - Longer rehab

➤ More complications
➤ Late surgery has good results.
■ Surgery may be necessary for
  ➤ Acute on chronic sprains
  ➤ Displaced osteochondritis dissecans
  ➤ Large avulsion fracture of the fibula
  ➤ Young athlete/dancer possibly

DISPOSITION
N/A

PROGNOSIS
N/A

CAVEATS AND PEARLS
■ Subtalar joint commonly injured with inversion injury
■ Look for bleeding on medial heel with subtalar joint injury, called "Battle's sign."
■ Instability is an anterior lateral rotatory instability since the lateral structures are torn and the medial structures intact.
■ Patients that go on to have chronic pain after an ankle sprain commonly have a missed diagnosis.
■ Patients that go on to have chronic instability after an ankle sprain commonly have had no or poor rehabilitation.
■ Literature reports residual symptoms in 20-40% of acute ankle sprains.
■ Most common reason for residual symptoms is incomplete rehabilitation.
■ Always check subtalar motion and proximal tenderness.

LATERAL CLAVICLE FRACTURES

JOEL SHAPIRO, MD
FRANCES CUOMO, MD

HISTORY
■ Mechanism: fall on outstretched arm or on point of shoulder
■ Commonly associated with contact and high-speed sports: rugby, bicycling, skiing, etc.
■ Epidemiology: M > F
■ Symptoms, acute fracture

➤ Pain over distal clavicle/fracture site
➤ Pain with shoulder range of motion
➤ Trapezius spasm
■ Symptoms, late with malunion/nonunion
➤ Chronic pain at nonunion site
➤ Pain with overhead motion or cross-body adduction
➤ Painful acromioclavicular (AC) joint with late degeneration
➤ Brachial plexopathy due to traction from lack of upper extremity suspension

PHYSICAL EXAM
■ Deformity over fracture site
■ Skin abrasions
■ Subcutaneous bone: requires careful exam for open fracture
■ Edema and ecchymosis, may extend down arm
■ Evaluate surrounding structures: neurovascular exam, pneumothorax (associated injury in 3% of fractures)
■ Attempts at shoulder range of motion will elicit pain and crepitus at fracture site and should be limited

STUDIES
■ Radiographs: AP of clavicle, AP view with 15° cephalic tilt (Zanca view), and shoulder trauma series, including axillary view to evaluate AP displacement

DIFFERENTIAL DIAGNOSIS
■ Diagnosis usually straightforward, confirmed with x-ray
■ Other anatomic disruptions may be confused with fracture: subluxation/dislocation of AC, sternoclavicular, or glenohumeral joints, acromial or coracoid fracture
■ Consider other injury with high-energy mechanism: floating shoulder, scapulothoracic dissociation, high rib fracture
■ Look for associated head/cervical spine injuries

TREATMENT
■ Based on anatomic classification of fractures
■ Originally classified by Neer into types I-III
■ Lateral-third fractures recently further subdivided into types I-V
➤ Type I: fracture lateral to coracoclavicular (CC) ligaments, extra-articular
➤ Type IIa: oblique fracture medial to CC ligaments
➤ Type IIb: fracture between conoid and trapezoid ligaments

- ➤ Type III: fracture extends into AC joint
- ➤ Type IV: periosteal sleeve fracture (pediatric)
- ➤ Type V: fracture of lateral third with extensive comminution
- ■ Treatment of types I, III, IV and V
  - ➤ Initially, nonoperative (sling/swath 6–8 weeks)
  - ➤ Failed nonoperative treatment may require late reconstruction
- ■ Treatment of type II
  - ➤ Controversial
  - ➤ Nonunion rates may be as high as 30% with nonoperative treatment
  - ➤ Options: primary reconstruction vs. treatment of symptomatic nonunions only
- ■ Reconstruction is ORIF (fragments often small) vs. modified Weaver-Dunn
- ■ Attempt should be made to retain distal fragment
- ■ All procedures include CC ligament reconstruction
- ■ Distal fragment excision with CC ligament reconstruction can also be used for late reconstruction if fragment is avascular/sclerotic
- ■ Other indications for ORIF: open injury (or impending open injury with severe skin tenting), associated neurovascular injury, floating shoulder, nonunion or malunion

DISPOSITION
N/A

PROGNOSIS
- ■ Types I, III, IV, V: nonoperative treatment has >90% union rate and >86% good result
- ■ Type II carries up to 30% nonunion rate with nonoperative treatment
- ■ Nonunions may be asymptomatic
- ■ Complications of nonoperative treatment include nonunion, malunion, subacromial impingement (callus), and posttraumatic degenerative joint disease of AC joint (type III)
- ■ Modified Weaver-Dunn may be used to manage these complications with good results reported
- ■ Return to sports 12–16 weeks, contingent on radiographic evidence of union

CAVEATS AND PEARLS
- ■ Lateral bone fragment often very small (ORIF challenging)

- Modified Weaver-Dunn with CC reconstruction is an option when distal fragment fixation is unobtainable
- ORIF – possible need for hardware removal
- Avoid transfixion of AC joint
- Protect repair with sling for 6 weeks
- Always include CC ligament reconstruction in acute and chronic cases

---

LATERAL CLAVICLE PERIOSTEAL SLEEVE FRACTURES

JAMES D. FERRARI, MD

HISTORY

- Mechanism: direct blow to the point of the shoulder
  - Sports and falls
- Distal clavicle splits through thick periosteal tube
  - Coracoclavicular (CC) and acromioclavicular (AC) ligaments remain intact
- Most injuries are not an AC separation or true dislocation
- Injury is usually a fracture or "pseudodislocation"
  - Can be a true AC separation in children >15
  - Lateral clavicular epiphysis ossifies and fuses in a short period around age 19
  - Most injuries are fractures that occur through this secondary ossification center
  - Tremendous remodeling potential
- Patients report pain, swelling, tenderness, +/– deformity
- Exceedingly rare for symptoms to persist chronically

PHYSICAL EXAM

- Swelling, pain, ecchymosis, tenderness at AC joint +/– deformity
- Patient supports elbow with other arm
- View clavicle from above to rule out posterior dislocation
- Proper neurovascular exam
- Check for tenderness in CC interval

STUDIES

- Preferably done standing
  - AP (Zanca view)
    - 15° cephalic tilt to avoid superimposition of AC joint on scapula

- Half as much exposure needed as in AP view of glenohumeral joint
- Axillary view
  - Rule out posterior displacement of clavicle
  - Rule out coracoid and acromion fractures
  - Film other side if questionable
- Standing AP view of both shoulders
  - Measure CC distances and calculate % increase on affected side
  - CC distance normally 1.0–1.3 cm
- Weighted views
  - Help distinguish type II from type III
  - Not needed, as they seldom change treatment plan or decision to perform surgery and inflict unnecessary pain on patient

DIFFERENTIAL DIAGNOSIS
- Acromion fracture
- Lateral-third clavicular fracture
- Coracoid fracture
- Septic arthritis

TREATMENT
- Classification
  - I: Mild sprain of AC ligaments without periosteal tube disruption; normal x-rays
  - II: Partial disruption of periosteal tube; CC interval increased up to 25%
  - III: Dorsal longitudinal split in periosteal tube; CC interval increased 25–100%
  - IV: Dorsal/posterior split in periosteal tube with displacement of clavicle posteriorly through deltotrapezial fascia
  - V: Dorsal split in periosteal tube and tearing of deltoid and trapezial fascial attachments; clavicle subcutaneous and CC interval increased >100%
  - VI: Subcoracoid dislocation of clavicle
- Nonoperative treatment for types I–III in adolescents up to age 16
  - Sling, ice, range of motion when pain allows
  - Isometric strengthening when pain allows
  - Tremendous remodeling potential within periosteal tube
  - Rarely any residual deformity

- Operative treatment favored for types IV–VI
  - Operative treatment consists of placement of clavicle back in periosteal tube and suturing of the tube
  - Temporary CC lag screw fixation or transacromial threaded Kirschner wires may be needed as well
  - Must be removed at 4–6 weeks
  - Sling until fixation removed
  - Begin mobilization at 6 weeks

DISPOSITION
N/A

PROGNOSIS
- Excellent results can be expected with type I–III injuries
- Limited series suggest good to excellent results seen with surgery as well
- Patients may return to sport when range of motion full and strength near normal
- Complication of nonoperative treatment of severe separations includes clavicular duplication

CAVEATS AND PEARLS
- True acromioclavicular separations probably don't occur in children <13
- CC ligaments are intimately bound to the inferior periosteal tube
- Tenderness in CC interval more likely to represent coracoid fracture than CC ligament tear in a child
- Stryker notch or axillary view best to identify coracoid fracture
- Apophysis of base of coracoid includes anterior-superior aspect of glenoid
- Grade IV injuries may look like grade II on AP views

LATERAL ELBOW INJURIES

CRAIG M. BALL, MD, FRACS
KEN YAMAGUCHI, MD

HISTORY
- Lateral elbow most common location of pain in general population
- Often history is not typical

- Overuse injuries more common than acute trauma
- Lateral epicondylitis
  - Related to chronic repetitive overload of wrist and finger extensors
  - Presents with pain centered on or just anterior to the epicondyle, worsened by activities involving resisted wrist extension
- Posterolateral rotatory instability (PLRI)
  - Related to a previous dislocation or lateral elbow surgery
  - Presents with clicking, catching, snapping, or a feeling that the elbow is slipping out of joint, worse with extension and forearm supination
- Radial tunnel
  - Related to compression of radial or posterior interosseous nerve, typically at the arcade of Frohse
  - Presents with pain in proximal extensor musculature, worsened by activities involving resisted supination
- Osteochondritis dissecans (OCD)
  - Related to repetitive compressive microtrauma with subchondral fatigue failure, usually in adolescents
  - Presents with lateral elbow pain in the midrange of motion during activities that involve a valgus stress; locking or catching can occur with loose bodies
- Plica
  - Becomes symptomatic following repetitive minor trauma
  - Subsequent fibrosis leads to persistent mechanical symptoms suggestive of a loose body
- Fractures – history of trauma

PHYSICAL EXAM
- Familiarity with injury patterns important
- Examination findings may not be typical
- Closely related structures can be involved in any pathologic process
- Lateral epicondylitis
  - Focal tenderness anterior and just proximal to epicondyle
  - Pain with grip and resisted wrist extension that is worse in elbow extension
- PLRI
  - Apprehension with full supination and extension
  - Lateral pivot shift apprehension test
  - Apparent valgus instability in supination but not pronation

- Radial tunnel
  - Tenderness well distal to epicondyle
  - Pain on resisted supination
- OCD
  - Lateral elbow pain with a valgus stress, swelling, and limitation of motion
  - Mechanical symptoms (catching, locking) from a loose body
- Plica
  - Lateral joint tenderness and swelling
  - Pain with repetitive flexion and extension of elbow
  - Mechanical symptoms
- Fractures
  - Localized tenderness
  - Painful limitation of motion

STUDIES
- Objective: rule out causes of similar pain around elbow
- Special investigations may be required
- Lateral epicondylitis
  - Usually a clinical diagnosis but selective local anesthesia injections helpful
  - Radiographs often normal
  - MRI may detect tendon degeneration
- PLRI
  - Varus stress test under fluoroscopic control may reveal instability
  - MRI can localize lateral collateral ligament (LCL) pathology but not usually necessary
- Radial tunnel – electrical studies typically normal
- OCD
  - Plain radiographs diagnostic in up to 75% if oblique views included
  - CT or MRI arthrography for defining lesion and presence of loose bodies
- Plica
  - Radiographs usually normal
  - MRI arthrography may demonstrate a meniscoid lesion in the radiocapitellar joint
- Fractures
  - AP, lateral, and oblique views (including radial head views) to delineate fracture pattern
  - CT helpful in complex cases

DIFFERENTIAL DIAGNOSIS
- Lateral epicondylitis (tennis elbow)
- LCL instability/PLRI
- Radial tunnel syndrome
- OCD
- Lateral synovial plica syndrome
- Fractures of the radial head or capitellum

TREATMENT
- Lateral epicondylitis
  - Conservative therapy mainstay of treatment (education, activity modification, NSAIDs, counterforce bracing, physical therapy, cortisone injections)
  - Surgery (open or arthroscopic extensor carpi radialis brevis debridement) only if this fails >12 months
- PLRI – reconstruction of ulnar LCL using a tendon graft
- Radial tunnel – initially conservative; surgical management controversial
- OCD
  - Initial rest until symptoms have subsided and radiographs improve
  - Arthroscopy for persistent symptoms or loose bodies (drilling for intact lesions, debridement if detached)
- Plica – arthroscopic excision of plica
- Fractures – stable anatomic ORIF to allow early motion

DISPOSITION
N/A

PROGNOSIS
- Lateral epicondylitis
  - >90% improve with nonoperative treatment
  - Of the remaining patients, 90% will improve with surgery but recovery is prolonged
  - Return to full-strength use of arm averages 5–6 months
- PLRI – with surgery, 90% will have a satisfactory result
- Radial tunnel
  - Conservative treatment usually successful
  - Results with surgery are mixed, and recovery can take up to 1 year

- OCD
  - On the whole, prognosis is good with minimal functional limitation
  - Minor extension losses can occur, and late degenerative change has been reported
- Plica – surgery is curative and recovery is prompt
- Fractures
  - Results determined by associated injuries and length of immobilization
  - For uncomplicated fractures, long-term outcome is generally good
- **Complications**
  - Surgical failures are certainly recognized
  - Reasons include improper patient selection, improper diagnosis, inadequate procedure, and surgically introduced pathology
  - Usually relate to incomplete recovery (need >6 months) or inadequate rehab
  - LCL insufficiency well recognized after lateral epicondylitis surgery
  - Recurrence following LCL reconstruction
  - Stiffness following surgery for OCD and especially fractures
  - Nerve injury with any arthroscopic procedure on the elbow

CAVEATS AND PEARLS
- Lateral epicondylitis the most common elbow affliction in adults
- Not all lateral elbow pain is lateral epicondylitis
- Common area of diagnostic confusion
- Different conditions can present in a similar manner
- Systematic approach required, dictated by history and physical exam
- Lateral epicondylitis and radial tunnel syndrome may coexist
- Plica may be more common than previously appreciated
- Suspect radial tunnel and plica in all cases of lateral epicondylitis
- PLRI being increasingly recognized
- When incompetent, the ligament does not become stable with time
- Ideal management of capitellum osteochondral lesions remains controversial
- No benefit of more complex procedures over simple debridement and loose body removal
- Rehabilitation critical in both surgical and nonsurgical treatment of lateral elbow injuries

LATERAL EPICONDYLITIS

CHAMP BAKER, MD
DAVID D. NEDEFF, MD

HISTORY

- Most commonly the result of work-related, repetitive strain injury
- Commonly called tennis elbow, although fewer than 10% of patients are tennis players
- 75% of cases occur in dominant extremity
- Direct or blunt trauma causes 10–15% of cases
- Peak incidence in fourth and fifth decades
- Slight male predominance
- Wide spectrum of theories on pathophysiology
- No significant inflammatory component to the disease; *tendinosis* more accurately describes condition than *tendinitis*
- Initiated as microtear, most often within origin of extensor carpi radialis brevis

PHYSICAL EXAM

- Point tenderness over anterior aspect of lateral epicondyle
- Pain with resisted wrist dorsiflexion is a key
- Grip strength frequently is diminished
- Grasping with elbow extended causes pain
- Elbow and wrist range of motion usually normal

STUDIES

- Plain radiographs usually normal
  - ➤ 10–25% may show calcification about lateral epicondyle
- Routine use of MRI not recommended
  - ➤ One study found MRI findings correlated with histopathologic findings at time of surgery
- EMG/nerve conduction velocity studies may be indicated if radial tunnel syndrome suspected
- Cervical spine radiographs or MRI if radicular complaints

DIFFERENTIAL DIAGNOSIS

- Radial tunnel syndrome is next most common cause of lateral elbow pain
- Radial tunnel syndrome can also coexist with lateral epicondylitis

- Tenderness from radial tunnel syndrome extends far distal to lateral epicondyle
- Diagnostic injection about common extensor origin should remove pain of lateral epicondylitis
- Effusion may indicate intra-articular pathology
- Rule out posterolateral rotatory instability
- Rarely, injury to lateral antebrachial cutaneous nerve can present as lateral elbow pain
- Don't forget cervical spine pathology

TREATMENT
- Nonoperative treatment is first line of treatment
- Cessation of offending activity and NSAID may be beneficial
- Strengthening, stretching, and retraining important for recovery
- Steroid injections may have benefit in patients with short duration of symptoms
- Steroid injections unlikely to help in the long term
- No good scientific evidence to support use of shock-wave, ultrasound, or laser therapy
- Counterforce bracing acts to lower extensor muscle activity
- Approximately 75% of patients respond to nonoperative treatment
- Operative treatment indicated after minimum 6 months of nonoperative treatment
- Several methods of surgical treatment
- Most methods involve excision of pathologic portion of tendon with or without reattachment of any elevated tendon
- Arthroscopic approach technically difficult but allows shortened rehabilitation period and common extensor tendon not violated
- Range of motion exercises started immediately with arthroscopic treatment (7–10 days later with open technique)
- Progressive strengthening started at 4–6 weeks after surgery

DISPOSITION
N/A

PROGNOSIS
- Approximately 75% good results with nonoperative treatment
- 85–90% good results with operative treatment
- Subjective results are often superior to objective findings, which often show persistent weakness

- Minimum 6 months after surgery before surgery deemed a failure
- Complications: persistent pain, residual weakness, posterolateral rotatory instability, synovial sinus formation
- Most common cause of continued pain: persistent extensor origin dysfunction

CAVEATS AND PEARLS
- Not an inflammatory process
- Pain with resisted wrist dorsiflexion crucial for diagnosis
- Must rule out radial tunnel syndrome
- Nonoperative treatment usually successful
- Key to surgery is removal of all pathologic tendon
- Arthroscopic technique allows quicker return to activity and/or sport

---

LATERAL LIGAMENT INJURIES

ROBERT F. LAPRADE, MD

HISTORY
- Sports or motor vehicle accident
- Mechanism – Varus injury, hyperextension injury, blow to antero-medial aspect of knee
- Most commonly occurs in combination with other ligament injuries so may be overlooked
- 15% of patients have injury to common peroneal nerve
- Chronic patients may have complaints of instability with every step (secondary to varus thrust gait)

PHYSICAL EXAM
- Often have minimal swelling on lateral side of knee (acute)
- May have lateral-sided joint line tenderness due to lateral capsular tearing
- Varus stress test – Do at 0° (full extension) and 30° flexion
  - ➤ 0° – If abnormal, usually significant multiligament injury
  - ➤ 30° – Increased varus opening is usually indicative of fibular collateral ligament and usually popliteus complex injury
- Positive posterolateral drawer test
  - ➤ Important to compare to contralateral knee as many patients have physiologic increase in their posterolateral drawer test

- Usually indicative of a combined lateral and posterolateral ligamentous injury
- Important to differentiate from a true posterior drawer test in neutral rotation; this test is performed with the foot externally rotated to approximately 15° and knee flexed 70–90°
- External rotation recurvatum test
  - Usually indicative of a significant concurrent anterior cruciate ligament (ACL) and/or posterior cruciate ligament (PCL) ligament injury in addition to posterolateral complex injury
  - Grasp the great toe and lift it off the table – Positive test when knee hyperextends and tibia externally rotates
  - Important to compare to contralateral knee to see how much increase in hyperextension occurs
- Dial test at 30° and 90°
  - One of most sensitive tests to assess for posterolateral corner injury
  - Performed either prone or supine
  - When performed supine, rotate the foot and ankle while stabilizing the thigh – Observe external rotation of tibial tubercle
  - Increased external rotation at 30° is indicative of a posterolateral corner injury
  - Dial test at 90° – An increase in external rotation at 90° indicates concurrent PCL injury. If no PCL injury, there should be less external rotation at 90° vs. 30°.
- Reverse pivot shift test
  - Very important to compare to contralateral knee; commonly positive in symptomatic patients
  - Perform with the knee flexed, foot externally rotated, and extend the knee to determine if the joint is subluxed and if it reduces
- Varus thrust gait
  - May be difficult to perform in acute situation
  - Can be very debilitating in chronic patients
  - Patients have a varus increase of lateral compartment at foot strike, results in thrusting with normal gait

STUDIES
- **Radiographs**
  - AP, lateral, infrapatellar view
  - Usually normal
  - Segond fracture (lateral capsular avulsion) commonly seen; usually present with concurrent ACL injury

➤ Arcuate fracture (avulsion fracture of fibular head/styloid) – Usually includes fibular attachment of fibular collateral ligament (FCL), biceps femoris, fabellofibular ligament, and popliteofibular ligament

➤ Chronic cases – Long leg standing x-ray – Assess for varus alignment in chronic cases because soft tissue reconstructions will stretch out if varus alignment is not corrected first

■ **MRI**
➤ Specific protocol necessary to look at posterolateral corner injuries
➤ Needs to include entire fibular head and styloid
➤ Thin-slice, coronal oblique views in line with popliteus tendon useful
➤ MRI useful in acute cases to determine location of pathology to assist with placement of surgical incisions
➤ MRI useful in chronic cases to assist in verification of posterolateral corner injury with combined knee ligament injuries

DIFFERENTIAL DIAGNOSIS
■ **Lateral-sided knee swelling**
➤ Lateral meniscus tear, Segond fracture with ACL injury, lateral meniscal cyst
■ **Common peroneal nerve injury**
➤ Direct contact contusion to nerve, herniated disc
■ **Instability**
➤ Quadriceps weakness
➤ Cruciate ligament injury
➤ Varus thrust gait: In chronic cases, may also be seen in patients with varus alignment and medial compartment arthritis

TREATMENT
■ **Acute injury**
➤ Establish diagnosis
➤ Assess motor/sensory status of common peroneal nerve
➤ Verify status of other ligaments of knee
➤ AP, lateral, and patellofemoral x-rays
➤ Strongly consider MRI scan using posterolateral knee protocol
➤ For partial injuries, consider immobilization for 3 weeks followed by ROM and therapy
➤ For complete injuries, plan for surgical repair (or reconstruction) within 2 weeks of injury (if possible)

- **Treatment considerations**
  - ➤ Partial vs. complete posterolateral corner injuries
  - ➤ Other concurrent ligament injuries of knee
  - ➤ Acute vs. chronic injuries
  - ➤ Common peroneal nerve deficits
- **Treatment options**
  - ➤ Nonsurgical
    - Immobilization in extension for 3 weeks for partial injuries, followed by ROM
    - Consider other concurrent ligament reconstructions or repairs as necessary based on examination
  - ➤ Surgical reconstructions
    - Acute injuries
      - Primary repair of structures from fibular head and styloid with suture anchors
      - Primary repair back to tibia of avulsed capsule
      - Recess procedure of popliteus and FCL avulsion off femur (with sutures tied medially over a button on the femur)
    - Chronic
      - If in varus alignment, perform proximal tibial osteotomy first to correct alignment
      - If in normal alignment (or postosteotomy) with instability, plan for surgical reconstruction with allograft (Achilles tendon) or autograft (hamstring tendons)
      - Need to reconstruct FCL for varus instability and popliteus/popliteofibular ligament for posterolateral rotation instability

DISPOSITION
N/A

PROGNOSIS
- Nonsurgical treatment
  - ➤ Grade 1 and 2 injuries usually heal with minimal instability
  - ➤ Complete (grade 3) injuries usually have problems with instability and develop medial compartment arthritis (medial meniscal tears)
  - ➤ Chronic cases often develop thrust gait, which inhibits all aspects of ambulation
- Surgical treatment
  - ➤ Recommended for complete (grade 3) injuries

➤ Acute cases do better than chronic injuries
➤ Perform surgical repair/reconstruction of posterolateral corner injuries concurrent with other ligament repairs/reconstructions
  Return to play
■ Nonoperative
  ➤ Usually 3–4 months
  ➤ Approximately 10–20% of patients with grade 2 injuries need ultimate surgical reconstructions.
■ Repairs/reconstructions
  ➤ Acute repairs – usually at 4 months after surgery
  ➤ Proximal tibial osteotomies – 6–9 months (if no underlying residual instability)
  ➤ Reconstructions (allograft or autograft) – 9 months
  ➤ Criteria: Normal knee stability and motion; motor strength as assessed by functional testing within 10–15% of normal knee
■ Complications of surgical treatment
  ➤ Infection (<2%)
  ➤ Deep vein thrombosis, pulmonary embolus (<2%)
  ➤ Arthrofibrosis (usually seen in combined ligament injuries, especially MCL)
  ➤ Recurrent laxity
  ➤ Common peroneal nerve neuroproxia (rare), usually in acute cases

CAVEATS AND PEARLS
■ Suspect posterolateral corner injury in patients with increased recurvatum
■ Patients with acute knee injury and common peroneal nerve sensory or motor deficits have a posterolateral knee injury until proven otherwise
■ Always obtain a full-length standing x-ray to assess for a varus alignment in a chronic posterolateral knee injury (AP and lateral views are not adequate to assess for this)
■ For acute cases, attempt to perform surgical repair within 2 weeks of injury. Scar tissue planes develop after this point and the tissues do not hold sutures well.
■ Evaluate for a posterolateral corner injury during the exam under anesthesia. It cannot be assessed once an ACL and/or PCL reconstruction has been performed.
■ Little controversy exists about acute repairs

- A standard method of performing posterolateral reconstructions has not been developed.
- In patients who have an arthroscopic "drive-through" sign (>1 cm of lateral joint line opening) during surgery, reassess thoroughly to verify there is no concurrent posterolateral corner injury
- Avoid hamstring exercises for 4 months after posterolateral corner reconstructions
- Use crutches with nonweight-bearing for 6 weeks after posterolateral corner repairs or reconstructions
- Consider posterior tibialis tendon transfer in patients who have common peroneal nerve motor deficits through 4 months after surgery

LATERAL MENISCAL TEARS

THOMAS L. WICKIEWICZ, MD

HISTORY
- Child
  - Snapping knee
  - Discoid meniscus – complete – incomplete
  - "Wrisberg" type
- Young adult
  - Usually history of trauma
  - Flexion – valgus – rotation (e.g., wrestlers)
  - Acute anterior cruciate ligament (ACL) disruption – lateral meniscal (LM) tears common with ski injuries
- Older
  - Degenerative; mass on lateral joint line
  - Horizontal cleavage tear of lateral meniscus with cyst formation
- Pain
  - Lateral joint line pain
  - Occasional referred pain down posterolateral calf with associated lateral compartment degenerative joint disease (DJD)
- Swelling
  - Locking – bucket tears of lateral meniscus – fascicle disruption
  - Mass – cyst (as above)

PHYSICAL EXAM
- Note ACL integrity on exam
- Joint line tenderness to palpation

- Pain with valgus compressive maneuvers
- Palpable mass (if cyst)
- Effusion
- Loss of terminal extension (if bucket tear)

STUDIES
- Double-contrast arthrograms – higher rate of inaccurate reading than medial secondary to anatomic issues around popliteal sleeve
- MRI: Imaging method of choice; must read both meniscal morphology (fascicle injuries) as well as meniscal signal on MRI

DIFFERENTIAL DIAGNOSIS
- Lateral meniscal tear
- Cystic torn lateral meniscus
- Ganglion cyst
- DJD
- Iliotibial band syndrome
- Patellofemoral syndrome
- Proximal tibial – Fibular joint DJD
- Osteochondritis dissecans, lateral femoral condyle

TREATMENT
- Excision vs. repair
  - Lateral meniscus more important than medial with regard to load transmission respective to its compartment (70% load vs. 50% for medial meniscus)
  - Consequently, total lateral meniscal excision associated with worse outcome (DJD) than total medial excision (amount and time course more rapid)
  - Treatment goal: preserve meniscal function
- Unstable "Wrisberg" type in child – attempt repair
  - Discoid – Adult – Degeneration tears – reshape and excise to stable meniscus tissue
- Tears with cyst: debride meniscus and decompress cyst inside-out
- Radial tears
  - Common in young athletes
  - Common in area of popliteal tendon hiatus
  - If incomplete, resect tear; must leave at least 3–4 mm of stable meniscal rim in front of tendon
  - If complete, radial split (all the way out to periphery/sleeve) – excision of tear will cause total excision of lateral meniscus
  - Consider repair – meniscus avascular – in front of sleeve

> Addition of fibrin clot may augment healing response and allow peripheral healing
■ Repair
  > Outside-in
  > Inside-out
  > All inside
    • Fascicle detachment – respond well to repair
    • Major issue – recognition of pathology

DISPOSITION
N/A

PROGNOSIS
■ Complications of repair
  > Neurovascular injury, especially peroneal nerve
  > Failure of repair
■ Success
  > Repairable tears have high success rates
  > Approach 90%
  > Higher rate of success with ligament surgery (ACL)
■ Return to play
  > Excision: when motion strength, proprioception allow; 2–4 weeks
  > Repair: 4 months

CAVEATS AND PEARLS
■ Significant anatomic issues
  > Unlike medial meniscus, the lateral meniscus does not have a complete capsular attachment around periphery (popliteal hiatus).
  > Popliteus tendon passes behind meniscus as the tendon comes to its femoral attachment.
  > The hiatus is spanned by a superior and inferior fascicle.
  > Lateral meniscus more mobile than medial
  > Area of meniscus in front of popliteal hiatus is avascular – implications for meniscal healing.
  > Fascicle disruption may allow "locking" of lateral meniscus – "bucket" tear without any abnormality of body of meniscus
  > Discoid variants
■ Special considerations
  > Vertical tears – posterior horn – complete; <10 mm in length or incomplete tears

> "ACL" pattern of LM tear – see with acute ACL disruption
> LM tear in proximity to tibial translation bone contusion seen on MRI
> These tears rarely cause symptoms if not unstable (cannot "bucket" tear at arthroscopy); may be left alone
> Fate: probably do not heal but do not progress; clinically silent
■ Meniscal transplantation
> Meniscal allograft viable technique
> Preoperative planning
> Not a treatment for osteoarthritis
> Coronal MRI – joint architecture to accept graft
> Insert transplant on common bone bridge between anterior and posterior horns
> Success can approach 75% with appropriate indications

LISFRANC INJURIES

SCOTT A. RODEO, MD

HISTORY
■ Also known as midfoot sprain
■ Common in football, soccer, basketball, rugby
■ Mechanisms of injury include axial load to midfoot or twisting injury to midfoot.
■ Injury occurs to dorsal tarsometatarsal ligaments, fracture of base of second metatarsal, or tear of Lisfranc's ligament (medial cuneiform to base second metatarsal).
■ Significant pain and morbidity can ensue.
■ Dislocation of the midfoot may occur, followed by spontaneous reduction.
■ Athlete complains of pain with prolonged standing and push-off.

PHYSICAL EXAM
■ Tenderness and swelling over dorsal aspect of tarsometatarsal joints
■ Midfoot deformity may be evident with higher-grade injury.
■ Assess stability of midfoot joints.
■ Squeeze test – Squeeze inwards at base of metatarsals: positive test produces pain or abnormal motion.

STUDIES
■ AP, lateral, oblique radiographs
■ Standing (weight-bearing) x-rays should be performed.

- Stress x-rays can demonstrate instability at tarsometatarsal joints.
- CT scan may show small fractures at base of metatarsals and cuneiforms.
- MRI useful to see tear of Lisfranc's ligament, but not routinely used
- Plain radiographic findings
  - Widening between medial and middle cuneiform
  - Widening between base of first and second metatarsals
  - Loss of colinearity between medial border second metatarsal and medial border of middle cuneiform (AP radiograph)
  - Loss of colinearity between medial border fourth metatarsal and medial border cuboid (oblique radiograph)
  - Fracture-dislocation: medial or lateral displacement of forefoot or divergent displacement (separation between first ray and lateral forefoot)

DIFFERENTIAL DIAGNOSIS

- Injury to extensor tendons/tibialis anterior tendon
- Navicular fracture/stress fracture
- Acute metatarsal fracture
- Stress fracture of second metatarsal

TREATMENT

- Mild sprain (no displacement, stability intact)
  - Control swelling, limit weight-bearing as indicated by pain
  - Semirigid foot orthosis to support arch
  - Can use bike for cross-training. Use heel weight-bearing only on injured side.
- Moderate sprain (small avulsion fractures, mild instability)
  - Cast or AFO for 6–8 weeks
  - Progression of activities depends on stability (recheck x-rays), pain
- Fracture/dislocation/unstable midfoot
- ORIF with 3.5-mm cannulated screws across tarsometatarsal joints
- Usually need to stabilize first, second, fifth tarsometatarsal joints
- Important to reduce gap between medial and middle cuneiform: use transverse screw
- Use Lisfranc screw: medial cuneiform into base of second metatarsal
- May also use percutaneous Kirschner wires, especially for fourth and fifth tarsometatarsal joints
- Interposed soft tissue can result in inability to achieve closed reduction.

- Verify stability and alignment with fluoroscopy in OR.
- Postop cast immobilization or removable AFO. Begin weight-bearing after 6–8 weeks.
- Remove screws at 10–12 weeks.
- Use molded semirigid foot orthosis for return to sports.

DISPOSITION
N/A

PROGNOSIS
- Chronic residual forefoot pain common after these injuries
- Return to play 2–6 weeks for mild injuries, up to 6 months if surgery required
- Repeated injury can result in midfoot collapse and eventual arthritis.
- Tarsometatarsal joint arthritis may require isolated tarsometatarsal joint fusions.

CAVEATS AND PEARLS
- Severity of "midfoot sprain" often not recognized
- Warn athlete of chance for chronic midfoot pain after this injury.
- Obtain standing x-rays to note widening between medial and middle cuneiform.
- Nonweight-bearing x-ray may be normal.
- Avoid fusion of fourth and fifth tarsometatarsal joints (mobile segment) – Fusion results in functional problems.

LITTLE LEAGUE ELBOW

GEORGE A. PALETTA, JR., MD
STEVE BERNSTEIN, MD

HISTORY
- Classic triad: medial elbow pain, diminished throwing effectiveness, decreased throwing distance
- Age
  - ➤ Childhood: pain about the medial epicondyle usually secondary to microinjury at the apophysis & ossification center
  - ➤ Adolescence: increase in valgus stresses on the elbow resulting in avulsion fractures of the medial epicondyle

> Look for partial avulsion in late adolescence as the epicondyle begins to fuse.
> Young adulthood: medial epicondyle fused, so injury more likely in muscular attachments and ulnar collateral ligament (UCL)
- Position
  > Pitchers inherently incur greater stresses across the elbow.
  > Pitchers > infielders > catchers > outfielders
- Pain
  > Most common complaint
  > Most often localized to the medial side
  > Pain before, during, or after throwing? Pain at all times is ominous.
  > Duration of pain (acute vs. chronic)
    - Child w/ acute onset following single throw: medial epicondyle avulsion
    - Young adult w/ acute onset following single throw: UCL injury
    - If pain chronic, think overuse.

PHYSICAL EXAM
- Look for loss of motion, muscle atrophy/hypertrophy, flexion contracture.
- Palpate for tenderness along medial epicondyle, lateral epicondyle, olecranon, radial head, collateral ligaments.
- Palpate flexor-pronator mass.
- Valgus stress test of Jobe
- Milking maneuver
- Palpate ulnar nerve in flexion & extension for subluxation.
- Complete neurovascular exam of upper extremity

STUDIES
- Standard AP & lateral radiographs, w/ comparison views
- If exam suggestive of ligamentous instability, obtain valgus stress views.
- Medial lesions:
  > Hypertrophy, fragmentation, avulsion fracture of medial epicondyle
  > Widening of medial epicondylar apophysis
  > Avulsion coronoid process at sublime tubercle
- Lateral lesions:
  > Osteochondrosis (Panner's disease) of capitellum or radial head
    - Typically younger children (age < 12 years)
    - Fragmentation, irregular ossification capitellum

➤ Osteochondritis dissecans of capitellum
  • Typically older children (age > 12 years)
  • Lucent lesion in the capitellum best seen on oblique view
■ Posterior lesions:
  ➤ Hypertrophy of the ulna causing chronic impingement, posteromedial osteophytes, loose bodies
■ Three-phase bone scan
  ➤ May be helpful for subtle changes in overuse injuries, stress fractures ulna
■ MRI
  ➤ Diagnostic test of choice for evaluating nonossified structures such as developing epiphyses & apophyses, UCL, cartilage, osteochondritis dissecans (OCD) lesions

DIFFERENTIAL DIAGNOSIS
■ Diagnosis often age-dependent
■ Childhood: Panner's disease, medial epicondyle apophysitis or widening, medial epicondyle avulsion fractures
■ Adolescence: OCD capitellum, medial epicondyle apophysitis or widening, medial epicondyle avulsion fractures, flexor-pronator injury, ligamentous injury
■ Early adulthood: flexor-pronator injury, UCL injury

TREATMENT
■ Medial tension injuries (medial epicondylitis, apophysitis)
  ➤ 6-wk course of abstinence from throwing
  ➤ Ice, NSAIDs, PT, modalities
  ➤ If resolution of sxs, gradual return to throwing
  ➤ For persistent symptoms, throwing is disallowed until the next season.
■ Medial epicondylar fractures
  ➤ If minimally displaced (<5 mm), treat with brief immobilization followed by gradual return to ROM & throwing at 6 wks.
  ➤ Displacement >5 mm will require closed reduction/internal fixation followed by brief immobilization & early ROM.
■ UCL injury
  ➤ If <2 mm side-to-side opening on stress views: 6–12 wks abstinence from throwing followed by gradual return to throwing
  ➤ If >2 mm side-to-side opening on stress views: treat as above; if no improvement will require reconstruction
  ➤ Acute complete tear of UCL in the elite throwing athlete requires reconstruction.

- Panner's disease
  - Typically loss of motion
  - Abstinence from throwing; may require prolonged avoidance of throwing
  - Restore ROM.
  - Serial radiographs until normal ossification
  - Resume throwing
  - Surgery not indicated
- OCD of the capitellum
  - Often assoc w/ loss of motion
  - If no mechanical symptoms, treat w/ abstinence from throwing, restoration of ROM, gradual return to throwing.
  - If persistent symptoms, may require drilling for stable lesion, internal fixation for unstable lesion
  - If loose body, remove fragment, drill OCD lesion bed.

DISPOSITION
N/A

PROGNOSIS
- Varies depending on diagnosis. OCD lesion has poor prognosis for return to pitching. Return to play w/o long-term sequelae is expected for most elbow injuries in the throwing athlete, even if surgical treatment necessary.

CAVEATS AND PEARLS
- Wastebasket term; make SPECIFIC diagnosis
- Medial side conditions: Medial epicondyle >>> medial collateral ligament injury
- Comparison radiographs critical

LITTLE LEAGUER'S SHOULDER (PROXIMAL EPIPHYSITIS)

GERALD R. WILLIAMS, JR., MD

HISTORY
- Typically male patient 12–14 years of age
- Usually occurs near the end of rapid growth phase
- Almost exclusively an injury of throwers, especially pitchers
- Mechanism – repetitive overuse, throwing; occasionally acute displaced fracture superimposed on chronic epiphysitis

- Complaints
  - Pain with throwing, progressive, associated with cocking or acceleration phase of throwing
  - Occasional night pain, ache
  - Acute pain with displaced fracture

PHYSICAL EXAM
- Acute fracture – severe tenderness over proximal humeral metaphysis, inability to raise arm
- Subacute or chronic
  - Moderate tenderness of metaphysis/physis circumferentially, even medially
  - Pain with resisted external rotation, especially at 90° of scapular plane abduction
  - Pain with passive abduction, external rotation, extension; usually not improved with relocation
  - Normal neurologic examination
  - Laxity examination may be misleading; throwers are typically lax in external rotation and tight in internal rotation

STUDIES
- Radiographs
  - Standard radiographs to include AP, scapular lateral ("Y"), and axillary views
  - Internal and external rotation views, comparison views of opposite shoulder, and serial radiographs at different points in time are often required
  - Findings
    - Subacute
      - Epiphyseal widening (comparison views important)
      - Juxtaphyseal periosteal elevation (internal and external rotation views important)
      - Physeal fracture with displacement (acute injury)
- MRI – helpful if x-rays normal and exam suspicious
  - Physeal widening
  - Juxtaphyseal edema
  - Early periosteal elevation
- Radionuclide scan will show uptake bilaterally; involved arm increased

DIFFERENTIAL DIAGNOSIS
- Anterior subluxation

- Superior labral tear (SLAP lesion)
- Rotator cuff tendinitis
- Metaphyseal osteomyelitis (typically in younger age group)
- Neoplasia, especially with persistent night pain

TREATMENT
- **Acute fracture**
  - Sling
  - Ice
  - Rest
  - **Nondisplaced** (<45° of angulation, translation <50% shaft width)
    - Pendulum exercises 7–10 days
    - Progressive passive mobilization 3–4 weeks
    - Overhead pulley 4–6 weeks
    - End-range stretching, strengthening 6–8 weeks
    - Resume submaximal throwing 4 months, progress over additional 3–6 months
    - Resume normal throwing 9–12 months
  - **Displaced** (>45° of angulation, translation >50% of cortex)
    - Closed reduction, percutaneous pinning – acute (<7 days)
    - Open reduction, percutaneous pinning – subacute, unattainable closed reduction
    - Cut pins below skin.
    - Postoperative rehabilitation
      - Immediate pendulum exercises
      - Pin removal 3 weeks
      - Progressive passive mobilization 3 weeks
      - Overhead pulley 4–6 weeks
      - End-range stretching, strengthening 6–8 weeks
      - Resume submaximal throwing 4 months, progress over additional 3–6 months
      - Resume normal throwing 9–12 months
- **Subacute or chronic epiphysitis**
  - Rest – absolute for 7–10 days
  - Ice for first 48 hours after acute flare
  - Nonsteroidal anti-inflammatories controversial
    - Growth plate disturbance
    - May interfere with early healing
  - Analgesic – acetaminophen
  - Pendulum exercises, progressive passive mobilization 7–10 days

> End-range stretch, strengthening – 4–6 weeks
> Resume submaximal throwing when end-range stretch and strengthening are pain-free (3–4 months)
> Resume normal throwing 6–9 months

DISPOSITION
N/A

PROGNOSIS
- Prognosis for return to throwing is good in both acute and subacute (chronic) cases.
- Reassess after return to sport to verify pain-free function
- Return to sport when range of motion is full and pain-free and strength is 80% (9–12 months)
- Complications
  > Growth arrest, deformity – very uncommon because of the little amount of growth remaining in the affected age group
  > Conversion of chronic epiphysitis to acute, displaced fracture – usually from unrecognized diagnosis
  > Postsurgical infection

CAVEATS AND PEARLS
- Diagnosis requires a high index of suspicion
- Significant tenderness along proximal humeral physis is key
- Oblique (internal and external rotation), normal side comparison, and serial radiographs important
- MRI is next-level test and may pick up cases in the early phases
- Rarely requires surgery
- Do not return to throwing too soon

LONG THORACIC NERVE INJURY

KEITH MEISTER, MD

HISTORY
- Sports, work-related, idiopathic, postsurgical
- Acute mechanisms
  > Crush injury
    - Erb's point between clavicle and second rib
    - Prolonged bed rest

➤ Stretch
  • Shoulder hyperabduction and/or extension
➤ Other
  • Postsurgical axillary dissection (mastectomy, first rib resection)
  • Acute serratus anterior rupture in rheumatoid arthritis
■ Chronic mechanisms
  ➤ Repetitive stretch
    • Sports: volleyball, gymnastics, golf, wrestling, archery, basketball
    • Other: backpacking
  ➤ Brachial neuritis most common cause
■ Acute/chronic complaints
  ➤ Scapular winging (chronic)
  ➤ Generalized shoulder weakness/pain
  ➤ Inability to elevate shoulder
  ➤ Difficulty lifting weight
  ➤ Scapular pain (chronic)

PHYSICAL EXAM
■ Complete evaluation of head and neck
■ Acute/chronic
  ➤ Postural scapular winging
  ➤ Altered scapulohumeral rhythm
  ➤ Decreased passive glenohumeral range of motion
  ➤ Active elevation to 130–140° only with scapular winging
■ Tests
  ➤ Scapular winging with resisted arm elevation, wall push-up

STUDIES
■ Routine shoulder radiographs (AP, axillary views) usually normal
■ **EMG confirms diagnosis**
■ Nerve conduction studies localize the lesion

DIFFERENTIAL DIAGNOSIS
■ Painful shoulder conditions
■ Trapezius palsy
■ Multidirectional glenohumeral instability
■ Voluntary winging

TREATMENT
■ Acute

➤ Cessation of inciting activity (sport)
➤ NSAIDs, physical therapy (scapular stabilization)
➤ High-dose steroids in acute brachial neuritis
■ Chronic
➤ Bracing: results are poor, may prevent trapezius stretching
➤ Physical therapy, scapular stabilization, plyometrics
➤ Functional rehab program (i.e., interval throwing in overhand athletes)
■ Surgical
➤ >1 year without EMG or clinical return
➤ Individuals unable to adapt
➤ Usually dominant shoulder only
➤ Sternal head transfer of pectoralis major, procedure of choice
➤ Pec minor, teres major, and rhomboids have also been used in transfers, but weaker function
➤ Scapulothoracic fusion not indicated, leads to shoulder dysfunction

DISPOSITION
N/A

PROGNOSIS
■ Usually good prognosis for nonoperative management of isolated lesions from closed trauma
➤ Reassess at 4- to 6-week intervals
■ Return to play
➤ Absence of clinical complaints
➤ Symmetrical muscle function and scapulohumeral mechanics
➤ Completion of functional rehab
■ Brachial neuritis
➤ 36% recovery at 1 year
➤ 75% recovery at 2 years
■ Surgical reconstruction restores scapular stability and shoulder elevation

CAVEATS AND PEARLS
■ Do not ignore head and neck as potential etiology of dysfunction
■ Voluntary/involuntary scapular winging in overhand athletes can result in associated lesions in throwers
➤ Rotator cuff tendinitis
➤ Internal impingement
➤ Instability

LUMBAR DISK HERNIATION

GUNNAR ANDERSSON, MD, PhD

HISTORY
- Often preceded by back pain
- Frequently sudden onset
- Occurs spontaneously or following physical activities such as lifting, bending, twisting
- Can be work-related, rarely vehicle accident
- Patient may recall "pop," "tearing," "knife in the back," "electrical" leg pain
- Leg pain is the dominating symptom, often radicular
- Back pain may disappear
- Mechanically sensitive: pain increases with activity, decreases with rest
- Sitting often painful

PHYSICAL EXAM
- Decreased spinal range of motion
- Positive straight-leg raise (or alternative root tension test) (herniations at L3/4, 4/5, 5/1): high sensitivity/low specificity
- Positive crossed straight-leg raise (well leg raise): low sensitivity/high specificity
- Reflex asymmetry (L3/4; patella; L5/S1; Achilles)
- Dermatomal sensory change (L3/4; anterior thigh; L4/5; lateral lower leg, dorsum of foot; L5/S1; posterior lower leg, lateral foot)
- Motor change (L5/S1 extensor hallucis longus; rarely drop foot)
- L1/2, L2/3 herniations are rare
- Straight-leg raise negative with L1/2, L2/3 herniations; femoral stretch test occasionally positive
- Cauda equina syndrome: bowel and/or bladder dysfunction, saddle anesthesia, variable leg weakness, weak or absent reflexes
- Upper motor neuron disorder: increased reflexes, sometimes clonus

STUDIES
- Diagnosis often made on history and clinical examination
- Studies confirmatory and necessary to identify level and location
- History, physical examination, and imaging must agree for diagnosis

- Radiographs (AP, lateral) are often normal; occasionally degenerative changes
- MRI: imaging test of choice
- Gadolinium-enhanced if previous spine operation
- CT, myelogram, myelo-CT alternative imaging tests
- Disk herniation present on imaging test (MRI, etc.) in 25–30% of asymptomatic pts
- EMG: test of nerve function: low specificity and sensitivity
- Distinguish between bulge (circumferential enlargement) and protrusion (focal enlargement)
- Disk degeneration is age-related and expected (normal)
- Laboratory (serologic) tests rarely helpful
- Sed rate, CBC if general illness, fever, weight loss
- Acute radiographs if external trauma
- Imaging rarely indicated during first 6 weeks
- Don't miss rare extraforaminal for lateral herniations

DIFFERENTIAL DIAGNOSIS
- Spinal stenosis (particularly lateral)
- Intraspinal disease process (tumor, infection): rare
- Fracture (dislocation)
- Upper motor neuron disorder
- Herpes zoster
- Extraspinal disease process (sciatic nerve tumor, compression)
- Sciatic nerve compression – pelvic area (abdominal, gynecologic, piriformis)
- Peroneal nerve compression – knee (internal: knee pathology, meniscal cyst; external: pressure, trauma to fibular head area)
- Aortic aneurysm
- Physical exam and imaging are critical and usually diagnostic
- EMG helpful with upper motor neuron and peripheral nerve disorders

TREATMENT
- Acute
  - ➤ Pain medication (rarely narcotics)
  - ➤ NSAIDs
  - ➤ Activity modification (avoid bed rest)
  - ➤ Information (see "Prognosis")
  - ➤ Epidural injections may be considered (variable response)

> Physical therapy after 2–3 weeks (conditioning, extension therapy)
> Modalities have no effect on herniation, but may "feel good"
> Spontaneous improvement expected
> Imaging usually unnecessary (consider patient expectations)
> Acute imaging and surgery if cauda equina syndrome
> Imaging at 6 weeks if clinically not improved
> Consider surgery if progressive muscle weakness, intractable pain
> Surgical procedure at 6–12 weeks if not improved
  • Microdiskectomy (limited approach diskectomy) is the gold standard procedure
■ Chronic
  > Reconditioning
  > Reduction of pain medication dependence
  > Pain management

DISPOSITION
N/A

PROGNOSIS
■ Excellent (80%+ improve over 4–6 weeks)
■ Free fragments (extrusions or sequestrations) have better prognosis than protrusions but may be more painful and cause greater neurologic deficits early
■ Surgical results better than 90% in patients with protrusions, extrusions, and sequestrations
■ Surgical results poor when findings small or questionable
■ Recurrence in 5–10% (same level or different level)
■ Uncomplicated excellent surgical results allow patients to return to full physical activity levels

CAVEATS AND PEARLS
■ Herniated nucleus pulposus (HNP) can be present without low back pain
■ Acute surgical treatment for cauda equina syndrome
■ Hyperreflexia associated with upper motor neuron disorder
■ HNP usually recovers within 6 weeks
■ MRI to confirm HNP
■ Imaging will show herniated disk in 25–35% of asymptomatic individuals

- Diagnosis requires concordance of symptoms, signs, and imaging
- Always consider nonorthopedic causes of back pain and sciatica
- Caveat: tumor, fracture, infection in older patient

LUMBAR FRACTURES

EDWARD GOLDBERG, MD
GREGORY BREBACH, MD

HISTORY
- Incidence: 10,000 new spinal cord injuries per year
- 80% male and <40 years old
- 200,000–500,000 lumbar compression fractures per year in the elderly population
- Detailed history, mechanism of injury, associated injuries must be sought
- Four basic mechanisms of spine trauma
  - Compression
  - Distraction
  - Rotation
  - Shear forces

PHYSICAL EXAM
- Follow trauma protocols
- ABCs
- Full examination of head/neck, abdomen, and GU system
- Inspection: clothing should be removed
- Palpation: systemic examination from head to toe
- Neurologic evaluation – Frankel scale
  - Motor, sensory, reflexes
  - Attention to dull discrimination, temperature, light and deep pressure
- Mechanism of injury
  - Axial compression – low energy results in compression fractures
    - Typically anterior wedging of vertebral body
    - Usually stable
    - Nearly 90% of all lumbar spine fractures
    - Rarely involves neurologic deficit
    - Osteoporosis predisposes the elderly population
  - Axial compression – high energy can result in burst fractures
    - Anterior and middle aspects of vertebral body

- May displace into neural canal, causing neurologic compromise
- Unstable 50–60% loss of anterior height, 25° kyphosis, 50% canal compromise

➤ Flexion – compresses vertebral body with additional tension forces posteriorly

➤ Flexion/distraction: chance fracture
- Common in motor vehicle accidents – seat belt injury
- Disruption of posterior spinal ligaments
- Commonly L1–L3
- Axial component – compression/burst fracture

➤ Fracture/dislocation
- Disruption of anterior, middle, and posterior spinal columns with distraction and rotation
- Highly unstable and associated with significant neurologic deficit
- Majority require surgery

➤ Lateral compression fractures
- Ligamentous injury must be assessed, or progressive deformity may develop

➤ Shear injuries
- Significant ligamentous injuries
- Produces anterior, lateral, or posterior listhesis (subluxation)
- Associated with neurologic injury
- Usually requires surgical stabilization

➤ Extension injury
- Hyperextension injury
- Anterior vertebral body avulsion fracture coupled with fracture of posterior columns
- Generally stable
- Stability often dictates surgical intervention (Denis)

➤ First-degree instability
- Severe compression fractures
- Seat belt injuries (flexion-distraction)

➤ Second-degree instability
- Burst fractures with late neurologic involvement

➤ Third-degree instability
- Fracture/dislocations
- Severe burst fractures with immediate neurologic involvement

STUDIES
- Radiographic evaluation
  - AP, lateral oblique views of the spine
  - Examine vertebral bodies for fracture
  - Focus on posterior aspect of vertebral body for retropulsion and translation
- MRI
  - Evaluation of spinal cord and soft tissues
  - Intervertebral disks
  - Posterior ligaments

DIFFERENTIAL DIAGNOSIS
- Centers on understanding mechanism of injury and correlation with physical exam
- Do not overlook ligamentous injury
  - Progressive deformity
  - Late neurologic deficit

TREATMENT
- Compression fractures
  - Generally stable
  - Rarely involve neurologic compromise
  - Hyperextension exercises and avoidance of compressive loading for 3 months
  - Hyperextension bracing/casting
  - If >50% compression, the fracture may be unstable
    - Ligamentous injury
    - ORIF with posterior instrumentation
    - Vertebroplasty
- Burst fractures
  - Management based on presence or absence of neurologic injury and stability
  - Neurologically intact
    - Nonoperative
    - Same conservative treatment as in compression fractures
  - Unstable
    - Anterior and posterior surgical stabilization with pedicle screw fixation
- Flexion/distraction (seat belt injury)
  - Chance fracture: anterior axial compression with involvement of posterior elements

> Bone only: hyperextension orthosis for 3 months
> With ligamentous disruption: posterior surgical spinal arthrodesis with posterior compression
> If 50% of height is lost, a ligamentous injury is often present
- Fracture/dislocation
  > Usually associated with severe neurologic impairment (50%+)
  > Requires surgical stabilization of the spine for early rehabilitation and mobilization
  > Posterior surgical stabilization with instrumentation and fusion
  > Shear fracture is the most unstable type

DISPOSITION
N/A

PROGNOSIS
- Complete injury: no motor or sensory function below the zone of injury
  > Poor prognosis for neurologic recovery
  > One- to two-root recovery may be attained
- Incomplete injury: partial preservation of motor and/or sensory function below the zone of injury
  > Intermediate prognosis
  > Brown-Sequard: ipsilateral motor and positional loss with contralateral pain and temperature loss
    • Significant room for recovery
  > Anterior cord syndrome: motor paralysis with loss of sensation at area of injury with preservation of posterior columns (positional, vibratory)
    • Poor prognosis for recovery
- Spinal cord recovery is better if bony impingement is recovered, especially in incomplete injury
- High-dose corticosteroids – methylprednisolone 30 mg/kg loading dose within 8 hours of injury, followed by 5.4 mg/kg/hr for 23 hours has been shown to improve outcome, especially in partial injury

CAVEATS AND PEARLS
N/A

LUMBAR SPONDYLOLISTHESIS

EDWARD GOLDBERG, MD
GREGORY BREBACH, MD

HISTORY

Definition
- Spondylolisthesis is the nonanatomic alignment of one vertebra on another
  - Anterior (most common)
  - Posterior
  - Lateral

History
- Like spondylolysis, commonly occurs in late childhood or adolescence
- Most commonly presents with low back pain
- Coincides with adolescent growth spurt
- Postural deformity – loss of lumbar lordosis
- Very few patients present with radicular pattern
  - Associated with high-grade slips
  - Nerve root compression is most commonly at the L5 nerve root in an L5-S1 slip

Classification
- Congenital: deficiency of superior sacral and/or inferior fifth lumbar facets
- Isthmic: most common in adolescents
  - Typical defect in the pars interarticularis
  - Acute fracture, fatigue fracture, or attenuation of pars
- Degenerative: most common overall
  - Found in adults
  - Secondary to segmental instability
- Traumatic: fracture of pedicle, lamina, or facets
- Pathologic: slip secondary to structural weakness of the bones
  - Osteogenesis imperfecta
  - Paget's disease
  - Tumor

Grading
- Meyerding grading systems for percentage of slippage

- Based on percentage of displacement of superior vertebral body on inferior vertebral body
- Grade I: 0–25%
- Grade II: 25–50%
- Grade III: 50–75%
- Grade IV: 75–100%
- Grade V: >100% – spondyloptosis

PHYSICAL EXAM

- Often asymptomatic
- Hamstring tightness, commonly insidious in onset
- May be unable to flex hip with knees extended
- Flattening of buttocks with high-grade slip
  - Palpable step-off between fifth spinous process and sacrum
- Phalen-Dickson sign: knee flexed, hip flexed gait
- Patients with grade I and II spondylolisthesis rarely have physical findings other than
  - Back pain
  - Back spasms
  - Hamstring tightness
- Abdomen may be thrust forward in high-grade slips
- Isthmic spondylolisthesis children and adolescents
  - Most common at L5-S1
  - L5 nerve root affected
  - Scoliosis present in about 20%
- Degenerative spondylolisthesis 65 years and older
  - Female > male
  - L4-L5 level most common, followed by higher lumbar levels
  - Secondary to segmental instability
  - Higher incidence of presentation with neurologic defect (40%)

STUDIES

- Radiographs: AP, lateral, and oblique views
- Isthmic: "Scotty dog" on oblique
  - Subluxation of superior vertebral body on inferior
  - Acute: irregular, narrow gap
  - Chronic: may be smooth and round with pseudoarthrosis
  - Bone scan: increased uptake in pars
  - Myelograph: seldom needed, will show typical hourglass deformity of thecal sac
  - CT
  - Single photon emission computed tomography

■ Degenerative: facet hypertrophy
> Disk space narrowing
> Osteophytes on vertebral bodies
> Subluxation – rarely >30%
> Myelograph: hourglass at level, usually L4-L5
> CT: degenerative change at facets
> MRI: compression of thecal sac
• Herniated disks
• Foraminal dimensions
• Spinal stenosis

DIFFERENTIAL DIAGNOSIS

■ Isthmic: osteoid osteoma, osteoblastoma, disk space infection, rheumatoid spondylitis, muscle or neurologic disorders
■ Degenerative: degenerative disk disease, spondylosis, spinal stenosis

TREATMENT

■ Isthmic spondylolisthesis
> Observation if <50% and asymptomatic
> Restrict activities and brace if <50% and symptomatic
> Fusion if >50% slip with documented progression in child, or those with slips of <50% who remain symptomatic despite conservative treatment
• In situ posterolateral fusion
• One-level fusion if <50% slip
• Two-level fusion if >50% slip
■ Adult spondylolisthesis (isthmic or degenerative)
> Pain relief primary concern
> Conservative treatment for >= 6 months
> Observation if asymptomatic, even with high-grade slip
> 15% of adults require surgery
• Decompressive laminectomy with likely foraminotomy
• Couple with posterolateral fusion
• Instrumentation decreases risk of pseudoarthrosis

DISPOSITION

N/A

PROGNOSIS

■ Progression during 10–15 years old, obtain radiographs every 6 months
■ Females more prone to slippage

- Greater slips (>30%) and higher slip angles generally represent a worse prognosis

CAVEATS AND PEARLS
- Degree of slip does not correlate to pain
- Degenerative spondylolisthesis is the result of long-standing segmental instability
  - Pars is intact
  - Rarely slips >30%
  - Adults can have either degenerative or isthmic spondylolisthesis
- Isthmic spondylolisthesis – acquired in childhood
  - Failure of pars
  - Activity and genetics both play a role

LUMBAR SPONDYLOLYSIS

GREGORY BREBACH, MD
EDWARD J. GOLDBERG, MD

HISTORY
- Definition
  - Pars interarticularis of L1, L2, L3, L4, or L5 is unilaterally or bilaterally disrupted
  - May or may not be associated with spondylolistheses
  - Most common L5-S1
- General questions: onset, location, frequency, duration, and intensity of symptoms
- Often asymptomatic
- 50% of cases associated with particular activity or traumatic event
- Hyperextension activities (repetitive loading)
- Common athletes
  - Divers
  - Gymnasts
  - Wrestlers
  - Football linemen
- May present as
  - Low back pain
  - Tight hamstrings
  - Buttock pain
- Can be acute, but usually insidious in onset
- Coincides with adolescent growth spurt (7–20 years)

- Incidence
  - 4.4% in 6-year-old children
  - 5.8% by adulthood
  - 18% intercollegiate football linemen
  - Male to female 2:1
- Spina bifida occulta occurs more frequently in patients with spondylolysis
- Positive family history often present

PHYSICAL EXAM
- General review of trunk balance, alignment, and posture
- Tight hamstrings: secondary to nerve root irritation?
- Phalen-Dickson sign – knee flexed, hip flexed gait
- Pain on palpation of posterior elements, especially if acute fracture present
- Lumbosacral low back pain, increased by hyperextension
- Referred back pain on single leg hops

STUDIES
- Radiographs: AP, lateral, and oblique
  - "Scotty dog" – fracture of neck of pars interarticularis on oblique x-ray
  - If defect is unilateral, contralateral pars may be sclerotic
- Acute fractures – bone scans may be useful
- Single photon emission computed tomography
  - More detail and localization
- CT
  - Not as helpful in impending stress fractures of the pars
  - Helps with differentiation from osteoid osteoma, osteoblastoma
- MRI
  - Assess nerve root compression
  - Unusual in patients without high-grade spondylolisthesis

DIFFERENTIAL DIAGNOSIS
- Spondylolysis
- Spondylolisthesis: decreased lumber lordosis, palpable step-off, radicular symptoms, diagnosis obvious on lateral radiographs
- Osteoid osteoma/osteoblastoma: common tumors of childhood – night pain
- Disk space infections
- Muscle or neurologic disorders
- Rheumatoid spondylitis

TREATMENT
- If symptomatic
  - Restrict activities
  - Followed by physical therapy
  - Back and abdominal strengthening
  - Hamstring stretching
- If continued symptoms, cast or brace – orthosis reduces lumbar lordosis

80% of patients have relief of symptoms with above treatments
- Surgical treatment
  - Direct repair of pars defect
    - Young patients without spondylolisthesis
    - Best in levels L1–L4
    - Healing less likely in patients >30 years old
    - Slip of 2 mm or greater also decreases chances of success
    - Degenerative disk disease by MRI a relative contraindication
  - Fusion in situ: rarely necessary
    - Symptomatic spondyloysis at L5-S1
    - Spans motion segment
    - Bilateral lateral spinal fusion with iliac crest bone graft

DISPOSITION
N/A

PROGNOSIS
- Monitor only if symptoms present
- Radiographs every 6 months
- Females more prone to develop spondylolisthesis
- Patients usually respond well to conservative therapy, without progression to olisthesis or disabling pain
- Most patients are asymptomatic and do not require activity modification or restriction of any kind

CAVEATS AND PEARLS
- Spondylolysis does not exist at birth; it is related to activity and has a genetic predisposition
- The shape of L5 and S1 may predispose the patient to listhesis
- Asymptomatic patients make up the great majority
  - No restrictions
  - Full sports participation
  - Follow-up only if symptomatic

LUMBAR STRAIN

GUNNAR ANDERSSON, MD

HISTORY
- Strain defined as muscular injury caused by voluntary contraction of muscle
- Sprain is ligament injury
- Usually occurs at myotendinous junction
- Most common after eccentric (lengthening) contraction
- Sport or work cause common
- Mechanism – lifting, bending, twisting, pushing, pulling, etc.
- Can occur following almost any activity involving the back
- Acute severe pain in back, occasionally buttocks
- Mechanically sensitive: pain with physical performance
- Difficulty moving when severe
- Improves when lying down
- Difficulty finding comfortable position
- Red flags: fever, general feeling of sickness, trauma, weight loss, night pain, history of cancer
- Most common in ages 25–44

PHYSICAL EXAM
- Decreased range of motion
- Acute muscle spasm (hard, prominent muscle)
- Often listing to one side
- Usually otherwise normal exam
- Palpate the back: red flag – intense local tenderness
- Palpate abdomen, renal area
- Stress sacroiliac joints
- Do brief neurologic exam: straight-leg raise, patella and Achilles reflexes, ankle and toe dorsiflexion

STUDIES
- Rarely indicated
- Usually normal except for degenerative spine changes
- Radiographs if red flags in patient history: fever, general feeling of sickness, trauma, weight loss, night pain, history of cancer, immunosuppression, steroid use, age >70

- X-rays are the first studies to consider
- CBC and sed rate if suspicious of tumor or infection

DIFFERENTIAL DIAGNOSIS

- Consider other spine condition if symptoms persist longer than 4-6 weeks
- Degenerative disk disease with annular tear (MRI, diskography)
- Spondylolisthesis (radiographs)
- Instability (flexion/extension radiographs)
- Spondylarthropathy (ankylosing spondylitis, etc.): morning stiffness, improvement with limbering
- Infection: severe unrelenting pain, night pain, fever, feeling of sickness, immunosuppression, IV drug use, corticosteroid use, tenderness
- Tumor: severe unrelenting pain, night pain, weight loss, history of cancer
- Fracture: trauma, osteoporosis (age, gender); age >70 years, tenderness, steroid use
- Nonspinal origin: kidney (stones, infection); gallbladder, intestines, pelvic organs
- Sacroiliac joints: pain location more distal and lateral; do provocation tests
- Fibromyalgia: pain in many locations, fatigue, sleeplessness, multiple tender points (trigger points)

TREATMENT

- Acute
  - Natural history is excellent: 90% recover in 3–4 weeks
  - Treatment, aimed at symptom control and prevention of functional loss
  - Analgesics (rarely narcotics)
  - NSAIDs
  - Consider muscle relaxants if severe muscle spasm (short period)
  - Most patients do well with analgesics only
  - NSAIDs probably as effective as muscle relaxants
  - No benefit to combining NSAIDs and muscle relaxants
  - About 1/3 of patients become drowsy with muscle relaxants
  - Do not use oral steroids
  - Do not use epidural injections
  - Do not use antidepressants for acute strains

- ➤ Modify activity (avoid prolonged sitting, lifting, bending, twisting)
- ➤ Do not prescribe bed rest
- ➤ Self-application of heat or cold may improve symptoms temporarily (ice acutely)
- ➤ Modalities are of questionable benefit (avoid pacifying the patient)
- ➤ Manual therapy can be beneficial (if no improvement, stop treatment)
- ➤ Do not prescribe traction
- ➤ Do not prescribe corsets or braces
- ➤ Do not consider surgery
- ■ Chronic
  - ➤ Exclude specific causes of back pain
  - ➤ Provide information about the benign nature and natural history
  - ➤ Avoid long-term drug treatment
  - ➤ Provide exercise therapy to improve functioning
  - ➤ Refer patients with severe, long-lasting low back pain and disability to a multidisciplinary treatment program (pain management, functional restoration, behavioral management)
  - ➤ Surgery unrewarding if no specific underlying cause is identified

DISPOSITION
N/A

PROGNOSIS
- ■ Excellent (90% recover in 3–4 weeks)
- ■ Early pain treatment and continued normal daily activities improve prognosis
- ■ Prognosis decreases as pain becomes more chronic
- ■ Workers' compensation cases present special problems (poorer prognosis)

CAVEATS AND PEARLS
- ■ Self-limiting problem with excellent prognosis
- ■ Stay active
- ■ Avoid medication dependence
- ■ Red flags for tumor or infection: history of cancer, recent infection, fever, IV drug abuse, prolonged steroid use, pain at rest (night pain), unexplained weight loss

- Red flags for fracture: recent significant trauma, any trauma in elderly, prolonged steroid use, known osteoporosis, patient >70
- If red flags: radiographs; if suspect tumor or infection, CBC, sed rate
- Consider work-related and psychosocial factors
- Do not overtreat

MALLET FINGER

JOHN FERNANDEZ, MD

HISTORY
- Most commonly closed/blunt injury
- Can be open
- Symptoms
  - Mild swelling
  - Little to no pain
  - Extension loss at distal interphalangeal joint (DIPJ)
  - Lag usually immediate; can be delayed
- Mechanism
  - Forced finger flexion against active extension
  - Usually blunt impact injury to fingertip
  - Terminal tendon avulsed
  - Fractured from insertion
  - Crushing injury: shoe cleat stepping on fingertip
  - May occur "spontaneously"
    - Little or no significant trauma
    - May develop on delayed basis
  - Ring/small finger most commonly affected
- Common in softball, basketball, football, volleyball

PHYSICAL EXAM
- Swelling at DIPJ dorsally
- Tenderness to palpation, dorsal DIPJ
- Usually mild; may have no pain at all
- Loss of active extension at DIPJ
- Passive extension intact
- Late findings
  - Flexion contracture at DIPJ
  - Hyperextension deformity at proximal interphalangeal joint (PIPJ; swan-neck deformity)

STUDIES
- Radiographs
  - AP, lateral, oblique of hand/finger
  - Usually normal appearance
  - 25% have dorsal fracture avulsion
  - Note percentage of articular surface involvement
  - Note any volar joint subluxation

DIFFERENTIAL DIAGNOSIS
- DIPJ dislocation
  - Instability, tenderness at joint
  - Radiographs show articular incongruity
- Phalangeal fracture
  - Tender at fracture
  - Radiographs show fracture on lateral
- DIPJ contracture
  - Passive extension not possible
  - Usually secondary findings at joint, arthropathy

TREATMENT
- Mallet finger classification
  - Type I
    - Closed/blunt injury of terminal tendon
    - With/without small avulsion fracture
  - Type II
    - Open injury/laceration of terminal tendon
  - Type III
    - Deep abrasion with loss of soft tissue and tendon
  - Type IV
    - A: transepiphyseal fracture, child
    - B: hyperflexion injury, 20–50% dorsal articular fracture
    - C: hyperextension injury, >50% fracture, volar subluxation
- Acute
  - Establish type of injury
  - Immediately treat based on injury type
- Type I
  - Place and maintain DIPJ in full extension
  - Avoid blocking PIPJ flexion
  - Avoid hyperextension
  - Disregard small fracture fragments (<20% articular surface), even if displaced

➤ Orthoplast volar gutter DIPJ splint (author's preference)
  • Fabricated by occupational therapist
  • Custom-molded, perfect fit
  • Held with Velcro straps
➤ Stack splint
  • Various sizes available "off the shelf"
  • May not fit many well, too loose/too tight
➤ Alumafoam splint
  • Place volar, avoid dorsal
  • Held with tape/coban wrap
  • Skin does not tolerate well
  • Foam padding wears out quickly
  • Detailed instructions necessary
➤ Splint is worn at all times including showers/baths.
➤ Remove splint 2–3 times per day to clean/dry finger.
➤ Remove only while supporting DIPJ in full extension.
➤ Place finger flat on table, then remove splint.
➤ Never allow finger to be without support in extension.
➤ Wear splint full-time 8 weeks.
➤ If at 8 weeks extension lag <15°, wean splint.
➤ Day: 2 hours on/2 hours off, night: all night
➤ Reassess after 2 weeks of weaning.
➤ If extension lag persist, wear 2 more weeks.
➤ Reassess again.
➤ Therapy for flexion ROM usually not needed
  • If at 3 months there is loss of flexion, begin passive ROM.
➤ Operative option: transarticular K-wire
  • Reserved for those who cannot wear splint
  • Dentist, surgeon, patient's choice
  • Local digital block
  • 0.035 or 0.045 K-wire
  • Place oblique/longitudinal across DIPJ
  • Fewer complications if oblique
  • Remove pin after 8 weeks and treat as above
■ Type II
➤ Open and repair with suture 5-0/6-0 monofilament
➤ Postoperatively treat as type I
■ Type III
➤ Soft tissue flap/reconstruction
➤ Tendon graft, if necessary
➤ Postoperatively treat as type I

- Type IV
  - ORIF large articular fragments (>20% articular surface)
  - K-wires, minifragment screws
  - Postoperatively treat as type I
- Late
  - Treat like acute injury up to 6 months in some cases.
  - Deformity has little or no functional impact; primarily cosmetic.
  - If deformity mild/no functional problem, do nothing
  - Note any secondary hyperextension of PIPJ
    - Usually predisposed with volar plate laxity
  - If deformity severe/secondary hyperextension of PIPJ
    - Spiral oblique retinacular ligament reconstruction
    - DIPJ fusion
  - Silver ring blocking splint if surgery not wanted

DISPOSITION
N/A

PROGNOSIS
- Early splint treatment
  - 80% good/excellent result
  - Good results decrease with lag in initial splint treatment
  - Return to play
    - Immediately with splint
    - 8–10 weeks without splint
  - Complications
    - Residual DIPJ extensor lag/droop
    - May lose some DIPJ flexion
- Transarticular wire
  - Similar result, greater morbidity
  - Return to play immediately
  - Complications
    - Infection
    - Pain at previous pin site
- Late repair/reconstruction
  - Fair/poor result
  - Return to play 6–8 weeks
  - Complications
    - Residual deformity
    - DIPJ/PIPJ stiffness

■ Fusion DIPJ
  ➤ Good result
  ➤ Return to play immediately with splint
  ➤ Complications
    • Loss of DIPJ motion
    • Diminished grip strength
    • Nonunion

CAVEATS AND PEARLS
■ Detailed instructions regarding splint use necessary
■ Splint cannot be removed without support
■ If pinning of joint preferred, place wire obliquely
  ➤ Less pin tract pain later
  ➤ If pin breaks, easily retrievable
■ Allow adequate time to heal; do not rush for ROM – 8 weeks minimum

---

MEDIAL ANKLE SPRAINS

CAROL FREY, MD

HISTORY
■ Anatomy
  ➤ Superficial deltoid ligament
    • Tibionavicular ligament
    • Calcaneotibial (sustentaculum) ligament
    • Posterior talotibial ligament
  ➤ Deep deltoid ligament
    • Deep anterior talotibial ligament
    • Deep posterior talotibial ligament
■ Mechanism
  ➤ Hindfoot and ankle eversion
  ➤ Abduction
  ➤ An isolated complete tear of the deltoid is rare.
  ➤ Partial tears of the anterior fibers are more common.
  ➤ A combination of pronation and abduction is more common.
    • Results in either an oblique lateral malleolus fracture or a syndesmosis injury
    • Medially either the deltoid ligament ruptures or there is an avulsion fracture of the medial malleolus

- Patient reports
  - Swelling
  - Medial ecchymosis
  - Pain on palpation over medial ligament structures
  - Rarely instability

PHYSICAL EXAM

- Swollen and tender at deltoid
- Palpate syndesmosis.
- Palpate entire fibula as there may be a high fibula fracture (Maisonneuve).
- Rare to see any laxity

STUDIES

Basic tests

- Radiographs
  - Standard AP, lateral, mortise
  - Usually normal
  - Observe syndesmosis width
    - 1 cm superior to the ankle joint line on AP
    - No more than 5 mm tibia-fibular space
  - Subtle lateral malleolar or Maisonneuve fractures
  - Medial joint space widening should be noted

Special tests

- External rotation/eversion stress tests on AP radiograph
  - Check for widening of syndesmosis.
  - Check for widening of medial clear space.

DIFFERENTIAL DIAGNOSIS

- Syndesmosis injury
- Posterior tibial tendon injury
- Tarsal coalition
- Sustentaculum injury
- Flexor digitorum longus tendon injury
- Flexor hallucis longus tendon injury
- Tarsal tunnel syndrome/neuropraxia
- Talonavicular joint injury
- Pes planovalgus

TREATMENT

- Isolated deltoid ligament injuries
  - Immobilize 4–6 weeks with weight-bearing.
  - Rehab

- Deltoid rupture associated with fractures or syndesmosis injury
  - ➤ Treat associated injury.
  - ➤ If joint does not reduce concentrically, open medial side and extricate deltoid.
  - ➤ Usually not necessary to repair deltoid

DISPOSITION
N/A

PROGNOSIS
N/A

CAVEATS AND PEARLS
- An isolated injury to the deltoid ligament is rare.
- Be very suspicious for a high fibula fracture.
- Be very suspicious for a syndesmosis injury.
- Rare to have instability with deltoid ligament injuries
- Rare to repair deltoid ligament
- Must rule out posterior tibial tendon injury
- The superficial ligament tears first, then the deep.
- The syndesmosis will tear if external rotation forces continue.

MEDIAL ELBOW INJURIES

CRAIG M. BALL, MD, FRACS
KEN YAMAGUCHI, MD
REVISED BY CHARLES NOFSINGER, MD

HISTORY
- Most medial elbow injuries related to overuse syndromes from activities such as throwing, golf, tennis, manual labor
- Some familiarity with stresses of and injuries unique to a particular sport is necessary
- Medial epicondylitis
  - ➤ Related to chronic repetitive overload of the flexor-pronator group at its origin
  - ➤ Presents with pain centered on or just anterior to the epicondyle, worsened by activities involving resisted pronation or wrist flexion
  - ➤ Associated ulnar nerve symptoms common
- Medial collateral ligament (MCL) instability
  - ➤ Acute rupture presents with acute medial elbow pain

➤ Persistent medial elbow pain with throwing suggests partial rupture from tensile overload

➤ Pain only when throwing >70% effort

- Flexor-pronator strain
  ➤ Partial rupture usually at the musculotendinous junction
  ➤ Presents with pain in proximal flexor musculature

- Medial epicondyle fractures – acute fracture secondary to chronic tensile overload, usually in adolescents

- Ulnar nerve injuries
  ➤ From compression by inflammation of MCL or traction from repetitive valgus loading
  ➤ Presents with symptoms related to the nerve

PHYSICAL EXAM

- Medial epicondylitis
  ➤ Focal tenderness just anterior to epicondyle
  ➤ Pain with resisted forearm pronation and wrist palmarflexion

- MCL instability
  ➤ Tenderness at insertion of anterior MCL
  ➤ Symptom reproduction with valgus stress test, milking maneuver, or moving valgus stress test

- Flexor-pronator strain
  ➤ Swelling and ecchymosis over medial forearm
  ➤ Tenderness distal to epicondyle over flexor-pronator muscles

- Medial epicondyle fractures – focal swelling and tenderness

- Ulnar nerve injuries
  ➤ Hypermobility of nerve (15% population)
  ➤ Positive nerve compression test
  ➤ Positive elbow flexion test
  ➤ Tinel's sign
  ➤ Objective sensory and motor dysfunction in hand

STUDIES

- Medial epicondylitis
  ➤ Usually a clinical diagnosis
  ➤ Radiographs often normal
  ➤ MRI may detect tendon degeneration
  ➤ Electrodiagnostic testing may show abnormalities with coexistent ulnar neuropathy

- MCL instability
  ➤ Plain radiographs for associated abnormalities (marginal osteophytes, loose bodies, ligament calcification)

- Valgus stress radiographs may show a side-to-side difference of >2 mm
- MRI arthrography for detection of complete ligament tears (less reliable for partial thickness)
- Arthroscopic valgus instability test also described

■ Flexor-pronator strain
- Pain radiographs may show ossification in the muscles near their origin
- MRI will show edema or partial origin detachment

■ Medial epicondyle fractures – AP and/or lateral radiographs to determine degree of displacement and rotation of fragment

■ Ulnar nerve injuries
- Plain radiographs (including epicondylar groove views) may show osteophytes or bone fragments
- Electrodiagnostic studies may show decreased amplitudes and conduction velocity slowing

DIFFERENTIAL DIAGNOSIS

■ Medial epicondylitis
■ MCL instability
■ Flexor-pronator strain
■ Medial epicondyle fractures
■ Ulnar nerve injuries

TREATMENT

■ Most injuries are treated nonsurgically
■ Treatment options should be related to rehabilitation plans in preparation for a return to sport
■ Medial epicondylitis
- Initially conservative (education, activity modification, NSAIDs, physical therapy program that emphasizes eccentric stretching and strengthening)
- Alterations in technique and/or equipment important
- Cortisone injections have higher risk than on lateral side
- Surgery (debridement) only as last resort
■ MCL instability
- Acute tears require reconstruction for return to sport
- Symptomatic chronic tears require reconstruction of anterior MCL using a tendon graft
- Postop rehabilitation very important
■ Flexor-pronator strain – rest followed by motion and strengthening exercises

- Medial epicondyle fractures – anatomic open reduction and internal fixation unless minimally displaced
- Ulnar nerve injuries
  - Avoid sustained or repetitive elbow flexion
  - Subcutaneous ulnar nerve transposition if symptoms warrant, as a submuscular transfer disrupts flexor-pronator integrity

DISPOSITION
N/A

PROGNOSIS
- Medial epicondylitis
  - >90% success rate with nonoperative treatment
  - Similarly high success rate in those requiring surgery
  - Recovery can be prolonged, with return to full-strength use of the arm averaging 6–8 months
  - Prognosis worse with ulnar nerve involvement
- MCL instability
  - With surgery, 80% will have a satisfactory result, with return to previous level of sport
  - Average time to competitive throwing 12 months
- Flexor-pronator strain
  - Return to sport as symptoms permit
  - Easier to prevent (strength and flexibility conditioning) than to treat
- Medial epicondyle fractures – long-term outcome generally excellent
- Ulnar nerve injuries – good results expected following anterior transposition
- **Complications**
  - Ulnar nerve involvement primary cause of surgical failure in epicondylitis
  - Chronic valgus instability from anterior MCL injury
  - Ulnar nerve injury following any surgical procedure on the medial elbow
  - Fracture of bone tunnels during MCL reconstruction
  - Medial antebrachial cutaneous nerve injury
  - Ossification (usually asymptomatic) near flexor-pronator muscle origin
  - Failure of ulnar nerve transposition due to incomplete release

CAVEATS AND PEARLS

- History and physical examination the cornerstones of diagnosis
- Nonoperative treatment for epicondylitis focuses on revitalization of the area of tendinosis by rehabilitation
- Cortisone injections should be used cautiously about the medial elbow
- Extension splinting for ulna neuropathy is poorly tolerated
- 2 years may be required following epicondylitis surgery
- High index of suspicion required to diagnose MCL injury
- MCL surgery required for return to sport only, as ability to perform ADLs is usually not affected
- Ulnar nerve not routinely transposed with MCL reconstruction
- Rehabilitation is prolonged because of forces generated during throwing
- Normal ulnar nerve EMG studies in the throwing athlete with significant symptoms do not preclude surgical treatment

MEDIAL EPICONDYLITIS

CHAMP BAKER, MD
DAVID D. NEDEFF, MD

HISTORY

- "Golfer's elbow"
- Much less common than lateral epicondylitis
- Highest incidence in fourth and fifth decades
- Equal male:female ratio
- Associated with activities that place repetitive valgus stress on elbow
- Pathology most commonly seen in flexor carpi radialis and pronator teres
- Microtears noted in flexor-pronator origin, which results in mucoid degeneration of the tendon
- Pain often insidious in onset

PHYSICAL EXAM

- Medial elbow pain worsened by resisted forearm pronation and/or wrist flexion
- Maximal tenderness usually over medial epicondyle
- Elbow and wrist range of motion usually normal

- Strength may be slightly decreased but often normal
- Ulnar nerve symptoms may coexist and cause decreased sensibility in little and ring fingers (elbow flexion test with wrist extension for >3 minutes)
- Important to assess ligamentous stability

STUDIES
- Plain radiographs usually normal
- Throwing athletes may have medial traction spurs or ulnar collateral ligament (UCL) calcification
- UCL calcification may indicate concomitant UCL insufficiency
- MRI may be indicated if suspicious of UCL tear or insufficiency
- EMG and/or nerve conduction velocity studies if ulnar nerve symptoms exist

DIFFERENTIAL DIAGNOSIS
- Ulnar neuropathy (elbow flexion test: maximal elbow flexion and wrist extension for >3 minutes)
- UCL insufficiency (valgus stress at 30° flexion)
- Cervical disk disease
- Median nerve compression syndrome (pronator syndrome)

TREATMENT
- As with lateral epicondylitis, most patients respond to conservative treatment
- NSAID, activity modification, rehabilitation program recommended
- Counterforce bracing and steroid injections may have a role
- Operative treatment recommended after minimum 6 months of conservative care
- Surgical goals similar to those of lateral epicondylitis
- Debride pathologic tendon, decorticate medial epicondyle, with or without reattachment
- Medial antebrachial cutaneous nerve at risk (neuroma formation)
- Medial epicondylectomy is out of favor
- If coexistent ulnar nerve symptoms, decompression of ulnar nerve may be sufficient
  - ➤ If symptoms more severe, anterior transposition of ulnar nerve may be required

DISPOSITION
N/A

PROGNOSIS

- Postoperative splint or sling for 7–10 days
- Wrist and hand range of motion exercises started immediately
- Passive and gentle active elbow range of motion exercises at 2 weeks
- Resisted wrist flexion and forearm pronation exercises started at 4–6 weeks after surgery
- Return to full activities by 4 months
- Some patients may require >6 months for full recovery
- High success rate for pain relief (85–95%)
- Coexistent ulnar neuritis carries worse prognosis
- Complications include ulnar nerve injury, medial antebrachial cutaneous neuroma, persistent pain, medial instability (primarily with medial epicondylectomy), and flexor pronator weakness

CAVEATS AND PEARLS

- *Tendinosis* more accurately describes condition than *tendinitis*
- Must rule out ulnar neuritis and UCL insufficiency
- Nonoperative treatment usually successful
- Key to surgery is removal of pathologic tissue and decortication of medial epicondyle
- Must decompress or transpose ulnar nerve if ulnar symptoms exist

---

MEDIAL KNEE LIGAMENT INJURY (MCL)

TIMOTHY S. BOLLOM, MD
ROBERT F. LAPRADE, MD

HISTORY

- Sports (contact or noncontact) or work-related injury (activity)
- Mechanism
  - Direct blow: lateral knee, lower thigh, upper leg
  - Noncontact: valgus, external rotation injury
- Pain, medial side
- Ability to ambulate/compete postinjury related to severity of medial collateral ligament (MCL) injury
- Sensation of pop/tear, presence of deformity
- Severe trauma – hx of knee dislocation, multidirectional instability
- Localized soft tissue swelling over medial knee
- Locking, catching, or mechanical symptoms (occasionally associated with meniscal pathology)

- History of previous injury, chronic instability
- Preseason physical findings (laxity on valgus stress)
- Common sports: football, skiing, gymnastics, volleyball, soccer, ice hockey

PHYSICAL EXAM

- Inspection – Ecchymosis, erythema, effusion (compare to contralateral knee)
- Palpation
  - Medial patellar tenderness
  - Patellar apprehension
  - Medial retinacular tenderness
  - Medial epicondyle
  - Meniscofemoral MCL
  - Joint line
  - Meniscotibial MCL
  - Hard mass – Chronics (Pelligrini-Stieda disease)
  - Patellar dislocation associated with valgus injuries, injured extensor mechanism (9–21%)
  - ROM (locked knee) – displaced meniscal tear
- Valgus stress testing (0°)
  - 0° – If abnormal, usually anterior cruciate (ACL) and/or posterior cruciate (PCL) combined injury
  - No instability if posterior capsule and PCL intact
  - Complete extension
- Gold standard – Valgus stress 30° (compare to contralateral knee)
  - Grade 0 (0 mm opening)
  - I (1–4 mm)
  - II (5–10 mm); grades I and II have definite end points
  - III (>10 mm) – No endpoint
  - Feel for joint line crepitation (underlying medial meniscus tear or articular cartilage damage)
  - Palpable clunk – associated with peripheral meniscal detachment
  - Assess for endpoint sensation
  - Compare to opposite knee
- Anterior drawer test in external rotation
  - 80°–90° knee flexion
  - Foot in 15° external rotation
  - May have combined ACL tear
- Associated ligament laxity tests
  - ACL (Lachman, anterior drawer, pivot shift)

> PCL (posterior drawer, posterior sag)
> Posterolateral (reverse pivot shift, external rotation recurvatum, varus laxity at 0° and 30°, dial test, posterolateral drawer test)
> Hip and ankle exam (document ROM)
> Distal neurovascular exam

STUDIES
■ **Radiographs**
> Generally normal
> AP, lateral, notch, skyline (four views)
> Fracture, lateral capsular avulsion sign (Segond), Pelligrini-Stieda lesions, evidence of patellar dislocation
> Valgus stress X-ray in adolescents to detect physeal (growth plate) fracture
■ **MRI**
> Sensitive and specific for MCL and associated ligamentous, meniscal injury
> Note location of tear
> Meniscofemoral – usually off medial epicondyle
> Midsubstance
> Meniscotibial – peel-off of tibial attachment
■ **Exam under anesthesia and arthroscopy**
> Usually necessary only to fully assess complex ligament injuries when MRI not available or contraindicated/inconclusive/inconsistent with exam

DIFFERENTIAL DIAGNOSIS
■ **Medial joint line laxity**
> Retinacular tear
> Lateral compartment arthritis (pseudolaxity), bicruciate ligament tears
■ **Decreased ROM and medial joint line tenderness**
> Medial meniscal tear
> Degenerative joint disease (DJD)
■ **Adolescent**
> Physeal fracture
> Osteochondritis dissecans

TREATMENT
■ **Acute injury**
> Proper diagnosis crucial
> Verify status of other knee ligaments

➤ AP, lateral, and patellofemoral x-rays
➤ For combined ligament injuries, strongly consider MRI

■ **Treatment considerations**
  ➤ Partial vs. complete MCL injury
  ➤ Isolated vs. combined ligament injury
  ➤ Acute vs. chronic injury

■ **Treatment options**
  ➤ **Acute isolated injuries and combined ACL/MCL tears**
  • Ice and elevation (first 0–48 hrs post injury), cold compression device
  • Crutches (until painless weight-bearing and no limp)
  • Isometric quadriceps contractions (several times daily)
  • Knee immobilizer (until able to perform a straight-leg raise without a sag)
  • Advance ROM as tolerated, exercise bike (20–30 minutes daily) as tolerated
  • Acute grade I and II injuries – Progress activities as tolerated
  • Acute grade III tears – Continue on crutches (weight-bearing as tolerated) until valgus at 30° returns to normal
  • Jogging progressing to sprinting and cutting
  • Full noncontact activity once 100% ROM and speed have returned
  • Full contact once all noncontact drills completed at 100%
  • Most grade I return to full activity in 1–2 weeks
  • Grade II return in 2–4 weeks
  • Grade III MCL sprains – Most return at 5–7 weeks
  • Good results with nonoperative treatment for isolated MCL lesions

■ Operative indications
  ➤ **Combined MCL and other ligament injuries**
  • Treat ACL/MCL (acute) as isolated MCL initially, plan for staged ACL reconstruction at 5–6 weeks
  • Combination of other ligament injuries (PCL, ACL/PCL, posterolateral)
    • Primary repair (suture anchors or drill holes)
    • Augment with hamstrings for midsubstance tears
  ➤ **Reconstruction: chronic**
  • If in valgus alignment, consider distal femoral osteotomy first to correct alignment to neutral
  • Normal alignment (or postosteotomy) – Surgical reconstruction with hamstrings or allograft tissue

DISPOSITION
N/A

PROGNOSIS
■ **Nonoperative treatment**
  ➤ Nonoperative treatment of acute grade III isolated MCL lesion, >90% excellent long-term results
  ➤ Nonoperative treatment for acute grades I and II MCL sprains, >95% excellent results
  ➤ Follow grade III meniscotibial MCL tears closely postoperatively to document healing
  ➤ Chronic MCL laxity generally does poorly with cutting/twisting activities

CAVEATS AND PEARLS
■ MCL tears may be associated with "triad" of ACL and medial meniscal tears
■ Many MCL sprains are never seen by physician (underreporting of grade I sprains)
■ MCL sprain diagnosis should be evident by history and physical
■ If ACL and MCL both torn, consider nonoperative rx of MCL for 4–6 weeks; once motion regained, reassess MCL, augment or reconstruct if medial laxity present at time of ACL reconstruction
■ Most meniscofemoral-based MCL lesions heal
■ Meniscotibial-based MCL lesions need to be followed more closely for healing
■ In combined MCL (+ ACL +/– PCL) – Caveat reduced knee dislocation.
■ In acute combined injuries, always check neurovascular status

MEDIAL MENISCAL TEARS

THOMAS L. WICKIEWICZ, MD

HISTORY
■ Young patients with traumatic injury
  ➤ Rotation – compression
■ Common with chronic anterior cruciate ligament (ACL)-insufficient knees

> "Bucket" tears/medial meniscus secondary stabilizer to anterior displacement in absence of ACL

■ Patient complaints
  > Pain localized to medial joint line
  > Locking
  > Swelling
  > Buckling – rule out giving way due to ACL
■ Older patients – usually atraumatic or minimally traumatic onset
  > Degenerative tears
  > Complaints typically similar but true locking uncommon

PHYSICAL EXAM
■ Medial joint line tenderness to palpation
  > Accurate finding in chronic meniscal lesions – not specific finding in young patients with acute ligamentous injury
■ Effusions common
■ Positive meniscal tests – many "named" tests exists; essentially all provide compression/rotation through compartment of knee
■ "Locked" knee – knee will not reach full extension, flexion minimally affected
■ "Bounce" test
■ Rule out collateral ligament injury – bone bruise

STUDIES
■ Double-contrast arthrograms – accurate test for medial meniscus if technically well performed
■ MRI currently most appropriate test if confirmation of diagnosis needed; more important in older population
■ Rule out intraosseous issues, especially avascular necrosis (AVN)
■ Diagnostic arthroscopy – allows treatment as well

DIFFERENTIAL DIAGNOSIS
■ Meniscal tear
■ Ligament injury
■ Loose bodies
■ Osteochondritis dissecans
■ AVN
■ Chondral injury
■ Patella dislocation
■ Lyme (regional)
■ Transient osteoporosis medial femoral condyle

TREATMENT
- Repair vs. excision
- Decision making
  - ➤ Age of tear
  - ➤ Location/type (meniscal anatomy/vascularity)
  - ➤ Vascularity
    - Red-Red
    - Red-White
    - White-White
  - ➤ Age of patient
  - ➤ Occupation
  - ➤ Meniscal tissue quality
  - ➤ Associated ligamentous issues – instability
- Goals
  - ➤ Preserve meniscal function vs. predictability of repair
- Excision – Arthroscopic
  - ➤ Portal selection
  - ➤ Adequate visualization
  - ➤ Technique (chondral damage)
  - ➤ Meniscal contour
- Repair
  - ➤ Open – peripheral tears
  - ➤ Arthroscopic
    - Outside-in
    - Inside-out
    - All inside

DISPOSITION
N/A

PROGNOSIS
- Repair predictability
  - ➤ Vascular zone > red-white > white-white
    - Overall clinical success 60–80%
    - Often higher with associated ligament surgery
  - ➤ Documented complete healing rates only about 50%
  - ➤ Partial healing accounts for other 10–30%
- Complications
  - ➤ Neurovascular injury – popliteal artery, nerve (saphenous, peroneal)
  - ➤ Failure of repair

- Return to play
  - Excision – when strength, motion, proprioception normal; allow 2–4 weeks
  - Repair – 4 months for torsional/contact sports

CAVEATS AND PEARLS
- Meniscal transplantation
  - Not a treatment for established arthritis
  - Viable technique if joint architecture not distorted (Fairbank's changes)
  - Preoperative MRI, especially coronal view
  - If compartment "squared off," meniscal transplant will extrude
  - If appropriate joint, success can approach 75%
  - Long-term efficacy: prevention or retarding progression of osteoarthritis still unproven
- Postmenisectomy patient
  - Persistent pain, often of different nature than preop
  - Beware of AVN; think MRI early to document in postop patients doing poorly

---

MERALGIA PARESTHETICA

WILLIAM E. GARRETT, JR., MD, PhD

HISTORY
- Numbness over lateral thigh
- Pain often absent
- Usually insidious onset
- Direct trauma to anterior superior iliac spine area (ASIS) may be cause of acute injury
- Chronic cases possibly due to belts or compression around waist
- May occur after surgery such as iliac crest bone graft with anterior incision
- Occasional history of prolonged ice use for groin injury

PHYSICAL EXAM
- Numbness isolated to proximal lateral thigh
- Numbness in distribution of lateral femoral cutaneous nerve (LFCN) of thigh
- Tenderness possible slightly inferior and medial to ASIS
- Percussion of tender area causes dysesthesias in area of numbness
- Surgical incision over anterior iliac crest near ASIS

STUDIES
- Usually not needed
- Diagnostic block of LFCN produces complete anesthesia and relief of any pain in area of numbness

DIFFERENTIAL DIAGNOSIS
- Hypesthesia due to CNS or peripheral nerve disease
  - ➤ Not usually isolated problem

TREATMENT
- Often none needed and improves with time
- Discontinue compressive clothing or equipment below ASIS
- Occasional steroid injection at point of injury
- Rarely neurolysis necessary

DISPOSITION
N/A

PROGNOSIS
- Excellent for functional recovery

CAVEATS AND PEARLS
- History and exam are characteristic.
- Look for clothing or equipment pressing ASIS.

METACARPAL FRACTURES

JOHN FERNANDEZ, MD

HISTORY
- Account for one third of hand/wrist fractures
- Symptoms
  - ➤ Pain at fracture site
  - ➤ Dorsal swelling
  - ➤ Deformity of hand/finger
- Mechanism
  - ➤ Direct
    - Impact injury metacarpal head/shaft
  - ➤ Indirect
    - Avulsion/rotation of digit
    - Flexion/extension bending
- Common in football, basketball

PHYSICAL EXAM
- Assess for associated injuries
  - Tendon ruptures/avulsions
  - Metacarpal joint (MPJ)/carpometacarpal joint (CMCJ) dislocations
  - Carpal fractures/dislocations
- Dorsal swelling
- Tenderness to palpation
- Crepitance with palpation/motion
- Deformity
- Malrotation of digit with flexion
- Overlap of fingers
- 5° of rotation-1.5-cm overlap
- Dorsal prominence/angulation
- Loss of metacarpal height/shortening
- Loss in range of motion
  - Extension loss at MPJ/proximal interphalangeal joint (PIPJ)
  - 2-mm shortening = 7° ext loss
- Extrinsic tightness
  - Adhesions of extensor tendons
  - Less PIPJ flexion with MPJ flexion
- Intrinsic tightness
  - Contracture of intrinsic muscles
  - Less PIPJ flexion with MPJ extension
- Late findings
  - Deformity
  - Loss of motion
  - Loss of grip strength

STUDIES
- Radiographs
  - AP/lateral/oblique of hand
  - Index finger/middle finger: 30° pronated lateral
  - Ring finger/small finger: 30° supinated lateral
- Points to assess
  - Shortening/loss of height
  - Angulation
  - Translation

DIFFERENTIAL DIAGNOSIS
- Contusion/soft tissue avulsion
- MPJ/CMCJ dislocation

TREATMENT
- Metacarpal fracture types
  - Spiral
    - Usually indirect rotational injury
    - Tend to rotate
  - Oblique
    - Usually impact injury
    - Blow to metacarpal head
    - Tend to shorten and rotate
  - Transverse
    - Usually impact injury
    - Dorsum of metacarpal
    - Tend to translate and angulate
  - Comminution
    - Proportional to energy of injury
    - Proportional to instability of fracture
  - Digits involved
    - Fracture "stabilized" by surrounding tissues
    - Intermetacarpal ligaments
    - Intrinsic muscles
    - Border metacarpals more likely to displace
      - Less soft tissue support
      - Thumb, index, and small metacarpal
    - Ring/small fingers
      - Compensatory CMCJ ROM
      - Increased deformity allowed
    - Index/middle fingers
      - Compensatory CMCJ ROM
      - Decreased deformity allowed
  - Fracture level
    - Shaft vs. neck vs. base
    - Neck fracture
      - Allows for greater angular deformity
      - Compensation through MPJ ROM
- Acute
  - Splint in "intrinsic plus" position
  - Wrist 20° extension
  - MPJ 70° flexion
  - IPJ full extension
  - Include adjacent uninjured digits
  - Strict elevation to limit swelling

➤ Treatment-dependent factors
  - Fracture type
  - Stability of reduction
  - Residual alignment
■ Criteria for acceptable alignment
  ➤ Index/middle finger
    - Angulation: <10°
    - Shortening: <3 mm
    - Rotation: none
  ➤ Ring/small finger
    - Angulation
    - Small finger: <30°
    - Ring finger: <20°
    - Shortening: <3 mm
    - Rotation: none
■ Nonoperative treatment
  ➤ Reduction
    - Anesthetic block
    - Wrist level
    - Fracture level (hematoma block)
    - "Three-point bending" technique
      - Hold hand/wrist
      - Apply pressure to metacarpal head
      - Use thumbs
      - Push dorsally from palm
      - Apply pressure to fracture apex dorsally
      - Use fingers
  ➤ Immobilize in "intrinsic plus" position
  ➤ Cast or splint
    - Control rotation
    - "Buddy strap"
    - Include adjacent uninjured digit
    - Shortening very poorly controlled
    - Recheck reduction every week, 3 weeks
    - After 3 weeks, recheck every 2–3 weeks
    - After first 3 weeks
      - Change splint/cast
      - Consider placing in orthoplast splint
      - Allow interval ROM
      - Cut down splint
      - Allow PIPJ ROM

- ➤ Fracture requires 6–8 weeks to heal
  - Radiographic healing may lag
  - Clinical healing occurs sooner
  - If no pain to palpation/ROM
  - Allow ROM/early light use
  - Allow normal use after radiographs healed
- Operative treatment
  - ➤ Indications
    - Unable to achieve acceptable reduction
    - Unable to maintain acceptable reduction
    - Unable to extend digit fully
    - Significant swelling
    - Open injuries
    - Associated injuries
  - ➤ Several options depending on fracture type
    - Percutaneous pinning
    - Interfragmentary screws
    - Dorsal plating
    - Tension/cerclage wiring
      - Allows for early ROM
  - ➤ Percutaneous pinning
    - Transverse/short oblique fractures
    - Intramedullary pin
    - 0.062/0.045 K-wire
    - Place through metacarpal head
    - Pull out proximal near wrist
    - Leave MPJ free to allow ROM
  - ➤ Cross-pinning
    - 0.045 K-wires
    - 1 pin proximal/2 pins distal to fracture
    - Pin to adjacent "intact" metacarpal
  - ➤ Dorsal plating
    - Transverse/short oblique fractures
    - Comminuted fractures
    - AO modular hand set
      - 2.7/2.5-mm plates
      - AO small fragment set
      - Quarter tubular plates
      - Interfragmentary screws
  - ➤ Long oblique/spiral fracture
    - Fracture 2× longer than bone diameter

- AO modular hand set
  - 2.7/2.0-mm screws
  - Use at least 2 screws
  - Place perpendicular to axis
- ➤ Tension/cerclage wiring
  - Transverse/short oblique fractures
  - Not comminuted
  - 0.045/0.035 K-wires/24-gauge wire
- ➤ Postoperative management
  - Splint 1 week
  - Begin therapy in 1 week
  - Edema modalities
  - Scar massage
  - Protected ROM
  - Removable orthoplast splint
- ■ Late
- ➤ Malunion
- ➤ Angular/rotational deformity
  - Osteotomy with ORIF
- ➤ Nonunion
  - Revision ORIF with bone grafting
- ➤ Loss of motion
  - MPJ release
  - Extensor tendon tenolysis

DISPOSITION
N/A

PROGNOSIS
- ■ Nonoperative treatment
  - ➤ 0–90% good/excellent result
  - ➤ Return to play immediately
    - Padded splint/cast
- ■ Complications
  - ➤ Loss of MPJ ROM
  - ➤ Loss of extension
  - ➤ Malunion/nonunion
  - ➤ Deformity
- ■ Operative treatment
  - ➤ Good results overall/25% complications

- ➤ Risks
  - Outweighed by risk of malunion
  - Infection
  - Tendon adhesions
  - Joint stiffness
- ➤ Return to play immediately
  - Padded cast/splint
- ■ Late repair/reconstruction
  - ➤ Fair/poor result
  - ➤ Complications
  - ➤ Residual deformity
  - ➤ MPJ/PIPJ stiffness

CAVEATS AND PEARLS
- ■ Begin ROM as soon as possible.
- ■ Refer to occupational therapist.
- ■ Removable orthoplast splint
- ■ Allow PIPJ ROM at very least.
- ■ Try to use pins/screws when possible.
- ■ Limit use of plates
  - ➤ More stripping necessary
  - ➤ Increased adhesions/loss of ROM
- ■ Increase threshold for surgery if extensor lag in finger.
- ■ Increase threshold for surgery if a lot of swelling.
- ■ Always inform patient of residual deformity even with good retained function.
  - ➤ Prominent dorsal bone
  - ➤ Loss of metacarpal head profile with fist
  - ➤ Mild rotational deformity

METATARSAL STRESS FRACTURES

MAYO A. NOERDLINGER, MD
BERNARD R. BACH, JR., MD

HISTORY
- ■ Recent change in:
  - ➤ Activity
  - ➤ Increased interval/frequency of exercise
  - ➤ Increased distance

➤ Shoe ware
➤ Prodromal aching
➤ Activity-related pain
➤ A twisting injury occurs that completes the fracture, causing severe pain
➤ Oligomenorrhea and amenorrhea

PHYSICAL EXAM

■ Most common in metaphysis and diaphysis of second and third metatarsal
■ Mild swelling
■ Exquisite point tenderness at fracture
■ Diffuse pain around fracture caused by tendinitis, bursitis

STUDIES

■ Plain radiographs often negative:
  ➤ Weight-bearing AP, lateral, and oblique views of the foot
  ➤ Delayed bone reaction (4–6 weeks)
  ➤ Subtle half-break in the cortex on one of the views
■ Technetium bone scanning
  ➤ With equivocal radiographs
  ➤ Not specific
  ➤ Also takes several days for the bone scan to become positive
■ CT scan
  ➤ Accurate for diagnosis of osseous lesions
■ MRI
  ➤ Evaluates soft tissue lesions
  ➤ Can reveal damage to articular cartilage or underlying bone

DIFFERENTIAL DIAGNOSIS

■ Interdigital neuroma
■ Metatarsalgia
■ Hallux rigidus
■ Hallux valgus
■ Turf toe
■ Sesamoidal pathology

TREATMENT

■ Stress fractures of the lesser metatarsals require rest
  ➤ Immobilization not necessarily needed
  ➤ Advance weight-bearing in 4–6 weeks when callus formed

- Return to activity that caused the injury cautiously
- Base-of-second-metatarsal stress fractures need prolonged immobilization
  - Electrical stimulation or ultrasound as adjunct

DISPOSITION

N/A

PROGNOSIS

- Excellent healing potential in diaphysis and metaphysis of lesser metatarsals
- Stress fractures of first and second metatarsals may require prolonged immobilization
- Electrical stimulation or ultrasound adjuncts

CAVEATS AND PEARLS

- "March fracture" is metatarsal stress fracture
  - Called because of its occurrence in military personnel
- Dancers prone to base-of-second-metatarsal stress fracture
  - Short first metatarsal and hypermobile first ray may predispose to this injury
- Suspect stress fracture in athlete who has recently had a change in training habits
- In female with stress fracture, suspect underlying oligomenorrhea/amenorrhea/eating disorders

MULTIDIRECTIONAL INSTABILITY

BRIAN J. COLE, MD
ROBERT A. SELLARDS, MD
REVISED BY CHARLES NOFSINGER, MD

HISTORY

- Instability pattern anterior and/or posterior with inferior component
- Pathology: global capsular laxity with or without a rotator interval lesion
- Mechanism
  - Inherent or congenital ligamentous laxity
  - Major trauma
  - Repetitive microtrauma

- Commonly atraumatic with bilateral laxity and generalized ligamentous laxity
- Seen in throwers, gymnasts, swimmers

PHYSICAL EXAM
- Bidirectional or greater instability
- Inferior instability: pain with carrying objects at the side, occasional numbness
- Posterior instability: arm flexed, internally rotated, adducted
- Posterior stress test
- Anterior instability: arm abducted, externally rotated
- Anterior stress test
- Relocation test
- Ligamentous laxity
  - Elbow and knee hyperextension
  - Thumb to forearm and hyperextensile metacarpophalangeal joints
- Sulcus sign
  - Hallmark of multidirectional instability
  - Downward traction of neutrally positioned arm; sulcus may remain with external rotation
- Examine contralateral shoulder for comparison
- Distinguish from voluntary dislocators
- Serial visits
- Rule out secondary gain

STUDIES
- Radiographs
  - Trauma series: true AP, scapular "Y" and axillary views
  - Usually normal
  - Look for head/glenoid defects
- MRI arthrogram
  - Evaluates capsular volume
  - Detects associated pathology
- Exam under anesthesia
  - Determine principal direction of instability
  - Grading (based on translation of humeral head)
    - 0: normal
    - 1: to glenoid rim
    - 2: over glenoid rim with spontaneous reduction
    - 3: locking over glenoid rim

- Abnormal: anterior translation of grade 2 or greater on affected side
- Abnormal: posterior translation of grade 3
- Normal: bilateral posterior translation of grade 2 or less
➢ Define secondary directions of instability
➢ Rotator interval: sulcus sign with inferior traction (space increases between lateral acromion and top of humeral head) in adduction that persists in external rotation
➢ Test in various arm positions

DIFFERENTIAL DIAGNOSIS
- Anterior instability
- Posterior instability

TREATMENT
- Nonoperative treatment
  ➢ Successful in majority of individuals (>80%)
  ➢ Deltoid, rotator cuff, scapular stabilizer strengthening
- Surgical indications
  ➢ Pain and disability
  ➢ Athlete who is unable to compete
- Surgery technique: open
  ➢ Determine principal direction of instability (exam under anesthesia) to determine corresponding surgical approach
  ➢ Anterior: laterally based selective capsular shift
  ➢ Posterior: if cannot stabilize through anterior approach
  ➢ Routine rotator interval closure
  ➢ May need combined approach
- Surgical technique: arthroscopic
  ➢ Lateral decubitus with traction for best exposure
  ➢ Suture plication of redundant tissue
  ➢ Thermal capsulorrhaphy is contraindicated
- Rehabilitation
  ➢ Weeks 0–6: orthosis or sling (favor neutral rotation, slight abduction)
  ➢ Weeks 0–6: gentle protected range of motion exercises
  ➢ Weeks 6+: begin range of motion out of brace
  ➢ Weeks 8–12: active range of motion as tolerated
  ➢ Months 6–9: sports

DISPOSITION
N/A

PROGNOSIS

- No long-term results on arthroscopic treatment
- Success with open procedures approximates 75% good and excellent
- Complications
  - Failure to diagnose instability
  - Voluntary instability with psychological component
  - Overly aggressive postoperative rehabilitation
  - Inappropriate patient selection
  - Axillary nerve damage
  - Thermal-associated capsular destruction

CAVEATS AND PEARLS

- Nonoperative treatment usually successful
- Serial examinations to arrive at correct diagnosis
- Nonaggressive postoperative rehabilitation

MYOSITIS OSSIFICANS

DAVID C. NEUSCHWANDER, MD

HISTORY

- Blunt trauma to anterior thigh, often associated with early return to play
- Often associated with more significant injuries (moderate and severe quadriceps contusions)

PHYSICAL EXAM

- Localized pain, exquisite tenderness and swelling, associated with loss of knee flexion
- May be associated with ipsilateral knee effusion
- Suspected if firm mass develops at 3–4 weeks at site of initial injury

STUDIES

- Plain x-rays are initially normal, but will show flocculated densities in soft tissues and underlying periosteal bone reaction at 3–4 weeks.
- Bony mass will stabilize and mature over approximately 6 months.
- Bone mass may be connected to femur by stalk, a broad-based connection, or no connection at all.
- Ultrasonography may demonstrate soft tissue changes of myositis prior to x-ray appearance.
- Technetium bone scan useful to monitor maturation of lesion

DIFFERENTIAL DIAGNOSIS

■ Periosteal osteosarcoma, parosteal sarcoma, and synovial sarcoma
■ Also osteochondroma, posttraumatic periostitis, and osteomyelitis
■ Combination of clinical history and x-rays will usually allow differentiation of myositis from above entities.
■ History of trauma, course of x-ray stabilization at 3–4 months, location, and a negative alk phos all help to differentiate from above entities.
■ CT scan used to determine size, density, and anatomic localization.

TREATMENT

■ Same treatment as quadriceps contusion
■ Centers around protection of involved area to avoid additional injury and minimize stiffness of involved muscles
■ Once myositis mature, most patients will be asymptomatic except for a few in whom surgical excision is performed when the lesion is mature.
■ En bloc excision of myositis if surgery undertaken
■ Hemostasis and atraumatic dissection and excision are necessary for successful surgical outcome.

DISPOSITION
N/A

PROGNOSIS

■ Return to play when pain-free and have at least 120° knee flexion (with hip extended) and do well with functional testing
■ Risk factors for development of myositis after quadriceps contusion include knee motion <120°, football injury, previous quad injury, delay in diagnosis >3 days, and ipsilateral knee effusion.

CAVEATS AND PEARLS

■ Can attempt to avoid by not returning to play prior to complete rehabilitation
■ Myositis has low morbidity and reflects a more severe injury, but does not require a specific change in treatment from a quadriceps contusion.
■ Does not alter the ultimate functional result as compared to quadriceps contusion
■ Surgical management prior to maturation of myositis can adversely affect result

- Intramuscular hematoma and repeated injuries appear to predispose to the formation of heterotopic bone.
- Myositis is more common in patients with moderate or severe injuries, but it does not correlate with the duration of disability.

NAILBED INJURIES

JAMES B. BENNETT, MD

HISTORY
- Sports or work fingertip/distal phalanx injury
- Most common hand injury
- Crushing or tearing injury
- Bleeding with subungual hematoma
- Common sports hand injury with trauma such as soccer, football, rugby, volleyball
- May have associated fracture/open vs. closed
- May have an associated tendon injury

PHYSICAL EXAM
- Nail anatomy
  - Nailplate or nail proper
  - Eponychium and proximal fold/paronychium and lateral fold
  - Extensor tendon insertion
  - Flexor tendon insertion
  - Nailplate intact with subungual hematoma
  - Nail avulsion with nailbed laceration
  - Fracture distal phalanx
  - Extensor tendon disruption
  - Flexor tendon disruption
  - Pulp of fingertip laceration
  - Flexion/extension against resistance for tendon integrity
  - Disrupted or lacerated nailbed or nailplate

STUDIES
- Radiographs
  - AP and lateral x-ray of the distal interphalangeal joint and distal phalanx
  - Flexion and extensor tendon testing
  - No CT or MRI required

DIFFERENTIAL DIAGNOSIS
- Finger pulp injury
- Tuft fracture
- Flexor/extensor tendon injury
- Infection

TREATMENT
- **Acute**
  - Evacuation of subungual hematoma
  - Heated paperclip
  - Disposable cautery Accu-temp, Concept
  - Nailbed repair with 6–0 or 7–0 absorbable suture
  - Loupe magnification
  - Use of removed nail reinserted as a stent
  - Artificial nail stent ("Inro" nail)
  - Nail matrix graft if nail matrix defect using like tissue – "toenail bed graft"
  - Remove entrapped nailbed at fracture site
  - Extensor tendon repair if indicated/K-pin
  - Flexor tendon repair if indicated
  - Fracture stabilization if indicated/K-pin
  - Fingertip reconstruction for soft tissue loss as indicated
- **Chronic**
  - Split nail deformity
  - Curved nail deformity
  - Infection/bacterial vs. fungus
  - Nail removal, scar removal and repair
  - Like tissue nailplate graft (toenail plate)
  - Wraparound toe free tissue transfer
  - Distal interphalangeal fusion for chronic extensor tendon or flexor tendon injury
  - Bone graft fracture nonunions or beak nail deformity

DISPOSITION
- Return to function 2–4 weeks non-operative, 6–8 weeks operative

PROGNOSIS
- Four to six months nail regrowth for healing
- Old nail is pushed off by new nail
- Some deformity is expected of the nail
- Nail deformity and shortening with amputation

- Return to sports activities: stable, noninfected with protective cover 7–10 days if nailbed repair
- Immediate return to sports if intact nail plate

Complications
- Nail deformity
- Nail loss
- Infection
- Fracture nonunion
- Tendon rupture

CAVEATS AND PEARLS
- Nail removed, repair nailbed, replacement of nail as stent
- Nail split-thickness vs. full-thickness graft from local nailbed tissue (like tissue finger or toenail)
- Mobilization remaining nail as a rotation flap
- Split-thickness and full-thickness toenail graft
- Artificial nail stent – "Inro nail"
- May be performed under digital block in the emergency room
- Loupe magnification
- Stack finger splint protection
- Absorbable suture repair nailbed

NAVICULAR STRESS FRACTURES

MAYO A. NOERDLINGER, MD
BERNARD R. BACH, JR., MD

HISTORY
- Repetitive stress in running or jumping athletes
  ➤ Athlete increases intensity of training too quickly
- Dorsomedial and medial arch pain
- Ill-defined pain
- Cramping

PHYSICAL EXAM
- Tender over dorsal medial navicular and medial longitudinal arch
- Swelling rare

STUDIES
- Obtain weight-bearing AP, lateral, and oblique views
  ➤ Location usually within central third of navicular

> Fractures sagittally oriented
> May initiate on dorsal surface
> Plain films often inconclusive
■ Establish diagnosis with bone scan or CT scan
> CT scan delineates severity and completeness of fracture line

DIFFERENTIAL DIAGNOSIS
■ Anterior tibial tendinitis
■ Acute navicular fracture
> Results from high-energy injury

TREATMENT
■ Early incomplete navicular stress fractures
> Short-leg nonweight-bearing cast for 6 weeks
> Gradual resumption of activity over weeks 7–12
■ Complete fractures or failed conservative treatment
> ORIF

DISPOSITION
N/A

PROGNOSIS
■ Pain resolves quickly with rest
■ Chance of nonunion and post-traumatic arthritis without prompt treatment
■ Chronic cases with separated fragments develop secondary changes
> Cystic degeneration
> Partial avascular necrosis of lateral fragment
> Sclerosis in margins of fracture
■ Secondary arthritis of talonavicular joint

CAVEATS AND PEARLS
■ The navicular is the keystone of the medial arch of the foot
■ Proximally, its concave surface articulates with the talus; the talonavicular joint is the key for pronation and supination
■ Distally, navicular articulates with all three cuneiforms
■ The posterior tibial tendon is the only muscle attaching to the navicular; inserts on inferomedial tuberosity
■ Strong calcaneonavicular (Spring) ligament attaches to inferior navicular

OLECRANON BURSITIS

CHRISTOPHER D. HAMILTON, MD
REVISED BY CHARLES NOFSINGER, MD

HISTORY

- Causes
  - Direct trauma – trauma to olecranon tip (i.e., falling)
    - Common in football
    - Associated with artificial turf
    - Common in ice hockey due to elbowing and checking
  - Traumatic overuse
    - Repetitive trauma
    - Leaning on elbows
  - Infectious or septic
    - May have local trauma with secondary infection
    - May coexist with other types of bursitis
  - Rheumatoid arthritis
  - Crystalline disease
    - Gout may predispose to infectious bursitis
    - Calcium phosphate deposition disease
- Symptoms and presentation
  - General symptoms
    - Swelling in olecranon bursa
    - Often acute change in size of bursa
    - Quite often painless, but annoying
  - Symptoms associated with infection, rheumatoid arthritis, or crystalline disease
    - Redness over olecranon
    - Swelling into forearm
    - May have fever or malaise
    - Elbow stiffness
    - Drainage from bursa

PHYSICAL EXAM

- Localized swelling over tip of olecranon
- Look for signs of external trauma
  - Folliculitis
  - Ecchymosis
  - Abrasions with surrounding cellulitis

- Especially important early
- Ice hockey players due to elbow pads
- Evaluate for signs of infection
  - Warmth
  - Pain more common in septic bursitis
  - Erythema
  - Cellulitis
  - Swelling
- Evaluate elbow range of motion
  - Loss of motion more common in infectious or rheumatoid causes
    - Pain limiting motion
    - Connection of bursa with joint in rheumatoid patients
- Compare contralateral elbow
  - Loss of motion due to arthritis
  - Presence of bony spurs
  - Prominent olecranon tip
  - Presence of thickened bursa
  - Gouty tophi or rheumatoid nodules

STUDIES

- Radiographs – helpful to exclude fractures in trauma
  - Soft tissue swelling
  - Chondrocalcinosis
  - Olecranon spur associated with traumatic bursitis
- Little role for other adjunctive studies
- Blood work – not overly helpful for infection unless late
- Aspiration and fluid studies helpful in causation and treatment
  - Gram stain
  - Cultures
  - Analysis of crystals from aspiration

DIFFERENTIAL DIAGNOSIS

- Olecranon bursitis – diagnosis usually easy and apparent
- Chondrocalcinosis involving bursa
- Infection
- Trauma and fractures to olecranon or radial head

TREATMENT

- Acute noninfectious bursitis
  - Many cases resolve spontaneously

- ➤ Local pads to prevent trauma
- ➤ Decrease use; sling may help
- ➤ Compressive wraps
  - Neoprene elbow sleeve
  - Ace wraps
- ➤ Aspiration to rule out infection if etiology in doubt, if symptoms significant, or if prolonged
- ➤ Corticosteroid injection after aspiration
  - More effective resolution
  - May unmask infection
- ➤ Presumptive antibiotics for *Staphylococcus aureus*
- ■ Acute septic bursitis
  - ➤ Aspiration and antibiotics
    - Aspiration for cell count, crystals, Gram stain, cultures
    - Oral antibiotics for mild cases
    - Cover for *S. aureus*
    - IV antibiotics for severe or nonresponsive cases
    - Generally need 10 days to 2 weeks treatment
  - ➤ Surgical drainage
- ■ Chronic olecranon bursitis
  - ➤ Serial aspiration
  - ➤ Treat for occult infection
  - ➤ Injection of corticosteroids into bursa
- ■ Rheumatoid olecranon bursitis
  - ➤ Bursa can communicate with elbow joint
  - ➤ Drainage can reflect infected joint
  - ➤ More drainage than usual
  - ➤ Need to treat aggressively
  - ➤ Recurrence rate very high
  - ➤ Differentiate from rheumatoid nodules where ulceration common, recurrence common after excision
- ■ Indications for surgical drainage
  - ➤ Failed aspiration and antibiotic treatment
  - ➤ Longstanding infections, either recurrent or resistant
  - ➤ Previous infection, drainage, or surgery
  - ➤ Desire for removal of bursa
- ■ Surgical treatment
  - ➤ Attempt to clear up severe infection
    - Antibiotics
    - Local decompression and drainage
  - ➤ Longitudinal incision in skin

➢ Excise all bursal tissue, which may extend proximally or distally
  • Skin can be thin – exercise care with dissection
➢ Immobilization at 45° flexion with compression for 7–10 days
  • If rheumatoid, consider longer immobilization
  • Consider drain use in rheumatoid patients, large bursae
  • Secondary aspiration of dead space occasionally necessary
■ Complications of surgical treatment
  ➢ Wound problems
  ➢ Infection
  ➢ Dehiscence
  ➢ Recurrence approximately 10%

DISPOSITION
N/A

PROGNOSIS
■ Many resolve spontaneously with local care and padding
■ If untreated, there are few long-term problems with chronic bursitis other than annoyance
■ Infection should be aggressively treated
■ Overall prognosis is excellent with symptomatic treatment of chronic bursitis and treatment of infection
■ Most surgical cases do well

CAVEATS AND PEARLS
■ In chronic cases, beware of occult infection and consider addition of oral antibiotics early on
■ *S. aureus* is isolated organism in >90%
■ Beware of a laceration over the bursa in ice hockey players, as infection rate is extremely high; cover with antibiotics
■ Careful surgical technique is critical due to poor blood supply of skin

OSGOOD-SCHLATTER DISEASE

JACK ANDRISH, MD
JAMES S. WILLIAMS, MD
REVISED BY CHARLES NOFSINGER, MD

HISTORY
■ Age

> Acute: skeletally immature girls 11–13, boys 12–15
> Chronic: skeletally mature; usually >18
- Incidence as high as 20% in adolescent athletes, 5% in nonathletic adolescents
  > Male:female 3:1
- Bilateral in 20-30%
- Anterior knee pain, aggravated by running and jumping
- Insidious onset, but usually associated with running sport
- Etiology
  > Pathoanatomy described as an apophysitis; biopsy study consistent with tendinitis and heterotopic ossification
  > Result of submaximal repetitive tensile stress at a time of rapid growth that results in minor avulsions and attempts at repair

PHYSICAL EXAM
- Acute
  > Tender bump ± soft tissue swelling corresponding to tibial tuberosity
  > Pain corresponds to location of tibial tuberosity
  > Tight hamstrings and tight quadriceps
- Chronic
  > Increased bony prominence of tibial tuberosity
  > Tender distal patellar tendon

STUDIES
- Plain radiographs
  > Skeletally immature
    - Lateral view – Fragmentation of tibial tuberosity apophysis (normal variant, not diagnostic of Osgood-Schlatter disease)
  > Skeletally mature
    - Lateral view – Ossicle within distal patellar tendon adjacent to tibial tuberosity (heterotopic ossifications)
  > Merchant view: Ossicle within distal patellar tendon gives the misleading appearance of a loose body

DIFFERENTIAL DIAGNOSIS
- Patellofemoral stress syndrome
- Internal derangement – plica syndrome, meniscus tear, osteochondritis dissecans
- Sinding-Larsen syndrome
- Iliotibial band syndrome
- Tibial tuberosity fracture

- Stress fracture
- Tumor

TREATMENT
- Acute
  - ➤ Follows the principles of extensor mechanism overload proposed by Henning
  - ➤ Stretching program for quadriceps, hamstrings, and heel cords
  - ➤ Hamstring strengthening
  - ➤ Cryotherapy
  - ➤ Neoprene counterforce brace vs. knee pad
  - ➤ Activity as tolerated; no need for immobilization
  - ➤ Consider NSAIDs
- Chronic
  - ➤ Same as for acute
  - ➤ NSAIDs
  - ➤ Surgical excision of patellar tendon ossicle

DISPOSITION
N/A

PROGNOSIS
- Excellent

CAVEATS AND PEARLS
- Perhaps most important function is to reassure family that the condition is self-limited, but may take up to 12–18 months to resolve.
- Benign process
- Focus on hamstring and quad flexibility.
- The bump will probably remain.
- Reported small but increased incidence of acute tuberosity physeal fracture in association

---

OSTEOCHONDRITIS DISSECANS (OCD) OF THE KNEE

JACK ANDRISH, MD

HISTORY

Definition
- A focal lesion of subchondral bone and articular cartilage that emulates avascular necrosis and may lead to osteochondral separation

Demographics

■ Usually presents in preteen or teenage years but can present later in life
■ Male:female incidence 3:1

Etiology

■ Most likely from trauma
  ➤ Repetitive microtrauma
  ➤ Macro-osteochondral fracture (but can also be the result of ischemic, genetic, or endocrine etiologies)
  ➤ Macro-(osteo)chondral fracture in the skeletally immature
■ Other considerations include
  ➤ Avascular necrosis
  ➤ Genetic disorder
  ➤ Endocrine abnormalities

History

■ Nonspecific knee pain, swelling, and stiffness that worsen with activity
■ Grinding, catching, or locking associated with loose or detached lesions
■ Bilaterally 30–40% in younger patients, 5% in older patients

PHYSICAL EXAM

■ Knee pain poorly localized, but tenderness often corresponds to the side of the lesion
■ Decreased ROM, often due to pain in extension and loss of flexion due to joint effusion
■ Atrophy and quadriceps weakness are later findings
■ Antalgic gait with external rotation of lower leg
■ Positive Wilson's sign for medial femoral condyle (MFC) lesions (knee flexed at 90° followed by internal rotation of the tibia and passive knee extension: pain at 30° [tibial spine abuts against MFC]; pain subsides with tibial external rotation)

STUDIES

■ Radiographs
  ➤ Get both knees for comparison
  ➤ AP best for MFC lesions, helpful for lateral femoral condyle (LFC), may help with patellar lesions
  ➤ Tunnel best for MFC lesions and for LFC

> Lateral best for LFC and MFC, helpful for femoral trochlea and patella
> Sunrise best for patella and trochlea
- MRI
  > Gives precise size of fragment
  > Can be used to stage the lesion and follow progression of healing
  > Increased signal on T2 behind the fragment is consistent with synovial fluid and instability of the fragment
- Arthroscopy
  > Ability to diagnose, stage, and treat OCD
  > Look for focal swelling of articular cartilage
  > Look for depression, blue-grayish color, fissuring, or cracking associated with edge of lesion
  > Guhl classification
    - Intact lesion
    - Early separation
    - Partially detached lesion
    - Crater ± loose body
- Miscellaneous studies
  > Bone scan for staging and prognosis
  > Arthrogram, tomograms, and CT imaging replaced by MRI technology

DIFFERENTIAL DIAGNOSIS
- Articular cartilage injury, acute or chronic
- Patellofemoral stress syndrome
- Plica
- Hoffa's disease
- Tendinitis (patellar tendon/quadriceps tendon)
- Iliotibial band syndrome
- Meniscus tear
- Ligamentous instability
- The deconditioned knee

TREATMENT
- Varies according to age of presentation, fragment size, fragment location, and fragment stability
- Nonoperative
  > Nonweight-bearing with crutches and optional use of knee immobilizer, with daily periods of ROM out of the immobilizer, for 6 weeks followed by 6 weeks or more of modified activity until radiographic and clinical evidence of healing

- Operative treatment options
  - ➤ Drilling to promote vascular ingrowth and healing (same rehabilitation as nonoperative regimen)
  - ➤ Excision
  - ➤ Internal fixation of in situ lesion
  - ➤ Reduction and internal fixation of displaced lesion
  - ➤ Bone grafting, antegrade vs. retrograde
  - ➤ OATS
  - ➤ Chondroplasty vs. osteochondral transplantation vs. autogenous chondrocyte transplantation
  - ➤ Osteotomy for realignment
- Fixation: may be open or arthroscopically assisted
  - ➤ Metallic: Headless compression screws (ACUTRAK and Herbert screws), cannulated AO screws (to be removed at 6–12 weeks)
  - ➤ Bioabsorbable: pins, screws (rehabilitation same as nonoperative)
- Open techniques
  - ➤ Osteoarticular allograft or autograft (rehabilitation same as nonoperative, return to sports at 6 months)
  - ➤ Autologous chondrocyte implantation (rehabilitation same as nonoperative, return to sports at 6–12 months)

DISPOSITION
N/A

PROGNOSIS
- Nonsurgical treatment
  - ➤ Works best for immature patients with stable lesions: >90% success rate
- Surgical treatment
  - ➤ Drilling ± compression (screw fixation) for young patients who fail conservative treatment
  - ➤ Fixation ± bone grafting for loose or unstable lesions
  - ➤ Allo/autografting/autologous chondrocyte implantation for larger lesions, LFC lesions, fragmented lesions, ± osteotomy or realignment procedure to unload lesion
  - ➤ Results vary according to age at presentation, fragment size, and location

CAVEATS AND PEARLS
- Poor prognosis
  - ➤ LFC lesions
  - ➤ Older age at presentation

> Fragmented lesions
> Large lesion in weight-bearing areas
> Unstable lesions
- Good prognosis
  > Younger age at presentation
  > Lesions not involving major load-bearing surfaces
  > Stable lesions
- Evaluation of the knee for pain should always include an evaluation of the hip.

OSTEOCHONDRITIS DISSECANS (OCD) OF THE PATELLA

MATTHEW SHAPIRO, MD

HISTORY
- Knee most common site for OCD
- Occurs rarely in patella
- Etiology is traumatic or vascular or combination
- May be associated with patellar subluxation
- Males affected more commonly than females
- Peak occurrence second decade of life
- May present with anterior knee pain, swelling, mechanical symptoms, or instability
- Bilateral 20%

PHYSICAL EXAM
- Retropatellar crepitation
- Effusion
- Patellar irritability

STUDIES
- Best seen on lateral x-ray as articular surface defect
- MRI and CT scan helpful in delineating anatomy

DIFFERENTIAL DIAGNOSIS
- OCD femoral trochlea even rarer
- Must be differentiated from other (more common) causes of anterior knee pain

TREATMENT
- Conservative treatment consists of symptomatic treatment and patellofemoral rehabilitation.

- In very young children, immobilization in a cast has been associated with healing.
- Surgical treatment consists of arthroscopic removal of fragment and curettage, if necessary.
- Larger fragments may be treated with fixation.

DISPOSITION
N/A

PROGNOSIS
- In very young children, cast immobilization has been associated with excellent results.
- Surgical treatment, with either removal or repair of the fragment, is commonly associated with persistent pain and dysfunction. Outcome is guarded.

CAVEATS AND PEARLS
N/A

OSTEOCHONDRITIS DISSECANS OF TALUS

GEORGE B. HOLMES, JR., MD

HISTORY
- Most patients have experienced a twisting injury to the ankle.
- Mechanisms: inversion, avascular
- Catching, grinding, instability, giving way
- Episodic swelling of ankle
- Pain localized to side of lesion
- Pain aggravated with activity
- May be associated with ligamentous injuries

PHYSICAL EXAM
- Often nonspecific
- Tenderness frequently associated to side of lesion
- Joint crepitation with range of motion
- Test for associated joint laxity.

STUDIES
- Radiographs
  - ➤ AP, lateral, mortise views
  - ➤ Plain radiographs of contralateral ankle

➤ For anterolateral lesions, AP view in dorsiflexion
➤ For posteromedial lesions, mortise view in plantarflexion
➤ In early stages films may be normal.
➤ Stress views if laxity is present on physical examination
■ Bone scan
➤ Helpful with persistent painful ankle, normal radiographs
➤ Timing: 2–3 months after injury
➤ Positive uptake in talar dome – Go to MRI or CT
■ MRI
➤ Useful for avascular changes, surrounding bone contusion
➤ Useful for assessment of chondral component
■ CT scan
➤ Helpful in assessment of bone component of lesion
■ Berndt and Harty classification
➤ Stage I: contusion, compression of subchondral bone
➤ Stage II: partially detached fragment
➤ Stage III: detached fragment remains in crater
➤ Stage IV: loose fragment

DIFFERENTIAL DIAGNOSIS
■ Ligamentous instability
■ Os trigonum
■ Sinus tarsi syndrome
■ Anterolateral impingement
■ Loose bodies

TREATMENT
■ Nonoperative
➤ Indications: asymptomatic lesions, teenagers
➤ Types of nonoperative treatment
  • Protected weight-bearing
  • Steroid injections (no positive effect)
■ Operative
➤ Open vs. arthroscopic
➤ Medial malleolar osteotomy, some posteromedial lesions
➤ Techniques
  • Drilling
  • Excision, curettage, abrasion, drilling
  • Bone grafting
  • Internal fixation
  • OATS procedure (previous failures)

- Rehabilitation
  - ➤ Primary goal: re-establishment of range of motion

DISPOSITION
N/A

PROGNOSIS
- Results of early surgical treatment better than those of later intervention
- Early results as good as 85%
- Late results: 50% may have some pain or swelling

Long-term complications
- Posttraumatic arthritis
- Limited ROM

CAVEATS AND PEARLS
- High degree of suspicion in patient with persistent pain after acute ankle sprain and with chronic ankle pain

---

OSTEOCHONDRITIS DISSECANS OF THE ELBOW

GEORGE A. PALETTA, JR., MD
STEVE BERNSTEIN, MD

HISTORY
- Insidious onset lateral elbow pain
- Typically adolescent age 13–16 years
- Chief complaints pain, loss of terminal extension
- Dull, aching, poorly localized pain aggravated by use, relieved by rest
- Pain with throwing, initially late cocking phase, then all phases
- Late symptoms include locking, catching, rest pain
- Strong association with throwing, typically dominant arm
- Also common in gymnasts
- Can occur in nondominant arm or nonthrowing athlete
- Etiologic theories include ischemia, trauma, genetic factors
- Currently no proven etiology; repetitive microtrauma most widely accepted
- Tenuous vascular supply to immature capitellum with end arterioles terminating at subchondral plate

- Repetitive microtrauma may produce focal end artery injury with subsequent bone death

PHYSICAL EXAM
- Pain/tenderness at radiocapitellar joint
- Flexion contracture common (average 15°)
- Pain with terminal passive extension
- Crepitance at radiocapitellar joint
- +/− pain with valgus compression
- Normal neurovascular exam

STUDIES
- Plain radiographs
  - AP/lateral/oblique/radiocapitellar views
  - Oblique view most sensitive
  - Initial radiographs may be normal
  - Typical appearance is rarefaction, irregular ossification, and radiolucent crater adjacent to articular surface
  - Loose bodies may be present in late cases
  - Deformity of capitellum or radial head can occur
- Tomograms
  - Rarely used
  - AP views may be helpful if x-rays negative
  - Can further define presence/extent of lesion
  - Use of contrast can help determine if articular cartilage/subchondral bone dissected from capitellum
- CT scan
  - Indicated if high clinical suspicion but x-rays negative
  - Can further define presence/extent of lesion
- Bone scintigraphy
  - Can be helpful if x-rays negative
- MRI scan
  - Gadolinium arthrogram technique helpful in determining status of joint surface and articular cartilage
- Arthroscopy
  - Excellent tool for determining lesion size, lesion stability, status of articular cartilage
  - Lesion often best seen from anconeus (posterolateral portal) with flexion of elbow
  - Should not be used as diagnostic tool only but as adjunct to definitive surgical treatment

➤ Lesion classification (based on arthroscopic appearance)
  • Type I
    • Intact lesion, no evidence of instability of subchondral bone, no disruption of articular cartilage
  • Type II
    • Open lesion with disruption (fissuring, fracture) of articular cartilage
    • Unstable lesion with impending collapse of subchondral bone (ballotable)
    • Partially detached lesion
  • Type III
    • Completely detached fragment, loose body

DIFFERENTIAL DIAGNOSIS

■ Panner's disease
  ➤ Typically younger children age <12 years
  ➤ Acute onset
  ➤ Fragmentation, irregular ossification entire capitellum
  ➤ Loose bodies typically absent
  ➤ Minimal residual deformity capitellum

TREATMENT

■ Type I
  ➤ Nonsurgical treatment
  ➤ Rest, avoidance of all throwing
  ➤ Splinting may be necessary if acute symptoms severe
  ➤ Range of motion as soon as possible
  ➤ Serial radiographs every 6–12 weeks until complete radiographic healing
  ➤ If no healing after 6 months consider arthroscopy, drilling of lesion
    • Drill in antegrade fashion from outside-in under arthroscopic visualization and fluoroscopic guidance
    • Do not violate articular cartilage
    • ?Promotes revascularization?
  ➤ Caution with respect to return to throwing
  ➤ Recommend no pitching for first 1 year upon return to throwing
■ Type II
  ➤ Determine status of lesion as stable, unstable, or partially detached

➤ If stable, consider trial of nonsurgical treatment as above
  • If nonsurgical Rx fails then drilling as above
➤ If unstable or partially detached, consider surgical treatment
  • Unstable but fully attached lesion
    • Arthroscopy and in situ pinning
    • Antegrade pinning under arthroscopic visualization/ fluoroscopic guidance
      • Protects articular surface
      • K-wires
      • Serial radiographs every 6–12 weeks until radiographic healing
    • Retrograde pinning via arthrotomy
      • Violates articular cartilage
      • K-wires vs. bioabsorbable pins
      • Serial radiographs every 6–12 weeks until radiographic healing
  • Partially detached lesion
    • If large lesion pin in situ
      • Open or arthroscopic (arthroscopic demanding)
      • Serial radiographs every 6–12 weeks until radiographic healing
    • If small lesion excise fragment
      • Drill/microfracture subchondral bed
      • Early range of motion
■ Type III
  ➤ Excision or ORIF
    • In most chronic cases fragment has hypertrophied or fragmented into several pieces so ORIF impossible
    • ORIF only if perfect fit into subchondral crater and adequate subchondral bone on fragment (>2 mm) to achieve anatomic reduction/solid fixation
    • If excision debride lesion bed and drill/microfracture
      • Early range of motion

DISPOSITION
N/A

PROGNOSIS
■ Type I
  ➤ Generally good
  ➤ Healing usually occurs

➤ Flexion contracture typically resolves
➤ Full functional recovery
➤ Guarded for return to throwing or gymnastics

■ Type II
➤ Guarded prognosis
➤ Healing unpredictable
➤ Fragment separation can occur
➤ If heals, then flexion contracture usually resolves and functional recovery occurs
➤ If fails to heal, may require fragment excision
➤ Recommend against return to pitching or gymnastics

■ Type III
➤ Short-term prognosis generally good for functional recovery
➤ Guarded long-term prognosis
➤ Typically recommend against return to throwing or gymnastics
➤ Late degenerative changes can occur
➤ Residual deformity of capitellum common

CAVEATS AND PEARLS

■ Focal involvement of capitellum
■ Most common in dominant arm of throwing athletes
■ Also common in gymnasts
■ Pain/loss of motion common presenting symptoms
■ Loose bodies in late cases
■ Amenable to arthroscopy in most cases if surgery required
➤ Must access posterior compartment
➤ Best visualized via posterolateral portal
➤ Accessory posterior portals may be necessary if drilling/microfracture/pinning
➤ Prefer pinning/drilling intact lesion from antegrade outside-in to avoid violating articular cartilage
  • Arthroscopic visualization/fluoroscopic guidance
➤ Prefer drilling/microfracture subchondral lesion bed from direct approach
■ Prognosis generally good for functional recovery
■ Guarded long-term prognosis in type III lesions
■ Careful counseling about return to throwing/gymnastics in most cases

OSTEOLYSIS OF THE DISTAL CLAVICLE

JAMES D. FERRARI, MD
REVISED BY CHARLES NOFSINGER, MD

HISTORY

- Etiology: most likely subchondral microfractures on clavicular side of acromioclavicular (AC) joint
  - Acromion and meniscal disk remain normal
- Can be precipitated by single traumatic event
  - Blow to shoulder
  - Swelling at AC joint
  - Pain recedes, then recurs as achiness
- Repeated traumatic episodes
  - Hockey player checked into boards
- Repetitive microtrauma
  - Weight lifting (bench press, military press, dips, push-ups)
- Vast majority are male

PHYSICAL EXAM

- Swelling
- Point tenderness at AC joint
- Pain at AC joint with cross-body adduction
- Pain with adduction of fully flexed arm
- Rarely a deformity
- O'Brien's (active compression) test helpful in delineating AC pain from SLAP pain
  - Arm forward flexed 90°, adducted 15°
  - Have patient resist downward displacement of arm in both fully pronated and fully supinated positions
  - Pain in shoulder much greater or only in the pronated position indicates SLAP tear
  - Pain at AC joint with both pronation and supination indicates AC joint pathology
  - Verify with cross-body adduction pain
- Injection of local anesthesia into AC joint helpful for diagnosis

STUDIES

- Zanca view (AP of AC joint with beam angled 15° cranial)
  - "Soft tissue" technique to prevent overpenetration (half the exposure of a shoulder film)

- Axillary to rule out posterior displacement of clavicle
- Compare to normal side if necessary
- Three phases of radiographic changes seen
  - Lytic: demineralization and loss of subarticular cortex in lateral clavicle +/− cystic erosions
    - Bone loss of 0.5–3 cm
    - Can last few weeks to 18 months
  - Reparative: eroded lateral clavicle reconstitutes
    - AC joint widening remains
    - Clavicle tapers
  - Burnt out: radiographic changes with resolution of symptoms
- In early stages, symptoms may be present without radiographic changes
- Bone scan not much help
- MRI may be helpful to rule out intra-articular pathology

DIFFERENTIAL DIAGNOSIS
- SLAP tear
  - O'Brien's test, crank test, biceps tenderness, MRI +/− gadolinium
- Multiple myeloma (>40 years old)
- Inflammatory arthritis
- Gout
- AC joint sepsis (IV drug abuser)

TREATMENT
- Nonoperative treatment: rest, avoidance of aggravating activities, NSAIDs
  - Single steroid injection may be helpful
- Surgery: distal clavicle resection of 8–12 mm
  - May be done arthroscopically or open
  - Probably no difference long term
- Postop rehab
  - Sling for 1–2 weeks
  - Active range of motion at 2 weeks
  - Strengthening when range of motion full

DISPOSITION
N/A

PROGNOSIS
- Natural history may be self-limiting over 1–2 years

➤ Difficult for athletes to rest that long
■ Surgery extremely successful
➤ Majority of athletes return to same level of play
■ Return to play when range of motion full and strength near normal
➤ Usually 6–8 weeks
■ Complications of surgery
➤ Infection
➤ Clavicular instability

CAVEATS AND PEARLS
■ Superior labral tears often mimic AC joint pathology
■ Infection of AC joint will mimic osteolysis of distal clavicle
➤ Will see changes on both sides of joint, not just clavicle
➤ Question hard about IV drug abuse
■ Injection diagnostic
■ Clavicular instability avoided by limited resection of clavicle not exceeding 2.5 cm when measured from acromion
➤ Small amount of AP instability seen early after open excision
➤ Need thorough repair of deltotrapezial fascia and superior AC ligament
■ Benefits of arthroscopic excision (small incisions, less AP instability in early postop period) unlikely to outweigh those of open excision (speed, less set-up time, less equipment)
■ If any question of intra-articular pathology, perform arthroscopy first

---

PATELLAR TENDINITIS

CHARLES A. BUSH-JOSEPH, MD

HISTORY
■ Anterior knee pain, gradual onset or after period of overuse
■ Common ages 15–40
■ Basketball or jumping sports
■ Often referred as jumper's knee or runner's knee
■ Recurrent symptoms based on activity

PHYSICAL EXAM
■ Occasional limp, pain with single-leg squat or jumping
■ Tender to palpation inferior pole of patella
■ Joint swelling uncommon, normal motion and stability

- No joint line tenderness
- Quadriceps/hamstring tightness

STUDIES
- Radiographs – Generally normal, may show calcification or ossification at inferior pole of patella
- MRI
  - Indicated only in refractory cases
  - Shows thickening of proximal portion of patellar tendon
  - May exclude intra-articular joint injuries

DIFFERENTIAL DIAGNOSIS
- Acute trauma – Meniscal or ligament injury, patellar dislocation
- Chronic – Chondromalacia patella or knee arthritis, chronic knee instability
- Prepatellar or pretibial bursitis
- Inflammatory knee arthritis – Rheumatoid, pigmented villonodular synovitis

TREATMENT
- Ice, quadriceps/hamstring stretching exercises
- Avoidance of impact and jumping activities
- Continue aerobic fitness and cross-training
- Neoprene knee sleeve
- Physical therapy in refractory cases
- Arthroscopic debridement in rare case with tendon degeneration noted on MRI

DISPOSITION
N/A

PROGNOSIS
- Acute symptoms resolve over 7–10 days, with complete resolution over 4–8 weeks typical
- Recurrences more common with objective tendon thickening

CAVEATS AND PEARLS
N/A

PATELLAR TENDON RUPTURES

CHARLES A. BUSH-JOSEPH, MD
REVISED BY CHARLES NOFSINGER, MD

HISTORY
- Sports or work injury
- Ages 20–45
- Men more common than women
- Sudden onset of pop in front of knee
- Inability to straighten or extend knee
- Acute onset of knee swelling and pain radiating into thigh
- Able to bear weight when supported or wearing knee immobilizer
- Rarely associated with knee ligament injury

PHYSICAL EXAM
- Acute knee and lower thigh swelling, ecchymosis common
- Palpable gap where patellar tendon would attach to patella
- Proximal migration of patella
- Patient unable to actively straight-leg raise
- Close exam of cruciate and collateral ligaments to rule out associated ligamentous injury

STUDIES
- Radiographs
  - Indicated in all patients
  - Reveal distal migration of patella
  - May show inferior pole avulsion fracture
  - Comparison lateral x-ray of normal knee may aid in diagnosis of partial injuries (rare) and helpful in surgical repair
- MRI
  - Not typically necessary (clinical radiographic diagnosis)
  - Distal migration of patella with loss of patella tendon signal
  - Can rule out associated meniscal or ligamentous injury

DIFFERENTIAL DIAGNOSIS
- Quadriceps tendon rupture – also with loss of active knee extension
- Patellar fracture – Radiographic diagnosis
- Acute hemarthrosis – Patient unable to extend knee due to pain and swelling associated with ligament injury, patellar dislocation, or peripheral meniscal tear

TREATMENT

- Surgical repair in all cases of complete tears
- Critical to restore proper patellar tendon length
- May require augmentation of repair with metallic wire, fiber wire or semitendinosus tendon graft
- Delayed repairs less predictable outcome than with acute repair
- Postoperative bracing to protect repair with ROM within safe limits
- Return to full sports and activities 4–8 months postoperatively

DISPOSITION

N/A

PROGNOSIS

- Majority of patients return to full activities without restrictions, although anterior knee pain common with impact sports.
- Long-term complaints of anterior knee pain and kneeling discomfort common

CAVEATS AND PEARLS

- Onset of joint swelling immediate – Suspect fracture
- Onset of joint swelling minutes to hours – Suspect tendon tear
- No visible swelling, only localized tenderness – Suspect tendinitis
- Patient able to actively extend knee – Suspect patellar or quadriceps tendonitis
- Patient unable to extend knee – Suspect quadriceps or patellar tendon tear, surgery indicated
- Palpable gap above patella – Suspect quadriceps tendon tear
- Palpable gap below tendon – Suspect patellar tendon tear
- X-rays indicated in all patients unable to extend knee or bear weight
- Results of early surgical repair or tendon tears better than delayed repairs
- Results of patellar tendon repairs (typically younger patients) generally better than quad tendon repairs (generally older patients)

PATELLOFEMORAL PAIN AND INSTABILITY

JOHN P. FULKERSON, MD

HISTORY

- Chief complaint: pain vs. instability

- Spontaneous onset vs. trauma?
  - Gradual onset
  - Relationship to training
    - Change in training intensity, frequency
    - Change in shoe wear
    - Isokinetic training
    - Open-chain quad strengthening
  - Traumatic
    - Blunt trauma (e.g., dashboard)
    - Sense of instability
- History of dislocation?
- Recent weight gain?
- Recent period of reduced activity/deconditioning?
- Location of pain
- Previous surgery?
  - Improved, no change, worse
  - Type of surgery
- Mechanical peripatellar symptoms?
  - Location
    - Medial peripatellar
      - Plica
      - Instability
    - Distal pole
      - Patellar tendinitis
    - Proximal pole
      - Quadriceps tendinitis
  - Knee flexion position (angle-specific)
- Sense of patella slipping out of position?
- What treatment modalities
  - Activity reduction
  - NSAIDs
  - Icing
  - Heat
  - Flexibility
  - Strengthening activities
- Provocative maneuvers
  - Pain with prolonged sitting
  - Pain ascending/descending stairs
  - Peripatellar pain with knees bent
  - Patellofemoral crepitation
  - Response to knee sleeve

- Closed
- Open patella type
- Open patella with lateral buttress

PHYSICAL EXAM

- Effusion
  - ➤ Occasionally noted with patellofemoral pain
- Hemarthrosis
  - ➤ Occurs with instability
- Generalized ligamentous laxity
  - ➤ Elbow recurvatum
  - ➤ Thumb-forearm laxity
  - ➤ Knee recurvatum
  - ➤ Pes planus
  - ➤ Hypermobile patella
- Position of patella
- Tracking of patella
  - ➤ Observe through flexion-extension.
  - ➤ Note "j" sign.
- Medial lateral patellar translation
- Localized tenderness
  - ➤ Fibrous nodules may mimic patellofemoral pain
  - ➤ Distal pole tenderness – Jumper's knee
  - ➤ Proximal patella – Quadriceps tendinitis
  - ➤ Tibial tubercle tenderness/prominence – Osgood-Schlatter
  - ➤ Medial peripatellar – Medial plica
- Fat pad hypertrophy
  - ➤ Peripatellar tendon soft tissue bulge with knee flexion
- Q angle
  - ➤ Measure from ASIS-patella-tibial tubercle
  - ➤ <20° considered normal
  - ➤ Dynamically increases with tibial external rotation and knee flexion
- Observe and measure for quad atrophy
- Patellar instability tests
  - ➤ Apprehension sign with attempt to displace patella laterally
  - ➤ Medial instability may occur with overextensive lateral release
- Ligament assessment
  - ➤ Anterior cruciate status – Mimics instability
  - ➤ Posterior cruciate status – Patellofemoral pain
  - ➤ Posterolateral corner – Mimics instability

➣ Medial collateral ligament status – Origin medial collateral tenderness with patellar dislocation
- General flexibility
  ➣ Quad tightness: >10° knee flexion difference prone vs. supine
  ➣ Hamstring tightness: Quantify in degrees of tightness
  ➣ Iliotibial band tightness: Ober test
- Foot alignment: Check for pronation
- Referred pain
  ➣ Check hip ROM – early degenerative joint disease
  ➣ Referred pain from back
- Caveat – RSD
  ➣ Skin hypersensitivity
  ➣ Temperature asymmetry
  ➣ Pain out of proportion
  ➣ Color changes

STUDIES
- Radiographs
  ➣ AP, lateral, Merchant, tunnel
  ➣ Assessment
    • Patellar osteophytes
    • Trochlear hypoplasia
    • Lateral tilt
    • Subluxation
    • Loose bodies
    • Patellar osteochondritis dissecans
- CT
  ➣ 0, 15, 30, 45° flexion standing
  ➣ Special studies to assess for instability
- MRI
  ➣ 15° knee flexion
  ➣ Assess for tilt/subluxation
  ➣ Assess for articular lesions
  ➣ Increased signal in subchondral bone
  ➣ Lateral femoral condyle bone contusion in acute instability
  ➣ Medial retinacular injury in acute instability
  ➣ Medial patellofemoral ligament injury

DIFFERENTIAL DIAGNOSIS
- Peripatellar pain
  ➣ Patellofemoral arthrosis

- ➤ Patellofemoral chondromalacia
- ➤ Patellofemoral pain secondary to posterior cruciate injury
- ➤ Patellar tendinitis
- ➤ Quadriceps tendinitis
- ➤ Plica syndrome
- ➤ Patellar osteochondritis dissecans
- ➤ Peripatellar nodules
- ➤ Referred pain
  - Hip
  - Back
  - Thigh
- ➤ RSD
- ■ Patellar instability
  - ➤ Quad weakness
    - Neurologic
    - Muscular
  - ➤ Anterior cruciate deficiency
  - ➤ Meniscal tears
  - ➤ Posterolateral corner injury

TREATMENT
- ■ Patellar pain – Nonsurgical
  - ➤ Strengthening
    - Closed-chain quad strengthening
      - Bicycle
      - Stair-stepper
      - Nordic Trak
      - Ellipticizer
      - Squats
      - Leg press
    - Straight-leg raises
      - With/without ankle weights (100 reps daily)
      - Females 6–8 # goal
      - Males 8–10 # goal
    - Avoid isokinetic strengthening/training.
    - Avoid open-chain quad strengthening.
  - ➤ Flexibility
    - Correct quad, hamstring, or iliotibial band tightness.
  - ➤ Reduce inflammation
    - Modify activities
    - Avoid provocative activities

- NSAIDs
- Ice
➤ Orthosis
  - Consider foot orthotics if pronation
  - Consider neoprene sleeve with patellar cutout
➤ Consider formal physical therapy
➤ Regain proprioception
■ Patellar pain – Surgical treatment
  ➤ Only considered if failure of prolonged nonsurgical treatment
  ➤ If lateral tilt, consider arthroscopic lateral release
  ➤ If symptomatic articular lesion, consider limited arthroscopic debridement
■ Patellar instability
  ➤ Acute
    - X-ray-positive loose body – Consider arthroscopic removal/replacement, size dependent
    - Short course of immobilizer/crutches
    - Begin early ROM, progress to weight-bearing as tolerated, & PT
    - Counsel on recurrences
  ➤ Recurrent instability
    - Normal Q angle: lateral release + medial imbrication
    - Increased Q angle: tibial tubercle anteromedialization ± lateral release + medial imbrication
    - Iatrogenic medial instability: lateral patellar tenodesis (Hughston-Deese procedure)
  ➤ Postop treatment
    - Mobilize quickly
    - Nonweight-bearing to limited weight-bearing for 6 weeks with tibial tubercle transfer; weight bearing as tolerated in all other patients
    - Consider graded ROM progression with soft tissue realignment

DISPOSITION
N/A

PROGNOSIS
■ Dependent on proper indications and correct surgical treatment
■ Poor prognostic indicators
  ➤ Diffuse articular changes

➤ Trochlear lesions >1.5 cm
➤ Workers' compensation issues
➤ Diffuse pain
➤ Poorly defined pain
➤ Hypersensitivity to pain
➤ Prolonged immobilization

CAVEATS AND PEARLS
■ Listen to patient.
■ Perform meticulous physical exam.
■ Conservative approach to patella surgically.
■ Avoid prolonged immobilization.
■ Beware RSD mimicking knee pain.
■ Beware referred pain from hip/back.
■ Don't overlook contributing factors
  ➤ Weight gain
  ➤ Open-chain quad training
  ➤ Pes planus with pronation
  ➤ Quad, hamstring, iliotibial band tightness
■ Rehab, rehab, rehab, and rehab!

PECTORALIS MAJOR RUPTURE

MARK BOWEN, MD

HISTORY
■ Uncommon injury
■ Mechanism
  ➤ Direct – blow to chest, injury to muscle belly
  ➤ Indirect – eccentric load to pectoralis muscle
■ Indirect – usually occurs in sports, bench press lifting
■ Symptoms – pain, pop, or tearing, swelling, ecchymosis, weakness, chest wall deformity
■ Most common – men 20s and 30s; rare in women
■ Complete injuries – avulsion from humerus muscle-tendon (MT) junction
■ Incomplete injuries – muscle substance + MT junction
■ Chronic tears may present with weakness and deformity
■ Question of anabolic steroid use may arise

PHYSICAL EXAM

- Swelling, ecchymosis
- Asymmetry of axillary fold and pectoralis muscle
- Palpable defect
- Pain with active or passive motion
- Weakness with adduction, forward flexion, internal rotation
- Defect accentuated by pressing palms together in midline – isometric contraction
- Chronic tears – defect and retracted muscle visible

STUDIES

- Radiographs
  - Plain x-rays, shoulder and chest – normal
  - Rare instance, bony avulsion from humerus is visible
- MRI
  - Sensitive for injury
  - Helpful for localization and extent of injury

DIFFERENTIAL DIAGNOSIS

- Biceps tendon tear
- Rotator cuff tear
- Clavicle or rib fracture
  - Direct trauma
  - Radiographic abnormality

TREATMENT

- Acute tear
  - Ice, protection for comfort
  - Establish diagnosis; degree and location by MRI
- Partial tendon tears, incomplete muscle injuries
  - Respond to conservative treatment
  - Mild deformity and strength deficit
  - Recover over 6–8 weeks
- Complete tear
  - Treatment directed by concerns over strength, cosmesis, discomfort
  - Athletes lose up to 50% horizontal adduction strength
  - Conservative results mixed
  - Surgical results excellent
  - Late repair possible, less predictable results
  - Avulsions – best surgical results

- Surgical repair
  - Humeral avulsions repaired direct to bone
    - Woven sutures in tendon, pass through drill holes, recess tendon into trough at attachment site
    - Suture anchors – weaker grasp of tendon
  - Repair of MT junction tears difficult due to placement of sutures in muscle tissue

DISPOSITION
N/A

PROGNOSIS
- Nonsurgical treatment
  - Deformity, weakness
  - High probability of sports participation, ? level
  - Less successful with complete tears
- Surgical treatment
  - More predictable outcome for complete tears and avulsions
  - Less deformity
  - Potential for near-normal strength and function
- Return to play
  - Nonsurgical
    - Few weeks is possible
    - Pain and swelling subside
    - Full motion and strength
  - Surgical
    - Progress strengthening over 3–4 months
    - 6 months
- Complications of surgery
  - Nerve injury
  - Incomplete repair only possible
  - Rerupture
  - Myositis – usually minor
  - Chronic weakness

CAVEATS AND PEARLS
- Suspect in patient with acute pain with bench press
- Physical exam diagnostic
- MRI localizes, determines extent of injury
- Avulsions – surgery recommended
- Secure anatomic repair possible with sutures and drill holes
- Suture anchors are reasonable alternative
- Incomplete and MT injuries may do well nonoperatively

- Early surgery easier than repair of chronic tear
- Poor quality of tissue in MT junction tears may dictate imperfect results

---

PELLIGRINI-STIEDA DISEASE

MICHAEL BROWN, MD
ROBERT F. LAPRADE, MD

HISTORY
- Posttraumatic disorder of the knee
- Heterotopic ossification of soft tissues in proximity to the medial femoral condyle in region of adductor tubercle/medial epicondyle
- Reaction to trauma to medial side of knee
  - ➤ Traumatic detachment of proximal origin of medial (tibial) collateral ligament
  - ➤ Injury to insertion of adductor magnus tendon
- Mechanism – Valgus force to the knee, knee dislocations
- Injury occurred at least 2–3 weeks prior to calcification or ossification
- Pain on medial side or anterior aspect of knee
- May have discomfort at extremes of flexion and extension

PHYSICAL EXAM
- Thickening of medial meniscofemoral capsule of knee
- Occasionally effusion present
- Limitation of knee ROM may be present
- Tenderness over medial femoral epicondyle
- May be tender over distal aspect of adductor magnus

STUDIES
- **Radiographs**
  - ➤ Full knee series
  - ➤ Plaque of calcification or ossification near medial femoral epicondyle/adductor tubercle region
  - ➤ Clear space (radiolucency) between calcification/ossification and femur (usually)
  - ➤ Calcification/ossification difficult to see on lateral film
  - ➤ Plaque not seen immediately after injury – Appears 2–3 weeks after injury
  - ➤ Posttraumatic arthritic changes may be present

- **Bone scan**
  - Increased tracer update at location of calcification/ossification in immature cases
  - Normal bone scan in mature cases
- **MRI scan**
  - Useful to demonstrate location of ossification and involvement of proximal medial collateral ligament (MCL) complex

DIFFERENTIAL DIAGNOSIS
- Osteochondroma

TREATMENT
- Nonsurgical
  - Surgical intervention rarely necessary
  - Physical therapy for ROM
  - Local heat may help cause some resorption of plaque
- Surgical
  - If mass is large enough to cause irritation, surgical resection may be warranted.
  - If surgery performed:
    - Must wait until area of calcification/ossification is mature on bone scan or else recurrence is likely
    - Take care to protect or reattach MCL attachment
    - Early ROM after resection to reduce scarring

DISPOSITION
N/A

PROGNOSIS
- Nonsurgical treatment
  - Usually minimal symptoms
- Surgical treatment
  - Usually return to near-normal motion

Return to play
- Nonoperative
  - Usually 2–3 months
- Surgical resection
  - Usually 2–3 months after resection
- Complications of surgical treatment
  - Infection (<1%)
  - Deep venous thrombosis; pulmonary embolus <5%

➤ Arthrofibrosis (usually combined with knee ligament and/or head injury patients)
➤ MCL laxity

CAVEATS AND PEARLS

- Strive for early knee ROM after a knee dislocation with MCL tear to prevent arthrofibrosis from Pelligrini-Stieda disease
- May consider prophylaxis with indomethacin in knee dislocation or head injury patients
- MRI is useful in planning surgical incisions, extent of ossification
- Usually safe to resect large lesions at 9–12 months after injury

---

PELVIC STRESS FRACTURES

WILLIAM E. GARRETT, JR., MD, PhD

HISTORY

- Insidious onset of groin or pelvic pain
- Usually in an athlete doing heavy routine of lower extremity
- Weight-bearing impact activity
- More common in females
- Females with eating disorders and amenorrhea more predisposed
- Pain worse during or after running
- Recent increase in exercise level often noted

PHYSICAL EXAM

- Tender usually over inferior pubis
- Range of motion and strength normal
- Few findings and characteristic history strongly suggest stress fracture

STUDIES

- Plain radiographs show fractures late but often not early in course
- Bone scan or MRI for early diagnosis
- Characteristic location is inferior pubic ramus

DIFFERENTIAL DIAGNOSIS

- Adductor strain
  ➤ More tender over muscle
- Pain with stretch
  ➤ Usually acute injury

- Athletic pubalgia
  - Tender over lower abdominal muscles
  - Usually not so painful with low-intensity jogging
- Femoral neck stress fracture
  - Very serious injury if undiagnosed
  - May lead to fracture, possible avascular necrosis
  - Distinguished by bone scan and MRI
- Gynecologic causes of lower pelvic pain
  - Often not exercise-related
- Get appropriate consult if needed

TREATMENT
- Rest, usually 3–6 weeks
- Exercise with pain delays healing
- Gradual return to sport based on pain
- Address issues of eating disorder and amenorrhea if present
- Primary care physician with interest in female athletic triad is extremely helpful
- Femoral neck stress fractures much more serious
  - Surgery if displaced
  - Rest if on compression side
  - Consider preventive surgery if on tension side

DISPOSITION
N/A

PROGNOSIS
- Healing of fracture predictable if patient is compliant
- Predisposing elements of eating disorders and menstrual disorders less predictable
- More serious complications possible in femoral neck stress fractures

CAVEATS AND PEARLS
- Strong index of suspicion is essential.
- Do not delay long in obtaining MRI or bone scan.
- Be very wary of femoral neck stress fractures.

PERONEAL TENDON INSTABILITY

CAROL FREY, MD

HISTORY

- ■ Anatomy
  - ➤ Brevis lies against the posterior lateral malleolus; longus lies lateral and posterior to the brevis.
  - ➤ Both become tendinous prior to ankle joint with common sheath.
  - ➤ Fibro-osseous tunnel formed by fibular sulcus anterior, calcaneofibular ligament (CFL) and posterior talofibular ligament (PTFL) medially, superior peroneal retinaculum (SPR) laterally and SPR/CFL posterior.
  - ➤ Each has a distinct sheath distal to fibula separated by peroneal tubercle.
- ■ SPR
  - ➤ Primary lateral restraint against peroneal instability
- ■ Fibula
  - ➤ Posterior aspect of lateral malleolus is the "fibular groove."
  - ➤ Large variation in depth of sulcus; 50% have bone ridge that augments sulcus
  - ➤ Fibrocartilage rim on lateral border consistently present and increases sulcus depth and aids stability.
- ■ Specific history
  - ➤ Acute vs. chronic
    - • Often history of inversion/supination sprain
    - • Occasionally repetitive with lateral instability
    - • Acute secondary to forced dorsifexion while pushing off
    - • Lateral ankle discomfort
    - • Snapping/popping
  - ➤ Subluxation
    - • Snapping/popping and pain as everts against resistance while palpating posterior border of fibula ("peroneal tunnel compression test")
    - • Beware of voluntary subluxators.
    - • Check hindfoot alignment; varus may promote.
    - • Check lateral ankle stability.
  - ➤ Dislocation
    - • Vague lateral ankle findings with chronic swelling

- May palpate tendon as "ridge" over lateral distal fibula
- Beware of associated tendon in acute dislocation.
- Easier to detect with patient in prone position

PHYSICAL EXAM
N/A

STUDIES
- Radiographs
  - Usually normal
  - "Fleck sign"
    - Avulsion fracture of posterior distal fibula
    - Represents injury to SPR
    - Possible peroneal dislocation
- Stress tests
  - If suspect lateral ligament injury
  - Instability of ankle
- MRI
  - May be used to check tendon pathology
  - Kinematic/Cine MRI may be useful for subluxation in future.
  - Check SPR.

DIFFERENTIAL DIAGNOSIS
- Tenosynovitis
- Tendinosis
- Split
- Rupture
- Subluxation
- Dislocation
- Fibula fracture
- Lateral process of talus fracture
- Ankle lateral ligament injury
- SPR injury
- Inferior peroneal retinaculum injury
- Cuboid subluxation
- Subtalar joint injury/instability

TREATMENT
- Nonoperative
  - If acute, can attempt cast immobilization
    - Plantarflexion and inversion for 4–6 weeks

- Followed by bracing
- Works 50% of the time
➤ Chronic types rarely improve with casting.
■ Operative
➤ Indications
- Failure of conservative treatment
- Pain
- Instability
➤ Contraindications
- Peripheral vascular disease
- Skin breakdown vasculitis
➤ In general
- Skin incision follows the line of the tendons.
- Develop full-thickness flaps.
- Beware of sural nerve and superficial peroneal nerve.
- Assess SPR.
➤ Subluxation
- Assess for splits/lateral instability.
- Incise SPR off fibular attachment; leave a cuff of tissue.
- Periosteal reflection of cuff, expose lateral cortex.
- Roughen lateral cortex to bleeding bone.
- Excise low-lying peroneus brevis muscle belly or peroneus quartus to make room.
- Excise redundant SPR tissue as necessary.
- Advance SPR and secure to bone with drill holes or suture anchors.
- "Pants-over-vest" repair of cuff
- Assess tension of SPR in both dorsiflexion and plantarflexion; avoid creating stenosis.
- If lateral ligament instability, add a modified Brostrum.
➤ Dislocation/acute
- Reduce tendons.
- If SPR avulsion with ORIF with mini-screws or suture
- If SPR ruptured then repair as for subluxation above.
➤ Dislocation/chronic
- Remove fibrous tissue within fibular groove.
- Fibular groove deepening
  - Use small curved gouge.
  - Avoid sharp distal edge.
  - Option for creating osteoperiosteal flap vs. bone wax on exposed surfaces

- SPR repair as per subluxation above
- Isolated soft tissue repair for chronic dislocation has a high failure rate.
- Options
  - Calcaneofibular ligament transfer
  - Bone block technique
  - Peroneus brevis tendon weave
  - Peroneus quartus reconstruction
➤ Postoperative management
  - Cast nonweight-bearing 2 weeks
  - Cast weight-bearing 4 weeks
  - Ankle brace for 6 weeks
  - Initiate active ROM at 6 weeks; avoid inversion.
  - Aggressive peroneal tendon strengthening and resistive exercises at 8–10 weeks

DISPOSITION
N/A

PROGNOSIS
N/A

CAVEATS AND PEARLS
- Always consider the possibility of peroneal nerve pathology in patient with history of recurrent ankle sprains but with negative anterior drawer and varus stress test.
- Often difficult to reproduce the subluxation on clinical exam
- Persistent pain/instability after lateral ligament reconstruction may be secondary to peroneal tendon pathology/subluxation.
- Chronic cases almost always require surgery if symptomatic.

PERONEAL TENDON TENDINITIS AND RUPTURES

CAROL FREY, MD

HISTORY
- Zones of injury
  ➤ Fibular groove
    - Site of most peroneus brevis (PB) injuries
    - PB in direct contact with sharp ridge of bone
    - 45° PB angulation of tendon in groove

- Peroneus longus (PL) overlies the PB in this location
- Cuboid tunnel
  - Site of PL injuries
  - PL in direct contact with lateral calcaneal wall, 45° course change at cuboid
  - In general, posttraumatic conditions in this zone are termed POPS (painful os peroneum syndrome).
- Injuries may occur at time of inversion ankle "sprain."
- PL lesions probably commonly missed
- Specific history/complaints if injured in fibular groove area
  - Acute vs. chronic
    - Often history of inversion/supination sprain
    - Occasionally repetitive with lateral instability
    - Acute secondary to forced dorsiflexion with push-off
  - Lateral ankle discomfort, retromalleolar, radiating
  - Consider inflammatory disorders in sedentary patient.
- Specific history/complaints if injured in cuboid tunnel area
  - Present with plantar-lateral foot pain, usually vague and chronic
  - Often posttraumatic from direct impact or supination/inversion force
  - Occasionally associated with paresthesia in sural nerve distribution
  - If acute, pain may worsen with weight-bearing or heel rise.

PHYSICAL EXAM

- Tenosynovitis/tendinosis
  - Fullness along tendon
  - Tenderness diffuse
  - Tendon intact but pain with stretch or resisted eversion
  - Weakness related to pain
- Splits
  - Localized tenderness at posterior ridge of fibula
  - Occasionally fullness in groove
  - Normal strength/excursion but pain
  - Pain with resisted eversion/plantarflexion
- Rupture
  - Diffuse tenderness
  - Fullness consistent with tenosynovitis
  - Weakness to eversion but often with little pain
- No instability on anterior drawer/varus tilt unless injury is associated with lateral ligament injury

■ In cuboid tunnel
  ➤ Localized tenderness in region of cuboid tunnel or peroneal tubercle
  ➤ May have swelling in this location
  ➤ Pain worse with heel rise, resisted plantarflexion of the first metatarsal, or forced inversion/supination/adduction
  ➤ Mild weakness to resisted eversion
  ➤ Check for lateral ligament instability.

STUDIES
■ Radiographs
  ➤ Usually normal
  ➤ "Fleck sign" = avulsion of posterior distal fibula; represents superior peroneal retinaculum injury and possible peroneal dislocation
  ➤ Stress test: to rule out ankle instability
  ➤ Assess for medial talar osteochondritis dissecans if lateral ligament injury.
  ➤ Assess for os peroneum fracture/diastases or proximal migration (oblique view).
  ➤ Assess for enlarged peroneal tubercle or lateral impingement from calcaneal prominence (Harris view).
■ MRI
  ➤ Very helpful in assessing peroneal pathology
  ➤ Delineates intrasubstance degeneration
  ➤ Kinematic/cine MRI for subluxation possible in the future
■ Ultrasound
  ➤ Inexpensive but technician-dependent
  ➤ Probably helpful only with frank ruptures
■ Tenography
  ➤ No longer common diagnostic test
  ➤ Can be useful if used with anesthetic for diagnosis/treatment
■ Tendonscopy may be more widespread in the future
■ Diagnostic injections
  ➤ Should relieve pain of POPS
  ➤ Inject sheath, not tendon.
  ➤ Can provide long-term therapeutic benefits

DIFFERENTIAL DIAGNOSIS
■ Tenosynovitis/tendinosis
■ Split
■ Rupture

- Subluxation
- Dislocation
- Fibula fracture
- Lateral process of talus fracture
- Superior peroneal retinaculum injury
- Inferior peroneal retinaculum injury
- Cuboid subluxation
- Subtalar injury
- Ankle lateral ligament injury

TREATMENT
- Nonoperative treatment
  - Tenosynovitis/tendinosis
    - Cast immobilization for 2–3 weeks
    - Peroneal strengthening exercises, NSAIDs
    - Physical therapy with dysinflammatory modalities
    - Lateral heel wedge
    - Shoe with firm heel counter and outflare heel
    - High-top shoe
    - Ankle brace
  - Ruptures
    - As above
- Operative treatment
  - Indications
    - Pain
    - Failure of conservative treatment
  - Contraindications
    - Peripheral vascular disease
    - Skin breakdown/vasculitis
  - In general:
    - Incision courses over posterior aspect of distal fibula and extends towards fifth metatarsal base
    - Develop full-thickness flap.
    - Beware of sural nerve/superficial peroneal nerve.
    - Check superior peroneal retinaculum.
  - Tenosynovitis
    - Decompress both PB and PL.
    - Maintain superior peroneal retinaculum.
    - Tenosynovectomy
  - Tendinosis
    - May present as flattening and attritional degeneration posterior to malleolus vs. intrasubstance thickening distally

- Tenosynovectomy
- Protect/maintain retinaculum.
- Elliptical excision of degenerative or attenuated tendon with side-to-side repair using nonabsorbable suture.
- Tubularize tendon.
- May resect up to 50% without weakening too much
- If total tendon involved, proceed with tenodesis of tendons and excision of necrotic tissue/segment.

➢ Split
  - Types
    - Longitudinal
    - Single
    - Multiple
    - Usually at or distal to lateral malleolus
  - If only peripheral portion of tendon involved (<50%), then excise and taper the edges.
  - If central split, excise edges and perform side-to-side repair.
  - Extensive involvement requires tenodesis and excision of diseased segment.

➢ Rupture
  - Debride the diseased segment.
  - Tenodesis to remaining tendon
  - If both tendons beyond repair/reconstruction, then consider free graft vs. flexor hallucis longus/flexor digitorum longus transfer.

➢ For cuboid tunnel and POPS
  - Incision extends distally from distal fibular to calcaneocuboid joint.
  - Surgery addresses pathology.
    - Decompress PL sheath.
    - Debride and repair diseased tendon.
    - If chronic rupture, then tenodesis to PB
    - Os peroneum pathology often requires excision followed by primary repair of PL.
    - Resect enlarge peroneal tubercle or perform lateral wall decompression.
    - Primary repair of acute tendon rupture is performed if proximal to os peroneum; otherwise, tenodese proximally.

■ Postoperative management
  ➢ Cast, nonweight-bearing for 2 weeks
  ➢ Short-leg walking cast × 4 weeks

> Ankle brace × 6 weeks
> Initiate active ROM exercises at 6 weeks; avoid inversion.
> Aggressive peroneal strengthening and resistive exercises at 8–10 weeks
- Complications
  > Sural nerve/neuritis
  > Superficial peroneal nerve injury
  > Recurrent pain
    - Inadequate debridement
    - Tenodesis may be necessary.
  > Refractory cases: if all else fails, may do subtalar fusion

DISPOSITION
N/A

PROGNOSIS
N/A

CAVEATS AND PEARLS
- Always consider the possibility of peroneal tendon pathology in patient with recurrent ankle sprains but with negative anterior drawer and varus stress test.
- May get stenosing PL tenosynovitis from enlarged peroneal tubercle, chronic os peroneum pathology, or exostosis off calcaneus.
- Acute os peroneum fracture/diastasis can occur with or without an injury to the PL.
- Remember, POPS does not require the presence of a bony os peroneum.
- Persistent pain after ligament reconstruction may be due to neglected rupture of peroneal tendons.

PLANTAR FASCIITIS

THOMAS O. CLANTON, MD

HISTORY
- Plantar fasciitis may be
  > Subcalcaneal or heel pain syndrome (proximal plantar fasciitis)
  > Midarch pain (true or distal plantar fasciitis)
- Risk factors for plantar fasciitis
  > Repetitive stress in athletes

- ➢ Obesity
- ➢ Middle age (40–70 years)
- ➢ Abnormal foot mechanics (pes cavus or pes planus)
- ➢ Prolonged standing (work-related)
- ■ Mechanism
  - ➢ Chronic repetitive stress on plantar fascia
  - ➢ Chronic degenerative/reparative process
  - ➢ Enthesopathy (example: ankylosing spondylitis, Reiter's syndrome)
- ■ Symptoms
  - ➢ Location of pain
    - Proximal plantar fasciitis
      - Subcalcaneal (plantar aspect)
      - At insertion of plantar fascia on medial calcaneal tuberosity
    - Distal plantar fasciitis
      - Midarch
      - Usually along medial edge
  - ➢ Characteristics of pain
    - Morning and startup pain may improve on ambulation
    - Recurs after prolonged, continued, or stressful activity

PHYSICAL EXAM
- ■ Point tenderness at origin of plantar fascia on calcaneal tuberosity
- ■ Pain on stretching the fascia (hyperextension of metatarsophalangeal joints) – primarily seen in distal plantar fasciitis
- ■ Look for heel cord tightness

STUDIES
- ■ If diagnosis is clinically obvious, no further studies are indicated
- ■ Studies are indicated if other diagnoses are suspected or patient does not respond to initial treatment
- ■ **Plain radiograph**
  - ➢ "Heel spur" ossification on plantar aspect of calcaneus
  - ➢ Association with plantar fasciitis may be coincidental
    - 50% patients with plantar fasciitis have heel spur
    - 16% asymptomatic patients have heel spur
  - ➢ Patient may focus on the spur, and this may negatively influence outcome
- ■ **Bone scan**
  - ➢ Very sensitive but nonspecific
  - ➢ Helpful in patients with equivocal diagnosis

- **MRI**
  - Not routinely indicated
  - Edema surrounding plantar fascia
  - Thickening consistent with chronic inflammation
  - Marrow edema at insertion site
- **EMG/Nerve conduction**
  - Indicated if compressive neuropathy suspected
  - Preoperatively to determine whether compressive neuropathy is present
  - Diagnoses include tarsal tunnel syndrome or compression of first branch of lateral plantar nerve

DIFFERENTIAL DIAGNOSIS
- Seronegative spondyloarthropathy (ankylosing spondylitis or Reiter's)
- Inflammatory arthritides (rheumatoid arthritis)
- Neuropathy (diabetes, alcoholism, compressive neuropathy)
- Calcaneal stress fracture (overuse, osteomalacia, osteoporosis)
- Plantar fat atrophy
- Infection (deep plantar abscess)
- HIV-related
- Other (sickle cell infarct, calcaneal apophysitis, Paget's disease)
- **Red flags to consider other diagnoses**
  - Bilateral symptoms
  - Associated symptoms (arthralgia, urethritis, uveitis, colitis)
  - No response to treatment

TREATMENT
- **Nonoperative**
  - Stretching exercises
    - Achilles tendon and plantar fascia
    - Home program or physical therapy
    - Must be done regularly and several times per day
    - 80% success rate
  - NSAIDs
    - 70% some improvement
    - Initial treatment for the inflammatory component
    - Not as beneficial in chronic phase
  - Heel pads/heel cups (multiple types available)
    - Controversial role
    - Success rates vary widely (2%–83%)

➤ Steroid and anesthetic injection
  - Useful in acute flare-up if pain is very localized
  - May make symptoms worse, especially with multiple injections
  - Rupture of plantar fascia has been reported after injection
➤ Orthoses
  - UCBL type or custom design
  - Useful in patients with coexisting biomechanical variation (cavus or planus foot)
  - Off-the-shelf orthoses do as well as custom-design orthoses
➤ Night splint
  - Useful in patients with startup pain
  - 5° dorsiflexion splint
➤ Casting
  - Provides continuous tension (stretch) on plantar fascia
  - Enforces rest
  - 50% success rate in recalcitrant cases
  - To be considered before surgery
➤ Combination protocol
  - Use multiple modalities together to optimize their effects
  - NSAIDs, stretching, pads or UCBL orthoses, maybe a steroid injection

■ **Operative treatment**
➤ Surgery for painful heel is rarely indicated until nonop treatment fails
➤ Before considering surgery, a detailed medical evaluation is necessary
➤ Open and endoscopic plantar fascia release
  - Open procedure includes
    - Medial release (one half to two thirds) of plantar fascia
    - Neurolysis and decompression of nerve to abductor digiti minimus
    - Removal of heel spur for nerve decompression and elimination as a focal point of attention
  - Endoscopic procedure
    - Good relief of pain reported (97%)
    - Main complication is related to complete release of plantar fascia, leading to lateral column overloading and pain
    - If nerve compression is coexistent, endoscopic procedure should not be attempted

DISPOSITION
N/A

PROGNOSIS
- \>90% of patients respond to nonsurgical treatment within 6–12 months
- Success rates for surgery 50–100%
- American Orthopaedic Foot and Ankle Society recommends a minimum of 6 months and preferably 12 months prior to considering surgery.
- Return to play
  - ➤ May continue to participate if symptoms can be controlled
  - ➤ If worsening with participation, then rest until startup pain improving and can ambulate without limp or severe pain
  - ➤ Return to sports activity should be done gradually while monitoring that the symptoms are not worsening

CAVEATS AND PEARLS
- Majority of patients who present to the office with heel pain have proximal plantar fasciitis
- When condition is bilateral, and especially if other sites of tendon or ligament attachments are associated with pain, think of inflammatory conditions and get appropriate tests
- If morning pain is the primary symptom, consider early use of a night splint
- Steroid injections sometimes help but often aggravate symptoms – use cautiously
- Main causes of treatment failure are failure of patient to follow regimen of rest, stretching, medication, and avoidance of irritating activities, failure to make correct diagnosis, impatience with nonoperative treatment program
- Sometimes the patients are worse after surgery

PLANTAR HEEL PAIN SYNDROME

THOMAS O. CLANTON, MD

HISTORY
- Acute or gradual onset (acute common only in traumatic etiology)
- Acute injury related to abrupt acceleration-deceleration stress

- Plantar heel pain aggravated by hard- or thin-soled shoes and stiff surfaces
- May be related to increase in body weight or change in activities
- Swelling uncommon in chronic condition
- More common in older individuals (>40 years)
- May be related to cortisone injections given for plantar fasciitis
- Common sports – long-distance running, basketball, soccer
- Pain characterized as deep and aching, aggravated by weight-bearing activity, usually relieved by rest

PHYSICAL EXAM
- Tenderness on plantar surface of heel
- Acute injuries may have swelling, ecchymosis, and limp – these are uncommon in chronic cases
- Most commonly the tenderness is plantar medial
- Tenderness to side-to-side heel compression more indicative of stress fracture of calcaneus
- Pain may accentuate with toe dorsiflexion through "windlass mechanism" – most commonly seen in mid or true plantar fasciitis
- Radiating pain at the lower edge of the abductor hallucis muscle near plantar medial heel should raise concern for entrapment of first branch of lateral plantar nerve going to the abductor digiti minimi
- Pain from fat pad atrophy more plantar central, easily palpable and tender calcaneal tuberosity; associated with weight loss behavior, lipodystrophy, or bowel resection/gastric stapling
- Positive Tinel's sign over tarsal tunnel associated with tarsal tunnel syndrome; symptoms may include heel, plantar foot, or ankle pain with burning or numbness in medial and/or lateral plantar nerve

STUDIES
- Radiographs
  - AP, lateral, oblique views of foot (usually normal – traction heel spur is not a source of pain)
  - Axial view of calcaneus
- Bone scan
  - Evaluate for stress fracture or infection
  - Often positive in proximal plantar fasciitis from periostitis
- MRI
  - Evaluate for plantar fasciitis or rupture

➤ Evaluate for flexor hallucis longus or flexor digitorum longus tendinitis
➤ Evaluate for tumor or other space-occupying lesion
■ ENG/nerve conduction velocity
➤ Evaluate for nerve entrapment
■ Laboratory tests
➤ Screening for seronegative arthropathies with sed rate, HLA-B27

DIFFERENTIAL DIAGNOSIS

■ Fat pad atrophy
■ Plantar fascia rupture
■ Plantar fasciitis
■ Flexor hallucis longus or flexor digitorum longus tendinitis
■ Tarsal tunnel syndrome
■ Entrapment of first branch lateral plantar nerve
■ Stress fracture of calcaneus
■ Tumor
■ Foreign body
■ Infection
■ Sever's disease (seen in children from calcaneal apophysitis during "growth spurt" years – pain usually posterior heel but occasionally plantar)
■ Seronegative arthropathy

TREATMENT

■ Acute
➤ Establish diagnosis
➤ Ice, elevation
➤ Early aggressive rest in a cast or removable boot
➤ Supportive insoles
➤ Stretching and strengthening exercises (except in plantar fascia rupture)
➤ NSAIDs
➤ Cortisone and anesthetic injection only for localized tenderness, failure of initial nonoperative management, no more than once in 3 months/three per year
➤ Surgery not indicated
■ Chronic
➤ Shoe modifications, supportive and well-cushioned, slight heel lift

➤ Heel cushions or heel cups; AOFAS study supports use of stretching and viscoelastic heel cushions in preference to initial use of custom orthoses

➤ Tendo Achilles and plantar fascia stretching exercises multiple times per day

➤ Morning pain often helped by use of dorsiflexion night splint, if not helped by morning/evening stretching alone

➤ Cortisone and anesthetic injection only for localized tenderness, failure of initial nonoperative management, no more than once in 3 months/three per year

➤ Cortisone injection near plantar fascia increases risk of plantar fascia rupture (avoid early loading)

➤ NSAID trial for at least 3 weeks; if no improvement, then switch meds or stop

➤ Surgery indicated only if diagnosis is determined and good nonoperative treatment program fails

DISPOSITION
N/A

PROGNOSIS
■ Acute injuries producing heel pain usually resolve within 2–6 months

■ Nonsurgical management of chronic heel pain is successful in 90% of patients

■ After failure of conservative treatment for 6–12 months, surgery may be considered for intractable plantar fasciitis

■ Postoperative recovery may be prolonged after plantar fascia release; heel pain may persist or recur

■ Complications include pes planus, lateral column overload from complete plantar fascia release, or pain/numbness from neuromas

CAVEATS AND PEARLS
■ Heel pain similar to back pain – multiple etiologies, hard to diagnose, mostly a soft tissue problem that responds to time and conservative measures

■ Diagnostic studies are necessary only for the atypical or nonresponsive case

■ Beware of surgical recommendation if diagnosis is unsure or no history of compliance with nonoperative treatment program

■ Beware of cortisone injections, especially multiple – may make heel pain worse from scar tissue or tissue damage

- Patients often focus on plantar heel spur, but spur is located in origin of flexor digitorum brevis and does not correlate strongly with presence of heel pain or relief from its removal; seen in 15% of normal population
- Newer treatment options of endoscopic plantar fasciotomy and high-intensity ultrasound (e.g., Ossatron) are as yet unproven, indicated only after failure of nonoperative treatment program

---

PLICA SYNDROME

WILLIAM R. POST, MD

HISTORY

- Etiology: blunt trauma/repetitive overuse
- Achy pain worse with prolonged knee flexion
- Nature of pain often described as burning but may be intermittently sharp
- Medial parapatellar location
- Anteromedial "bandlike" distribution
- Anteromedial "snapping"

PHYSICAL EXAM

- Hallmark: maximum tenderness over medial femoral condyle proximal to joint line
- Plica often palpable in full extension
- Strength and flexibility deficits common
- Prone quad flexibility assessment critical
- Patellar mobility limited
  - ➤ Both factors exacerbate problem
- Pathophysiology
  - ➤ Medial parapatellar plica is a normal synovial fold
  - ➤ Remnant of embryologic development
  - ➤ Other plical folds
    - Ligamentum mucosum
    - Suprapatellar plica
    - Lateral plicae extremely rare
  - ➤ Medial plica involved in practically all symptomatic plica syndromes
  - ➤ Synovium densely innervated
  - ➤ May become thickened and inflamed as result of localized blunt trauma or repetitive microtrauma

➤ Associated lateral patellar retinacular tightness may contribute by stretching plica tight.
➤ Quad inflexibility may compress plica beneath vastus medialis oblique (VMO).

STUDIES
■ Standard knee radiographs to rule out underlying pathology
■ Other studies not indicated

DIFFERENTIAL DIAGNOSIS
N/A

TREATMENT
■ Avoid provocative activity.
■ Correct strength and flexibility deficits.
■ Ice, tissue mobilization, NSAIDs
■ Phonophoresis over plica region
   ➤ Follow-up: 4–6 weeks
   ➤ Continue with program until asymptomatic or plateaued
■ Corticosteroid/local anesthetic injection (once) may be necessary to resolve symptoms
   ➤ Use after failure to progress
   ➤ Treats inflammation
   ➤ Diagnostic value too; if no acute relief, reconsider diagnosis
■ Arthroscopic plica resection for refractory patients
   ➤ Findings include:
      • Plica thickening
      • Synovitis around plica
      • Impingement of plica between patella and medial trochlea, chondromalacia of medial trochlea at site of impingement
      • Not all findings present in every patient

DISPOSITION
N/A

PROGNOSIS
■ Nonoperative treatment often successful
■ These patients overlap with anterior knee pain patients.
■ Surgical treatment in properly selected patients is highly effective.

CAVEATS AND PEARLS
■ Diagnosis made by history and physical examination

- Avoid plica resection found at arthroscopy if no clear pathologic changes.
- As a general rule, if you did not consider the diagnosis preoperatively, think twice.

POSTERIOR CRUCIATE LIGAMENT INJURIES

CHRIS HARNER, MD

HISTORY

- Posterior cruciate ligament (PCL) injuries 1/20 as common as anterior cruciate ligament (ACL) injuries
- Controversies regarding treatment
- Few surgeons perform >10 PCL reconstructions annually
- Multiple injury mechanisms
  - Fall on hyperflexed knee
  - Hyperextension
  - Hyperextension + varus
  - Hyperextension + valgus
- Suspect with dashboard injury (e.g., motorcycle, motor vehicle accident)
- Spectrum of pathology dependent on forces
  - High energy (e.g., motorcycle, motor vehicle accident, fall from height)
  - Low energy (e.g., sports)
- PCL injury can be isolated, combined, or associated with knee dislocation
- Initial complaints
  - Acute
    - Pain
    - Mild/moderate effusion
    - Posterior knee ecchymosis
    - Rule out associated knee dislocation
  - Chronic
    - Pain ± disability
      - Medial compartment pain
      - Patellofemoral pain
    - Instability if associated with posterolateral corner (PLC) injury
  - Isolated PCL may be asymptomatic

PHYSICAL EXAM
- Acute and chronic
  - Assess neurovascular status
  - Loss of motion
  - Effusion (usually less than ACL)
  - Posterior drawer test
    - Knee flexed 90°
    - Posterior force applied to tibia
    - Grade 1 – Medial tibial plateau step-off visible/palpable anterior to medial femoral condyle
    - Grade 2 – No step-off, flush with medial femoral condyle
    - Grade 3 – Step-off visible/palpable posterior to medial femoral condyle
  - Posterior sag test (Godfrey test)
    - Hip and knee flexed to 90°
    - Assess effect of gravity
    - Look for posterior "sag" of tibial plateau (compare contralateral)
  - Rule out associated ACL injury
    - Lachman
    - Anterior drawer
    - Pivot shift test
  - Assess for medial collateral/lateral collateral ligament laxity
    - Instability at 0° – Suspect ACL or PCL + collateral injury
    - Instability at 30° – Most sensitive for collateral ligament injury
  - Assess PLC
    - ACL and PCL injury often occur together
    - Most common associated ligamentous injury
    - Posterolateral spin at 90° > 30° – PCL
    - Posterolateral spin at 30° > 90° – PLC
    - Dial test/thigh foot angles
      - Perform supine or prone to compare side-to-side tibial external rotation
      - Increased with PLC injury
      - Minimally increased with isolated PCL injury
      - Greatest with combined PCL + PLC injuries
  - Extension-recurvatum test
    - Excessive asymmetric hyperextension
    - Implies PLC injury

➤ Reverse pivot shift
  • Knee is subluxed in flexion (~90 degrees)
  • Knee reduces in extension (~0–10 degrees)
  • Opposite of ACL pivot shift
  • Greatest with combined PCL + PLC injuries
➤ Gait analysis
  • Most critical in chronic situation
  • Assess knee alignment
    • Chronic varus malalignment + PCL
      • Surgical Tx – Consider osteotomy
    • Check for hyperextension

STUDIES
■ Radiographs
  ➤ AP and lateral most critical
  ➤ Flexed weight-bearing PA
    • Chronic PCL injury may show early degenerative joint disease (DJD)
  ➤ Merchant (skyline)
    • Chronic PCL injury may show patellofemoral DJD
  ➤ Mechanical axis/full length
    • Assess alignment, especially in chronic setting
■ MRI
  ➤ Can identify location of injury
  ➤ May demonstrate interstitial injury
  ➤ Very helpful in combined ligament injuries
■ Bone scan
  ➤ Used to assess early DJD
  ➤ Recommended for monitoring patients
■ Arteriogram
  ➤ Order if knee dislocation suspected
■ Stress radiographs
  ➤ Uncommonly used
  ➤ Little benefit

DIFFERENTIAL DIAGNOSIS
■ Acute
  ➤ ACL vs. PCL
  ➤ R/O combined ligament knee injuries
  ➤ MRI very helpful

- Chronic
  - Instability
    - R/O ACL injury
    - Combined PLC injury
  - Pain
    - Medial compartment/patellofemoral compartment DJD
    - Medial meniscus pathology (be aware that posterior sag displaces the medial meniscus and can create medial joint line pain)

TREATMENT
- Based on severity of injury and activity level of patient
- Acute/chronic
  - Determine if isolated versus combined injury
    - Grade 1 – Most treated conservatively
      - PCL may undergo partial healing
      - Some grade 2 injuries do not do well
      - Quad rehab
    - Grade 2/3
      - Splint in full extension for 1 month
      - Quad rehab
    - Combined – usually surgically treated
  - PCL surgical treatment
    - Open or arthroscopic techniques
    - Controversies regarding best methods
      - Single vs. double bundle
      - Transtibial vs. tibial inlay
    - Controversies regarding graft choices
      - Autograft vs. allograft
      - Patellar tendon vs. hamstring vs. quad tendon vs. Achilles tendon
    - In chronic PCL – address other patholaxities
    - If varus malalignment
      - Think osteotomy
      - Sagittal plane osteotomy to decrease posterior translation
  - Residual loss of flexion – 5–10° loss of flexion common following surgery
  - Graft laxity – at best, most knees will be a trace to 2+ posterior drawer
  - Graft failure

- Few long-term studies – Spectrum of severity, acute vs. chronic, and isolated vs. combined makes comparison difficult
- Post-op rehabilitation
  - ➤ Concept – Avoid posterior sag
  - ➤ Immobilize in full extension for 2–4 weeks to protect PCL repair
  - ➤ Delay active knee flexion to reduce posterior forces
  - ➤ Some surgeons use prone passive or active assisted flexion early
  - ➤ Quad rehab program ~3 months
  - ➤ Consider knee manipulation if knee flexion not progressing beyond 10–12 weeks

DISPOSITION
N/A

PROGNOSIS
- Return to play
  - ➤ Insolated nonsurgical
    - Grade 1 or 2 – 2–4 weeks
    - Grade 3 – 4–6 weeks
  - ➤ Combined injuries requiring surgery: 9–12 months post-op
- Complications
  - ➤ Neurovascular injury with initial injury or surgical treatment
  - ➤ Avascular necrosis medial femoral condyle rare
  - ➤ Arthrofibrosis
  - ➤ If "anterior drawer" > Lachman translation, suspect PCL
  - ➤ Patellofemoral symptoms may be initial complaints of unrecognized PCL
  - ➤ Chronic medial compartment pain may be related to PCL
  - ➤ Major concerns: ACL, PLC

CAVEATS AND PEARLS
- Suspect PCL injury in patient with "dashboard" type of mechanism
- Always rule out associated ligamentous injuries
- Obtain radiographs to rule out avulsion fracture
- In combined injury, always suspect possible knee dislocation
- PCL reconstructions should be performed by experienced ligament surgeons
- Surgical patients must be apprised of severity and difficulty of procedure
- Inform surgical patients of potential for neurovascular injury

POSTERIOR SHOULDER INSTABILITY

BRIAN J. COLE, MD
ROBERT A. SELLARDS, MD
REVISED BY CHARLES NOFSINGER, MD

HISTORY

- Less common shoulder instability: 2–4% of all glenohumeral dislocations
- Common in football lineman
- Mechanism
  - Direct: posterior-directed force at proximal humerus
  - Indirect: flexion, internal rotation, adduction
  - Other: 3 E's: ethanol, epilepsy, electricity
- Associated with laxity and may be voluntary
- >50% undiagnosed at initial presentation and may present late
- Associated findings
  - Reverse Bankart: posterior inferior labrum torn from glenoid
  - Posterior capsular attenuation or damage
  - Reverse Hill-Sachs: anterior medial humeral head and cartilage injury

PHYSICAL EXAM

- Symptoms (i.e., pain) recreated with arm flexion and internal rotation
- Locked posterior dislocation: fixed internal rotation, prominent coracoid
- Posterior subluxation: positive posterior stress test
- Voluntary positional and/or muscular instability (rule out psychological)

STUDIES

- Radiographs
  - Trauma series: true AP, scapular "Y" and axillary views
- CT scan
  - Identify associated fractures (glenoid, humeral head)
  - Rule out excessive glenoid retroversion
- MRI
  - Less commonly needed
  - Detect labral lesions

- Exam under anesthesia
  - ➤ Determine principal direction of instability
  - ➤ Grading (based on translation of humeral head)
    - 0: Normal
    - 1: To glenoid rim
    - 2: Over glenoid rim with spontaneous reduction
    - 3: Locking over glenoid rim
    - Abnormal: anterior translation of grade 2 or greater on affected side
    - Abnormal: posterior translation of grade 3
    - Normal: bilateral posterior translation of grade 2 or less
- Define secondary direction of instability
- Rotator interval: sulcus sign with inferior traction (space increases between lateral acromion and top of humeral head) in adduction that persists in external rotation
- Test in various arm positions

DIFFERENTIAL DIAGNOSIS
- Other instability patterns (i.e., bidirectional, multidirectional)
- Voluntary instability
- Laxity – excessive (but normal) asymptomatic passive glenohumeral translation

TREATMENT
- Dislocation <6 weeks
  - ➤ <20% head defect – closed reduction and immobilization 3–4 weeks
  - ➤ >20% head defect – closed reduction, consider subscapularis transfer
- Dislocation >6 weeks
  - ➤ Closed or open reduction as needed with immobilization 3–4 weeks
  - ➤ If >20% head defect, consider subscapularis transfer
  - ➤ If >40% head defect, consider arthroplasty
- Nonoperative treatment: rehabilitation
  - ➤ Strengthening of external rotators and posterior deltoid
- Surgical indications
  - ➤ Inability to achieve reduction
  - ➤ Recurrence
  - ➤ Pain
  - ➤ Loss of function

- Surgical technique: open
  - Posterior vertical incision centered at glenohumeral joint
  - From spine to axillary fold
  - Interval: between infraspinatus and teres minor
  - Deltoid split, partial release of infraspinatus and teres minor laterally
  - Avoid dissection below teres minor (quadrilateral space)
  - Medial labral repair with capsular shift as needed
- Surgical technique: arthroscopic
  - Lateral decubitus with traction
  - Suture anchors, single-point fixation device (i.e., Suretac), knotless anchors
  - Repair labrum lesion anatomically
  - Identify and address all pathology
  - Evaluate rotator interval (anterosuperior capsule)
  - Capsular plication
  - Thermal shrinkage can lead to posterior capsular destruction
- Rehabilitation
  - Handshake orthosis 0–6 weeks
  - Protected range of motion in external rotation, full extension after 6 weeks
  - Active range of motion as tolerated after 12 weeks
  - Sports at 6–9 months

DISPOSITION
N/A

PROGNOSIS
- Results
  - Higher recurrence rates vs. anterior instability
- Complications
  - Recurrence
  - Loss of internal rotation

CAVEATS AND PEARLS
- Axillary view to determine direction of dislocation
- High index of suspicion in acute setting with appropriate mechanism
- Examination with comparisons to contralateral shoulder
- Evaluate for voluntary instability with psychological disturbance

POSTERIOR TIBIAL TENDON INJURY

CAROL FREY, MD

HISTORY

- Dysfunction of the posterior tibial tendon (PTT) due to tendinosis or rupture results in:
  - ➤ Pain over the tendon
  - ➤ Loss of tendon function
  - ➤ Progressive pes planovalgus deformity
- Possible etiology
  - ➤ Pes planus/pronation and ligament laxity
    - Chronic stress on the PTT
    - EMG shows increased duration and intensity of PTT activity in pronated feet
  - ➤ Intratendinous shear stress
    - Multiple insertion sites
    - Independent motion of insertion sites creates shear stress
  - ➤ Seronegative inflammatory disease
  - ➤ Attritional tendon degeneration
  - ➤ Trauma
  - ➤ Iatrogenic
    - Steroid injection into tendon
    - Cortisone weakens collagen fibers

PHYSICAL EXAM

- Stages of clinical presentation
  - ➤ Stage I
    - Pain with activity
    - Swelling, tender along tendon
    - Single-leg heel rise may be positive
    - No deformity
  - ➤ Stage II
    - Pain along PTT
    - Flexible pes planovalgus foot
    - Single-leg heel rise is positive
    - May have lateral impingement of subtalar joint or calcaneofibular abutment
  - ➤ Stage III
    - Stiff, fixed deformity of subtalar or transverse tarsal joint

- Lateral abutment
- Degenerative joint disease in hindfoot

STUDIES

- Standing AP radiograph
  - ➤ Lateral subluxation of talonavicular joint
  - ➤ Abducted forefoot
- Standing lateral radiograph
  - ➤ Midfoot sag (talonavicular, navicular cuneiform, and cuneiform metatarsal joints)
- Standing AP ankle radiograph
  - ➤ Demonstrate calcaneofibular abutment
  - ➤ Rule out valgus tilt at tibiotalar joint
- Tenography
  - ➤ Invasive
  - ➤ Difficult to interpret
  - ➤ Poor correlation with surgical findings
- MRI
  - ➤ Sensitive
  - ➤ Anatomy well defined
  - ➤ Order if diagnosis in question
- Ultrasound
  - ➤ Tendon size
  - ➤ Fluid
  - ➤ Intratendinous changes
  - ➤ Cheap
  - ➤ Fast
  - ➤ Under investigation

DIFFERENTIAL DIAGNOSIS

- Subtalar dysfunction
- Medial ankle sprain
- Tarsal tunnel syndrome
- Flexor hallucis longus tendinitis
- Flexible pes planus
- Tarsal coalition
- Plantar fasciitis/rupture

TREATMENT

- Stage I (tendinitis with no deformity)

➤ Nonoperative
- Rest
- Short-leg cast
- NSAIDs
- Physical therapy
  - Achilles tendon stretch
  - PT resistive strength
  - Modalities
- Extradepth shoe, firm medial heel counter
- Total contact insert with medial post and firm arch support
- Short custom AFO

➤ Operative
- No response to nonoperative treatment in 3–4 months
  - Tenosynovectomy, debridement
  - Tendon repair
  - Tendon transfer augmentation
  - May add medial displaced calcaneal osteotomy if flexible flatfeet with hindfoot valgus (reduces stress on tendon repair)

■ Stage II (tendon degeneration with elongation, flexible deformity)
➤ Nonoperative
- NSAIDs
- Orthotic with medial post and firm arch support
- UCBL orthotic device
- Extradepth shoe with firm medial heel counter
- Medial flare to heel
- Custom AFO

➤ Operative
- Tendon repair and transfer with flexor digitorum longus; may fail if used alone
- Arthrodesis
  - Subtalar
  - Talonavicular
  - Double arthrodesis (T-N, C-C)
  - Triple arthrodesis
  - Lateral column lengthening with arthrodesis at C-C joint
  - Combination of limited arthrodesis with tendon reconstruction
- Medial displacement calcaneal osteotomy with tendon reconstruction

- Evans-type calcaneal lengthening osteotomy with tendon reconstruction
- Evans-type calcaneal osteotomy with medial displacement calcaneal osteotomy and tendon reconstruction

■ Stage III (fixed deformity)
- ➤ Nonoperative
  - Orthotic medial post with arch support
  - Extradepth shoe with extended firm medial heel counter
  - AFO
- ➤ Operative
  - Arthrodesis
    - Subtalar
    - Double (C-C, T-N)
    - Triple – Usually required

DISPOSITION
N/A

PROGNOSIS
N/A

CAVEATS AND PEARLS
■ Medial displacement calcaneal osteotomy contraindicated with significant fixed forefoot varus (needs triple)
■ If marked forefoot abduction, may need lateral column lengthening
■ If stiffness or degenerative joint disease of the hindfoot joints, do not do medial calcaneal displacement osteotomy.
■ Medial shift of calcaneus reduces valgus moment arm of gastrocsoleus muscle.
■ Heel valgus corrected with medial displacement calcaneal osteotomy and subtalar motion preserved
■ Posterior tibial tendon dysfunction is the most common cause of an acquired flatfoot deformity.
■ Loss of PTT function causes rotatory subluxation of calcaneus in relation to the talus.
■ Achilles tendon usually contracted with PTT dysfunction

POSTEROLATERAL KNEE INJURIES

ROGER V. LARSON, MD
REVISED BY CHARLES NOFSINGER, MD

HISTORY

- Sports, work, or motor vehicle injury
- Often considerable trauma involved
- Rarely an isolated injury
- Often associated with other injured ligaments – anterior cruciate ligament (ACL), posterior cruciate (PCL)
- Mechanism includes varus, hyperextension, or external tibial rotation
- Can include major lateral disruption with peroneal nerve injury
- If chronic may include
  - Hyperextension "give way" (functional instability with knee in extension)
  - Posterolateral pain
  - Varus "thrust"
  - Occasional peroneal nerve symptoms
- More symptomatic with varus knee alignment
- "Give way" when pivoting (especially away from involved knee)

PHYSICAL EXAM

- Increased external tibial rotation at all flexion angles (thigh/foot angle)
- If acute, lateral and posterolateral tenderness and possibly ecchymosis
- If isolated will have slight increase of posttibial translation near 30° but not at 90° flexion
- Frequent increased varus laxity
- Occasional increased hyperextension
- Positive posterolateral drawer test
- Positive reverse pivot shift
- Occasionally positive external rotation/recurvatum test (Hughston)
- In varus knee and chronic instability may have "varus thrust" with ambulation
- Commonly will have associated ACL or PCL laxity

STUDIES

- Radiographs

➤ AP, lateral, tunnel, Merchant (four views)
➤ May be normal
➤ May have associated intra-articular fracture (plateau)
➤ May have ligament avulsions (fibular head, Gerty's tubercle) or proximal fibular fracture
■ MRI
➤ Excellent for evaluation of lateral/posterolateral structures
➤ Lateral collateral ligament (LCL), biceps, lateral capsular structures accurately defined
➤ Popliteofibular ligament less well defined
➤ Associated ligament and meniscal pathology well defined
■ Stress radiography
➤ Helpful in documenting and quantitating varus laxity
➤ Helpful in document and quantitating associated PCL laxity

DIFFERENTIAL DIAGNOSIS
■ Lateral injury without disruption of major restraints to posterolateral rotation (i.e., biceps tendon avulsion, iliotibial band avulsion)
■ Anteromedial instability (need to observe to determine which tibial plateau is translating with external rotation)
■ Isolated ACL or PCL tear (will not have increased external tibial rotation)
■ Anterolateral instability (will have positive pivot shift)

TREATMENT
■ Acute
➤ Establish diagnosis and define injured structures.
➤ Splint
➤ If isolated, posterolateral rotatory injury (PLRI) and minor instability may be treated with bracing and rehabilitation
➤ If major lateral disruption, will likely need early operative intervention (within 3 weeks) for direct anatomic repair, possible augmentation
➤ If peroneal nerve involved may need early exploration/decompression
■ Treatment Considerations
➤ Age and activity level
➤ Varus or valgus mechanical alignment
➤ Degree of laxity
➤ Associated instabilities

- Treatment options (chronic)
  - Advancement and reefing of existing structures (usually bone block recession at epicondyle)
  - Creation of static restraint in position of popliteus tendon (popliteus bypass procedure)
  - Creation of restraint in position of LCL and popliteofibular ligament
    - Biceps tenodesis (entire or partial)
    - Reconstruction with free grafts (autograft or allograft)
    - Combinations of above
    - Valgus osteotomy as initial procedure if varus alignment and lateral thrust

DISPOSITION
N/A

PROGNOSIS
- Frequently missed diagnosis that leads to chronic functional instability
- With acute severe disruptions best results with early intervention (within 3 weeks) for anatomic repair and augmentation
- Many factors involved in prognosis since rarely isolated injury

CAVEATS AND PEARLS
- Isolated PCL tear does not create increased external tibial rotation at 30° and 90° of knee flexion. If present there is combined injury involving posterolateral corner.
- If combined injury (PCL, posterolateral corner), treating only the PCL will not correct abnormal rotation (PLRI).
- With acute severe lateral disruptions, early (within 3 weeks) repair/augmentation provides best results.
- Reconstructions should include tissue in position of popliteofibular ligament (i.e., attach to fibular head).
- Varus alignment with PLRI should be corrected with osteotomy before soft tissue reconstruction.

POSTTRAUMATIC ULNAR WRIST PAIN

ARTHUR RETTIG, MD
RON NOY, MD

HISTORY
- Mechanism of injury
  - Fall on outstretched arm with wrist dorsiflexed and radially deviated (intercarpal pronation)
  - Results in triquetrolunate ligament injury
  - May result in triangular fibrocartilage complex (TFCC) tear
  - May result in distal radioulnar joint (DRUJ) sprain or dislocation
- Complaints
  - Pain ulnar aspect of wrist and stiffness
  - May complain of click
  - May hear or feel pop
  - Chronic cases may report
    - Ulnar wrist pain
    - Click
    - Pain with pronation/supination (TFCC, DRUJ injuries)
    - Pain with ulnar deviation of wrist
- Frequently presents remote from injury
- If midcarpal instability, frequently no history of injury

PHYSICAL EXAM
- Acute
  - Tenderness of lunotriquetral (LT) ligament, TFCC, or DRUJ
  - Swelling, decreased range of motion
  - For LT ligament injury, Reagan shuck test or Klineman shear test helpful
  - For TFCC injuries and DRUJ
    - Pain at extremes of pronation and supination
    - May demonstrate catching in TFCC injures
  - Demonstrate pain with passive ulnar deviation
  - Check two-point discrimination
- Chronic
  - Tenderness at site of injury (LT ligament, TFCC, or DRUJ)
  - Decreased grip strength
  - For LT injury, Reagan shuck test or Klineman shear test

➤ For TFCC injuries, pain at extremes of pronation/supination and ulnar deviation
➤ Piano key sign for DRUJ instability
➤ Catch-up clunk for midcarpal instability

STUDIES
■ Radiographs
  ➤ Usually plain radiographs normal
  ➤ If grade II-III LT ligament injury (with associated palmar radial lunate triquetrum) dorsal radial triquetrum
  ➤ VISI pattern present on lateral view (palmar-flexed lunate-scaphoid)
■ Arthrogram helpful to rule out TL perforation and TFCC perforation
■ Bone scan helpful to localize pathology if other studies negative – nonspecific
■ MRI with contrast may be helpful in TFCC tears and TL tears (unreliable)
■ Cinefluoroscopy helpful in midcarpal instability
■ CT scan helpful to rule out bony injuries such as hook of hamate fractures
■ Arthroscopy
  ➤ Gold standard for TFCC tears, LT ligament tears
  ➤ Advantage of combining diagnosis with treatment

DIFFERENTIAL DIAGNOSIS
■ LT ligament injuries – clinical – MRI, arthroscopy
■ TFCC injuries – clinical – MRI, arthroscopy
■ DRUJ instability – clinical – dynamic axial CT scan
■ Hook of hamate fracture – bone scan, CT scan
■ Midcarpal instability – exam, cinefluoroscopy
■ Hypothenar hammer syndrome (Guyon's canal) – Doppler, arteriogram
■ Chondral lesion proximal pole hamate – clinical injection, arthroscopy
■ Ulnar carpal impingement syndrome – x-ray, exam
■ Ulnar styloid carpal impingement syndrome – x-ray, injection

TREATMENT
■ Acute
  ➤ TL ligament injuries (grade I) – no x-ray changes
    • Rest, splint for 3 weeks
    • If symptoms after 6–8 weeks, arthroscopy, pinning

➤ TFCC injuries – if DRUJ stable
  • Rest, splint
  • If symptoms after 6 weeks, arthroscopy, debridement vs. repair
➤ TFCC injury if unstable DRUJ
  • Arthroscopy, repair
➤ Midcarpal instability
  • Usually not seen acutely
  • Rest, splint – no reliable surgical treatment other than four-corner fusion
➤ Chondral lesion proximal hamate
  • Arthroscopy, debridement

■ Chronic
➤ TL ligament injuries
  • If symptomatic, TL arthrodesis (if no ulnar impaction)
  • Beware of ulnar impaction (ulnar + variance) – may do ulnar shortening to enhance stability of TL joint
➤ TFCC injury – if symptomatic
  • If radial tear – debridement
  • If peripheral tear, may repair with arthroscopically assisted suture technique
  • If ulnar + variant, may require ulnar shortening (either Felden wafer or shortening osteotomy)
➤ Midcarpal instability
  • Rest, splint, special splint for sports to support ulnar aspect of carpus
  • If nonoperative treatment fails
  • Accept and modify activity
  • Reconstruction ulnar link of V ligament (unpredictable)
  • Four-corner (ulno-capitate-lunate-triquetral) arthrodesis
  • Results in decreased range of motion – radial deviation/ulnar deviation and flexion/extension
➤ DRUJ instability
  • If no arthrosis – reconstruction
  • Many procedures, none predictable, ulnar shortening if ulnar + variance
  • If arthrosis, DRUJ arthrodesis and ulnar osteotomy (Suave Kapandji), hemiresection arthroplasty (Bowers)

DISPOSITION
N/A

PROGNOSIS

- TL ligament – if grade I – good results with rest, splinting
  - ➤ Results of TL pinning or arthrodesis unpredictable
  - ➤ Rehab: short-arm cast for 6 weeks
  - ➤ Return to sports 4–6 months
- TFCC tear
  - ➤ Good results with debridement radial tear if ulnar neutral or negative variance
  - ➤ Return to sports 6–8 weeks
  - ➤ Good results if repair peripheral tear if performed <3 months
  - ➤ Poorer results with ulnar carpal impingement
- Midcarpal instability – usually do well with modified activity, splinting
  - ➤ Results of surgery variable
  - ➤ Must inform patient range of motion will be decreased after arthrodesis
- DRUJ instability
  - ➤ Surgical results variable

CAVEATS AND PEARLS

- Ulnar wrist pain very common
- Important to find anatomic point of tenderness if possible
- Obtain PA 0 rotation x-rays of both wrists to assess ulnar variance
- Beware of ulnar + variance as underlying cause of symptoms
- Wrist arthroscopy excellent diagnostic tool if all tests negative and patient fails adequate nonoperative treatment
- Clinical exam most important
- Be familiar with all possible differential diagnoses

PREPATELLAR BURSITIS

MATTHEW SHAPIRO, MD

HISTORY

- Usually the result of a direct blow to front of knee (dashboard mechanism)
- May be the result of repetitive injury from kneeling ("housemaid's knee")
- Consider possibility of septic bursitis

PHYSICAL EXAM
- Swelling anterior to patella, or overlying tibial tubercle
- Aseptic bursitis often painless
- Severe tenderness or erythema may be indicative of septic process

STUDIES
- In chronic cases stippled calcification may be visualized on x-ray.

DIFFERENTIAL DIAGNOSIS
- Dashboard mechanism also associated with patellar fracture, retro-patellar traumatic chondromalacia, and posterior cruciate ligament rupture.
- Consider other causes of anterior knee pain.

TREATMENT
- Symptomatic treatment with ice, NSAIDs, activity avoidance, and protective pad
- Consider aspiration and instillation of corticosteroid in trouble-some cases.
- In recalcitrant cases, surgical excision may be considered.
- Arthroscopic treatment has been recommended.

DISPOSITION
N/A

PROGNOSIS
- Rarely disabling, often simply troublesome
- May be cured with conservative treatment
- Surgical treatment for recalcitrant cases most often curative

CAVEATS AND PEARLS
- Beware of septic bursitis.
- Injection of steroid into a septic bursa can be disastrous.

PROXIMAL BICEPS TENDINITIS AND TENDON RUPTURE

FRANK A. CORDASCO, MD
REVISED BY CHARLES NOFSINGER, MD

HISTORY
- Mechanism of injury etiology
  - Concurrent impingement most common

> Primary bicipital tendinitis less common
> Acute traumatic: biceps dislocation (shallow groove or sub-scapularis tear)
> Acute traumatic: biceps disruption (narrow groove)
> Acute traumatic: biceps partial tear with SLAP tear
> Calcific tendinitis
■ Initial complaints
> Anterior shoulder pain
> Nocturnal discomfort
> Activity-related pain
> Inability to participate in athletic activity
> "Popping" (instability of biceps tendon)
> Asymmetry (instability vs. proximal disruption)
■ Complaints in chronic case
> Chronic anterior shoulder pain
> Nocturnal discomfort
> Limited use of arm overhead

PHYSICAL EXAM
■ Observation and inspection
> Proximal biceps asymmetry: instability vs. proximal disruption – "Popeye" muscle
■ Palpation
> Bicipital groove tenderness (humerus – 10° of internal rotation)
■ Special tests
> Speed's test: shoulder flexed, elbow extended (positive if pain with resisted flexion)
> Yergason's test: elbow flexed, resisted supination (positive if pain in groove)
> Ludington's test: hands behind head, isometric contraction biceps – subluxation
> De Anquin's test: arm rotated while examiner palpates anteri-orly (pain in groove)
> Heuter's sign: resisted elbow flexion in pronation and supina-tion (positive if pronation strength is greater)
> Selective injection tests: biceps sheath vs. subacromial space
   • Consider ultrasound-guided (radiology) lidocaine injection of biceps sheath

STUDIES
■ Plain radiographs
> Bicipital groove view

- Specific tests:
  - ➤ Obtained to identify degree of injury, associated pathology
  - ➤ Arthrography: may reveal biceps dislocation
  - ➤ Ultrasonography: accurate, technician-dependent
  - ➤ MRI: assess presence of associated pathology

DIFFERENTIAL DIAGNOSIS
- Impingement syndrome
- Glenohumeral instability
- SLAP tear
- Adhesive capsulitis
- Coracoid impingement

TREATMENT
- Nonsurgical management
  - ➤ Biceps tendinitis
    - Rest and modification of activity
    - NSAIDs
    - Corticosteroid injection: biceps tendon sheath – consider ultrasound-guided
    - Exercise and rehabilitation
      - Phase I: decrease inflammation, begin range of motion exercises
      - Phase II: active range of motion and progressive strengthening
      - Phase III: sport-specific adaptations, plyometrics, medicine ball rehabilitation
    - Adjunctive modalities
      - Ultrasound: thermal and nonthermal properties
      - Phonophoresis: ultrasound-enhanced delivery of topical medications
      - Iontophoresis: Uses electricity to introduce ions into skin
  - ➤ Long head biceps tendon rupture
    - Rest and modification of activity
    - NSAIDs
    - "Benign neglect"
  - ➤ Long head biceps tendon instability
    - Often associated with subscapularis tears
    - Does not generally respond well to nonoperative measures
- Surgical management
  - ➤ Biceps tendinitis

- Primary treatment: associated pathology – arthroscopic subacromial decompression and debridement
- Long head biceps tendon rupture or partial tear
  - Arthroscopic debridement of partial tear if good-quality tissue remains
  - Arthroscopic debridement of stump in complete tear and subacromial decompression
  - Tenodesis for complete rupture or large partial tear
  - **Transfer long head biceps tendon to short head biceps tendon**
  - Arthroscopic release for large partial tear: controversial
  - Arthroscopic repair of SLAP tear when present
- Long head biceps tendon instability
  - Tenodesis and treatment of any associated pathology
  - **Transfer long head biceps tendon to short head biceps tendon**
  - Reconstruction of transverse humeral ligament (mixed results)
  - Arthroscopic release: controversial

DISPOSITION
N/A

PROGNOSIS
- Nonsurgical treatment
  - Biceps tendinitis/long head biceps tendon rupture
    - Success: 70–85% if rotator cuff tendons intact
    - Success: 33–65% if rotator cuff tear present
  - Long head biceps tendon instability
    - Poor results unless instability and associated pathology (subscapularis) corrected
- Surgical treatment
  - Tenodesis: recent studies 60–88% success
  - Insufficient data regarding results of reconstruction of transverse humeral ligament, transfer long head biceps tendon to short head biceps tendon and arthroscopic release
- Return of play
  - 6 weeks to 3 months following arthroscopic debridement and decompression
  - 4–6 months following tenodesis or transfer
  - 4–6 months following SLAP repair (sport-specific)

➤ Criteria: no pain, full range of motion, strength within 90% of contralateral shoulder/elbow
■ Complications
  ➤ Failure of biceps tenodesis
  ➤ Failure of biceps tendon following debridement of partial tear

CAVEATS AND PEARLS
■ Biceps tendon pathology is rarely isolated
■ Impingement syndrome is the most common concurrent problem
■ Long head biceps tendon disruption: often associated with rotator cuff tears
■ Long head biceps tendon instability: often associated with subscapularis tear
■ Treatment of biceps tendon pathology must include treatment of associated pathology
■ Long head biceps tendon disruptions that are spontaneous and occur in the presence of an intact rotator cuff rarely require surgical intervention
■ Biceps found just distal to pectoralis major insertion in complete disruptions

PROXIMAL HUMERUS FRACTURES

GERALD R. WILLIAMS, JR., MD

HISTORY
■ Young patients: high-energy trauma
■ Older patients: fall from height
■ Mechanism – single-event trauma, direct blow to shoulder or indirect trauma to distal arm
■ Complaint – pain, inability to raise or use arm
■ May be associated injuries – complaints of pain in same arm or distant site

PHYSICAL EXAM
■ Swelling, ecchymosis subacutely
■ Marked tenderness of proximal humerus
■ Subtle deformity unless associated with dislocation
■ Do not move arm until after x-ray if fracture or dislocation suspected

- Vascular examination – radial and brachial pulses should be present and symmetrical
- Collateral circulation extensive – vascular injury may be subtle
- Sensory examination around shoulder is unreliable
- Must document motor function of five major peripheral nerves (axillary, musculocutaneous, radial, median, ulnar)
- Most common neurologic injury – mixed brachial plexus injury
- Most common single peripheral nerve injury – axillary nerve

STUDIES
- Radiographs
  - Radiographs are essential and often all that is necessary
  - Radiographs should include AP view, scapular lateral ("Y") view, and axillary lateral view
  - Axillary view essential for documenting associated dislocation, especially posterior
- CT scanning: secondary test to aid in quantitating tuberosity displacement or planning surgery
- MRI: not usually indicated; may show nondisplaced greater tuberosity fracture if x-rays are normal
- Arteriogram indicated if absent or asymmetrical pulses
  - Most common arteriographic abnormality: damage to third portion of axillary artery at origin of posterior humeral circumflex artery
- EMG not useful acutely
  - Used to clarify injury and follow recovery subacutely

DIFFERENTIAL DIAGNOSIS
- Contusion
- Dislocation with or without spontaneous reduction
- Subluxation
- Rotator cuff tear, especially in patients >40
- Adjacent fractures (clavicle, scapula)

TREATMENT
- **Acute**
  - Rule out dislocation
  - Reduce dislocation if present; beware of nondisplaced fracture lines
  - Sling, ice
- **Treatment considerations**
  - Age

➤ Associated injuries or medical problems
➤ Activity level
➤ Fracture displacement

■ **Treatment options**
➤ **Nonoperative**
  • Indicated in nondisplaced fractures and medically debilitated patients
  • Pendulum exercises within 7–10 days
  • Range of motion of elbow, wrist, and hand immediately
  • Progress passive mobilization – 3 weeks
  • Overhead pulley – 4–5 weeks
  • End-range stretching, strengthening – 6–8 weeks
  • Return to sport – pain-free, 80% strength (3–6 months)

➤ **Operative**
  • Closed or percutaneous reduction, percutaneous pinning
    • Young patient, good bone, little comminution
    • Two-part surgical neck, valgus-impacted four-part
    • Pins should be cut under the skin
  • Open reduction, internal fixation (blade-plate, percutaneous pins, sutures, intramedullary devices)
    • Comminuted surgical neck, isolated tuberosity fractures, three-part and standard four-part fractures in patients <40
  • Hemiarthroplasty – four-part fracture in patient >40
    • Cement standard
    • Tuberosity reconstruction to shaft and to one another
  • Postoperative rehabilitation
    • Immediate pendulum exercises
    • Progressive passive mobilization within 7–10 days
    • Pin removal at 3–4 weeks
    • Overhead pulley – 4–5 weeks
    • End-range stretching, strengthening – 6–8 weeks
    • Return to sport – pain-free, 80% strength (3–6 months)

DISPOSITION
N/A

PROGNOSIS
■ Any fracture with intra-articular component, even nondisplaced, will have greater stiffness
■ Functional result most correlated with residual displacement, especially tuberosities

■ **Nonoperative treatment**
  ➣ 80–90% good or excellent if rehabilitation started early (7–10 days)
  ➣ Return to sport when motion is pain-free and strength at least 80% (3–6 months)

■ **Operative treatment**
  ➣ Surgical neck – 80–90% good or excellent if rehab started early
  ➣ Isolated tuberosity – 80–90% good or excellent if rehab started early
  ➣ Three- and four-part – 10–15% good or excellent, 65–70% satisfactory (loss of motion), 15–20% unsatisfactory
  ➣ Return to sport if result is satisfactory, motion is pain-free, strength 80% (3–6 months)

■ **Complications**
  ➣ Nonunion – highest in surgical neck
  ➣ Malunion
  ➣ Avascular necrosis – 10–15% in three-part and valgus-impacted four-part; 60–80% in standard four-part
  ➣ Infection
  ➣ Neurovascular injury

CAVEATS AND PEARLS
■ Take adequate x-rays, especially an axillary view
■ Do not miss posterior dislocation
■ When using percutaneous pinning, cut pins under the skin
■ Try to obtain anatomic reductions whenever possible
■ Any treatment should allow early or immediate passive motion
■ Use intraoperative x-rays or fluoroscopy liberally to confirm fracture reduction and implant placement.

QUADRICEPS CONTUSIONS

DAVID C. NEUSCHWANDER, MD

HISTORY
■ Blunt trauma to anterior thigh
■ Exact injury may not be apparent in cases of mild injury and may not have precluded athlete from further play
■ Athlete usually notices localized pain, tenderness, and swelling with associated loss of knee flexion

PHYSICAL EXAM
- Hallmarks of exam are tenderness, swelling, and limited knee flexion
- Mild cases – Knee flexion >90°, localized tenderness, and no gait alteration
- Moderate cases – Knee flexion <90°, swollen tender muscle mass with antalgic gait
- Severe
  - Markedly tender thigh with marked swelling
  - Contour of muscle not defined by palpation
  - Usually need crutches for ambulation
  - Frequently associated with effusion of ipsilateral knee

STUDIES
- Initial x-rays negative
- X-rays at 3–4 weeks show localized densities within soft tissues
- Underlying bone may show evidence of periosteal reaction
- Both the soft tissue densities and periosteal reaction are early findings of myositis ossificans.

DIFFERENTIAL DIAGNOSIS
- Acute compartment syndrome – uncommon
  - Blunt trauma with progressively increasing swelling and pain out of proportion to that which would be expected
  - Must rule out bleeding diatheses, use of coumadin, or vascular injury
  - Often associated with continued play after initial contusion, but usually not associated with sensory deficit
  - Active quadriceps contraction and passive knee flexion significantly increase pain
  - Massive thigh swelling and complaint that leg feels better in dependent position than in elevated position
  - Paresthesia, if present, found over anterior knee (femoral nerve) and medial aspect of lower leg and foot (saphenous nerve)
  - Diagnosis made by anterior compartment measurements with pressure within 10–30 mm Hg of diastolic blood pressure
  - Treatment is anterior compartment fasciotomy
- Myositis ossificans
  - Occurs with compression of muscle tissue against underlying bone with injury to muscle fibers and blood vessels

TREATMENT

- R.I.C.E. (rest, ice, compression and elevation)
- Treatment in three phases
- Immobilize in knee flexion to limit hemorrhage
- Early restoration of pain-free motion
- Gradual functional rehabilitation for strength and endurance
- Avoid heat modalities including ultrasound, and avoid massage and stretch
- Usual return to activity after 1–3 weeks for mild injury and 5–10 weeks for moderate to severe injury
- Aspiration of hematoma and use of injectable proteolytic enzymes or use of acetic acid iontophoresis reported
- Rarely surgery necessary at 6 months after injury to remove mature myositis ossificans

DISPOSITION
N/A

PROGNOSIS

- May return to activity when pain-free with at least 120° knee flexion with the hip extended, and performing well with functional testing
- Wear circular wraps or thigh sleeve when returning to activity
- Majority of athletes able to return to activity 2–3 weeks

CAVEATS AND PEARLS

- Muscle of anterior thigh that lies in contact with bone throughout length of thigh is especially vulnerable to external compressive forces.
- Heat modalities including ultrasound should not be used; also, massage and stretch are contraindicated.
- Immobilization with knee flexion, along with thigh compression, increases tension in the anterior compartment and limits extent of intramuscular hematoma.
- Do not have athletes return to activity before completely rehabilitated; may easily reinjure and have higher risk of complications with reinjury.

QUADRICEPS STRAINS

DAVID C. NEUSCHWANDER, MD

HISTORY

- Acute anterior thigh pain caused by violent contraction against excessively forced stretch
- Commonly seen in track and field, football, basketball
- Symptoms may not be present until athlete finishes activity.
- Any active contraction of the quadriceps will exacerbate symptoms.
- If knee flexion is more painful with the hip extended than with it flexed, then there is greater involvement of the rectus femoris (only quadriceps muscle that crosses both hip and knee joints).
- If hip extension does not exacerbate pain and loss of knee flexion, then the vastus medialis, vastus intermedius, and vastus lateralis are most involved.

PHYSICAL EXAM

- Deep palpation can usually determine the site of injury (usually at rectus insertion into quadriceps tendon).
- May have palpable defect or mass that occurs only with muscle contraction

STUDIES

- Plain x-rays are generally normal.
- X-rays are helpful in chronic cases to rule out myositis ossificans.
- CT scan will have areas of low density near injury site, corresponding to the inflammation and edema of an acute injury.
- MRI T2-weighted images can delineate injury site and probably severity of injury, but not believed to be cost-effective or practical unless a complete tear is suspected.

DIFFERENTIAL DIAGNOSIS

- Femoral shaft or a femoral neck stress fracture (in case of rectus strain)
  - ➤ Would need high index of suspicion as x-ray would usually be normal and would need bone scan or MRI to aid with diagnosis
- Myositis ossificans in chronic cases

TREATMENT

- R.I.C.E. (rest, ice, compression, elevation)

- Grade I strains represent small area of muscle involvement with little hemorrhage and localized pain.
  - Have knee flexion of 90° or greater with mild symptoms and no functional loss with recovery in a few days
- Moderate or second-degree injury has partial tear of musculotendinous unit.
  - Knee flexion measured prone is usually <90°
  - Pain is more acute with loss of function
  - Swelling present and active contraction and passive stretch cause pain
  - Athlete will often use crutches in grade II or III injury.
  - Often difficult to differentiate grade II and grade III injury (complete tear of musculotendinous unit).
- Grade III injury usually with knee flexion <45°
  - Rehab program includes early motion and adjunctive modalities (ice, electrical stimulation, TENS, and compressive wraps and sleeves).
  - Surgical treatment recommended for complete musculotendinous tears of rectus femoris in the middle or lower third of the thigh.

DISPOSITION
N/A

PROGNOSIS
- Quadriceps reinjury more common than reinjury of a hamstring (but less common than reinjury of the adductors)
- Serial examination very important in determining athlete's progress through rehab process.
- Athlete may return to play when pain-free and has regained full knee motion and strength within 10% of contralateral leg.
- Recommend use of circular wrap or sleeve and protective pad when athlete resumes competition.
- Majority of grade I injury patients return to play in a few days; grade II injury patients return in 2–3 weeks.
- Potential complications of complete grade III tears include rerupture, weakness of knee extension, and lack of full knee flexion.

CAVEATS AND PEARLS
- Muscle strain injury occurs at the musculotendinous junction regardless of strain rate and architecture of the muscle.
- Strength and warm-up can protect against injury.

- Quads are type II (fast twitch) muscle fibers and are best trained by high-intensity and rapid activity.
- Early motion during healing phase desirable (high-speed, low-force isometric exercise) done concentrically
- Strains occur in musculotendinous junction; muscle contusions can occur anywhere along muscle.

RADIAL COLLATERAL LIGAMENT INJURY OF THE THUMB (REVERSE GAMEKEEPER'S)

GERARD GABEL, MD

HISTORY
- One-tenth to one-third as common as gamekeeper's
- Sports < work injury, home injury
- Mechanism: forceful ulnar deviation of thumb, usually a fall on out-stretched arm/adducted thumb
- May feel "pop" – tear of radial collateral ligament (RCL)
- Immediate pain
- Dysfunction due to pain and instability
- Weakness of grasp, with pushing
- Swelling along radial aspect of metacarpophalangeal joint
- Chronic cases complain of pain with use, mostly pushing activities
- Common sports: football, basketball
- May be acute superimposed on chronic
- May have dorsal capsular or volar plate injury (but RCL injury primary issue)

PHYSICAL EXAM
- Swelling, tenderness to palpation along radial > ulnar aspect of metaphalangeal (MP) joint
- No Stener's lesion equivalent
- Occasional mild interphalangeal (IP) or carpometacarpal (CMC) level tenderness
- Obtain plain x-rays prior to stress testing (if nondisplaced avulsion fracture, don't do stress exam)
- Ulnar deviation stress exam of RCL
  ➤ Usually requires Xylocaine block – 5 cc 2% Xylocaine, inject along radial metacarpal neck
  ➤ Hold MP joint in neutral deviation, 30° of flexion (to relax volar plate)

➤ Ulnarly deviate MP joint
➤ Check for degrees of laxity as well as firm end point
➤ Check in full extension to assess involvement of volar plate
➤ Check opposite thumb stress exam
➤ >25–30° of increased laxity indicative of complete RCL avulsion
➤ <25° of asymmetry, incomplete lesion
■ Chronic cases (>6 weeks postinjury)
➤ Less tenderness, but similar laxity findings
➤ May have firm end point
➤ Thumb rests in adducted position, radial metacarpal head prominent

STUDIES
■ Plain radiographs
➤ True AP/lateral of thumb centered at MP joint
➤ Findings: Avulsion fracture (displaced or nondisplaced), volar subluxation, ulnar deviation of MP joint
➤ Specific tests: stress AP x-rays (postblock)
  • To quantify/document degrees of angulation, to rule out Salter I or II growth plate fracture
  • Obtain on all patients except those with nondisplaced avulsion fractures
■ Arthrogram may show leak along RCL, may outline RCL; rarely used
■ MRI – excellent visualization in acute cases, less so in chronic cases

DIFFERENTIAL DIAGNOSIS
■ Salter fractures – Salter I fractures, if nondisplaced, may mimic RCL injury on exam and nonstress x-ray
➤ Must do stress x-ray on all patients with open growth and negative initial x-ray
■ Volar plate injuries – hyperextension injury, tender to extension stress, negative ulnar deviation stress exam
■ Metacarpophalangeal dislocation – hyperextension injury, plain film diagnosis; no stress exam

TREATMENT
■ Incomplete injuries
➤ Stable
  • Splint protection
  • Immediate active and passive range of motion
  • No varus/valgus
  • Resume sports as tolerated

➤ Unstable
  • Splint or cast immobilization 3 weeks
  • Active and passive range of motion
  • No varus/valgus
  • Return to sports as tolerated with or without thumb-based MP protective splint
■ Complete injuries: operative – some controversy as no Stener's lesion present, but still recommended
  ➤ 2.0-cm incision along radial MP joint
  ➤ Split abductor, reduce/pin MP in 15° of flexion/slight radial deviation
  ➤ Minisuture anchor repair of RCL to proximal phalanx margin (anatomic)
  ➤ Cast, start protected range of motion at 3 weeks
■ Chronic cases – ligament reconstruction using palmaris longus (or partial strip of radial wrist extensor or flexor)
  ➤ Same exposure as in acute cases
  ➤ Split remaining RCL longitudinally, identify/prepare anatomic origin and insertion, pin joint
  ➤ Harvest palmaris longus graft
  ➤ Minisuture anchors at origin and insertion double-strand graft reconstruction

DISPOSITION
N/A

PROGNOSIS
■ >90% good and excellent results (stable with good range of motion)
■ Mild to moderate loss of motion common (10–30°) – minimize with early/protected range of motion
■ Prognosis dependent on MP stability
■ Return to play
  ➤ If stable, return as pain permits
  ➤ If unstable/operative, return with abduction splinting/taping at 6–8 weeks

CAVEATS AND PEARLS
■ Don't misdiagnose Salter injury
■ Frequently overlooked; may be more disabling than gamekeeper's thumb

RADIAL HEAD FRACTURES

GEORGE A. PALETTA, JR., MD
STEVE BERNSTEIN, MD

HISTORY

- Indirect trauma
  - Fall on outstretched arm, axial force along radius
- Anatomy
  - Intra-articular
  - Articulates w/ capitellum
  - Governs forearm rotation
  - Provides secondary valgus stability
  - 60% of axial load at elbow through radiocapitellar joint
  - Radial head surface concave, capitellum convex
  - No actual contact until 135° elbow flexion

PHYSICAL EXAM

- Tenderness at radial head
- Effusion (hemarthrosis)
- Pain on active/passive forearm rotation
- Limited active/passive ROM
- MUST examine distal radial-ulnar joint (DRUJ)
  - R/O disruption DRUJ (Essex-Lopresti lesion)
- Examine medial side to R/O medial collateral ligament (MCL) injury
  - Valgus stress test
- Possible aspiration of hemarthrosis, injection local anesthetic
  - Facilitates exam of passive ROM

STUDIES

- Radiographs
  - Overlapping structures make interpretation difficult.
  - True lateral essential
  - Oblique (Greenspan views) may be helpful.
  - Nondisplaced fractures difficult to see
  - Posterior fat pad sign
  - R/O associated capitellum fractures
  - Ipsilateral wrist views to R/O Essex-Lopresti lesion
- CT scan
  - Helpful to assess comminution, displacement, fragment size
  - Helpful if considering ORIF

DIFFERENTIAL DIAGNOSIS
- Fracture classification
  - Modified Mason classification
    - Type I
      - Nondisplaced/minimally displaced (<2 mm)
      - No block to passive rotation
    - Type II
      - Marginal fracture with displacement (>2 mm), impaction, angulation
      - Good potential to achieve rigid internal fixation
    - Type III
      - Comminuted fracture of entire head
      - Poor potential to achieve rigid internal fixation
    - All types may have associated injuries:
      - Elbow dislocation
      - Interosseous ligament injury of forearm
      - Disruption DRUJ
      - Triangular fibrocartilage complex (TFCC) tear
  - Schatzker classification
    - Type I
      - Wedge fracture +/− displacement
    - Type II
      - Impaction fracture
      - Part of head/neck intact
    - Type III
      - Comminuted fracture

TREATMENT
- Based on Mason classification
- Type I
  - Splinting
  - Pain medication
  - ?Aspiration + injection local anesthetic
  - Early ROM as soon as comfort allows
- Type II
  - If limited motion
    - Aspiration + injection local anesthetic to assess mechanical block
  - If no block to motion
    - ?Closed reduction, splinting, early ROM
    - Most require ORIF

➤ If block to motion
- ORIF if amenable to fixation
  - Herbert/Acutrack screws, wires, bioabsorbable pins
  - Place fixation in "safe zone"
    - 110° arc on lateral side, 65° anterior, 45° posterior from mid-radial head w/ forearm in neutral
  - 50% radial head should be intake for ORIF.
  - Early ROM if stable fixation
- Excision if not amenable to fixation
■ Type III
➤ Excision radial head
- Just proximal to annular ligament
- Direct lateral approach
- Beware posterior interosseous nerve.
- Average 2 mm proximal radial translation (except DRUJ disruption)
- Early postop ROM
➤ Prosthetic replacement if MCL instability/DRUJ disruption
➤ MCL/DRUJ injuries must be addressed.
■ Late excision radial head
➤ Indications
- Pain, malunion, nonunion type II or III
- 80% good results
■ Radial head replacement
➤ Improve elbow stability
➤ Prevent proximal translation radius
➤ Silastic, metal, allograft implants
- Poor long-term using Silastic
➤ Indications
- Type III fractures w/ assoc elbow dislocation + gross instability
- Associated Essex-Lopresti lesion
- MCL/DRUJ disruption must be repaired.

DISPOSITION
N/A

PROGNOSIS
■ Complications:
➤ Radiocapitellar arthrosis
➤ Nonunion
➤ Proximal radial migration (>1 cm)
➤ Chronic valgus instability

CAVEATS AND PEARLS

- Examine DRUJ for Essex-Lopresti lesion
- Rule out associated MCL injury/valgus instability
- Consider hemarthrosis aspiration/local anesthetic injection
- True lateral radiograph critical. Oblique views may be helpful.
- If excision required, consider concomitant prosthetic replacement if associated MCL instability or DRUJ disruption
- Late radial head resection for painful malunion or non-union

---

RIB INJURIES

ROBERT A. SELLARDS, MD
BERNARD R. BACH, JR., MD

HISTORY

- Mechanism of injury
  - Direct – football tackle
  - Indirect – repetitive muscular contraction
- Child abuse possible in pediatric population
- Classification
  - First rib fractures
  - Rib fractures
  - Slipping rib syndrome
  - Stress fractures
  - Avulsion injuries
- Rib fractures
  - Direct – blunt force contacting chest wall
  - Indirect – repetitive muscular contraction
- First rib fractures
  - Direct
    - Etiology – high-energy trauma such as car crash
    - Think intrathoracic trauma
  - Indirect
    - Repetitive overhead sports or trunk rotation
      - Basketball players – rebound rib
      - Baseball players – throwing and nonthrowing arms
- Stress fractures
  - Golfers – fourth and sixth ribs of side with leading arm
  - Rowers – pain in posterolateral thorax around scapula
  - Swimmers, surfers, gymnasts, swinging athletes

- Slipping rib syndrome
  - Pediatric patients
  - Trauma to eighth, ninth, tenth ribs
  - Rib "slipping out of place"
- Avulsion injuries
  - Occur in lower ribs
  - Seen in baseball pitchers, heavy laborers

PHYSICAL EXAM
- Observation
  - Shortness of breath
  - Pain with deep inspiration
  - Deep breathing – spasm and pain
  - Bruising on thorax
  - Flail chest – paradoxical chest movement with inspiration
- Palpation
  - Palpate each rib to evaluate tenderness
  - Costovertebral angle tenderness – think renal injury
  - Auscultate lung fields to rule out pneumothorax
- Hooking sign
  - Slipping rib syndrome exam
  - Finger beneath costal cartilage of distal ribs
  - Pull anteriorly – if pain recreated, diagnosis confirmed

STUDIES
- Chest x-rays with coned-down view of painful area
  - Evaluate presence of pneumothorax
- Bone scan
  - Obtain if x-rays negative and pain persists
  - Good for stress fractures

DIFFERENTIAL DIAGNOSIS
- Renal injury with costovertebral angle tenderness
- Pneumothorax
- Rib contusion (no splinting with deep inspiration)
- Costochondritis

TREATMENT
- Usually nonoperative
- Ice, rest, NSAIDs, analgesics

- Intercostal nerve block
  - ➤ Administer when pain and spasms do not resolve
  - ➤ Infiltrate intercostal nerve and fractured rib
  - ➤ Bupivacaine effective
- Return to sport
  - ➤ May participate once pain has resolved
  - ➤ Early return places patient at risk for serious injury
- Other treatments
  - ➤ Chest binders – physician's discretion
  - ➤ Polyurethane jackets for football players – preventive
- Physical therapy
  - ➤ Strengthen serratus anterior and external oblique
  - ➤ Modify body movements (i.e., golf swing, rowing form)

DISPOSITION
N/A

PROGNOSIS
- Excellent with conservative treatment
- Rare nonunions may require rib excision versus open reduction and internal fixation

CAVEATS AND PEARLS
- Prolonged thorax pain in upper-body athlete – think stress fracture
- Coned-down radiographic views of painful ribs
- Rib problems in children – hooking sign

ROTATOR CUFF PATHOLOGY

FRANK A. CORDASCO, MD
REVISED BY CHARLES NOFSINGER, MD

HISTORY
- Mechanism of injury/etiology
  - ➤ Anatomic and mechanical
    - Acromion and coracoacromial arch (extrinsic)
      - Prominent coracoacromial ligament
      - Acromial morphology (types I, II, III)
      - Anterior acromial spurs (acquired)
      - Os acromiale (unfused acromial epiphysis)

- Acromioclavicular (AC) osteophytes
- Congenital subacromial stenosis
- Intrinsic cuff pathology
➤ Vascular factors
- "Critical zone" – tendon hypovascularity 1 cm medial to insertion
- "Watershed area" – anastomosis osseous and tendinous vessels
- Vascularity: bursal surface > articular surface
➤ Overuse syndrome
- Repetitive microtrauma
- Fatigue of scapular stabilizers: secondary impingement
➤ Glenohumeral instability
- Increased humeral head translation: tension overload of cuff
- "Internal impingement"
➤ Trauma: single event
➤ Scapulothoracic instability
- Long thoracic nerve injury: forward scapular tilt/secondary impingement
- Chronic AC separation: loss suspensory mechanism/secondary impingement
■ Initial complaints
➤ Pain
- Nocturnal discomfort
- Activity-related
➤ Loss of function
➤ Weakness
■ Complaints in chronic case
➤ Swelling "fluid sign"
➤ Progressive weakness
■ Classification
➤ Neer: three stages
- Stage I: edema and hemorrhage, <25 years old
- Stage II: fibrosis and tendinosis, 25–40 years old
- Stage III: partial or complete tears, >40 years old
➤ Post: size of tear
- Massive, >5 cm
- Large, 3–5 cm
- Medium, 1–3 cm
- Small, <1 cm

PHYSICAL EXAM
- Observation and inspection
  - Atrophy of spinati and/or deltoid (chronic)
  - Long head of biceps tendon disruption (chronic)
  - Scapular winging (long thoracic nerve injury)
- Palpation
  - AC joint tenderness (may be associated)
  - Bicipital groove tenderness (may be associated)
  - Greater tuberosity tenderness (acute)
  - Posterior glenohumeral joint line tenderness (chronic cuff tear arthropathy)
  - "Fluid sign" (chronic)
- Range of motion and strength testing
  - Four planes: forward elevation in scapular plane, external rotation neutral, external rotation 90° ABD, and internal rotation
  - Discrepancy between passive and active motion
  - Arc of pain (60–120°)
  - Weakness forward elevation in scapular plane and external rotation
- Special tests
  - Neer impingement sign: pain forward elevation in scapular plane >120°
  - Hawkins impingement sign: pain flexion to 90° and internal rotation
  - Impingement injection test: positive if impingement sign negative after injection
  - Jobe test: "empty can sign" – pain with resistance (also "full can sign")
  - External rotation lag sign (infraspinatus)
  - Drop sign (supraspinatus)
  - Lift-off test, Gerber (subscapularis)
  - Internal rotation lag sign (modified lift-off test, subscapularis)
  - Belly-press test "Napoleon's sign" (subscapularis)

STUDIES
- Plain radiographs
  - AP glenohumeral joint in the scapular plane external rotation & internal rotation – evaluate for:
    - Calcific deposits

- Excrescences of greater tuberosity
- Acromiohumeral interval (<7 mm): suggestive of full-thickness tear
- Early signs of cuff tear arthropathy (arthritis)
➤ Axillary view – evaluate for:
  - Os acromiale (unfused acromial epiphysis)
  - Joint space narrowing
  - Humeral head centering on glenoid
➤ Supraspinatus outlet view (Neer)
  - Acromial morphology
➤ AP 30° caudal tilt view (Rockwood) – evaluate for:
  - Anterior acromial spur and calcification of coracoacromial ligament
■ Specific tests:
➤ Evaluate integrity of rotator cuff tendons when marked loss of function occurs after acute injury or when conservative measures (see below) fail to improve symptoms
■ Arthrography
➤ Inexpensive and invasive
➤ Single/double contrast
➤ "Geyser sign" – erosion into AC joint
■ Ultrasonography
➤ Inexpensive and noninvasive
➤ Technician-dependent
■ Subacromial bursography (historical)
■ MRI
➤ Expensive and noninvasive
➤ Midsubstance and bursal surface tears
➤ Peribursal fat plane – loss of normal high signal – tear
➤ Size, retraction, specific tendons, muscle wasting and fatty substitution
➤ Can detect clinically insignificant pathology
➤ Surgical decisions should not be based on MRI alone

DIFFERENTIAL DIAGNOSIS
■ Instability
■ AC arthritis or osteolysis
■ Calcific tendinitis
■ Adhesive capsulitis
■ Coracoid impingement

- Cervical spine
- Suprascapular nerve palsy
- Parsonage-Turner syndrome
- Pancoast tumor

TREATMENT
- Nonsurgical management
  - Rest and modification of activity
  - NSAIDs
  - Exercise and rehabilitation
    - Phase I: decrease inflammation, begin range of motion
    - Phase II: active range of motion, progressive strengthening
    - Phase III: sport-specific adaptations, plyometrics, medicine ball rehabilitation
  - Adjunctive modalities
    - Ultrasound: thermal and nonthermal properties
    - Phonophoresis: ultrasound-enhanced delivery of topical medications
    - Iontophoresis: uses electricity to introduce ions the skin
- Surgical management (failure of nonoperative treatment)
  - Partial-thickness tears
    - Arthroscopic subacromial decompression
    - Open subacromial decompression
  - Full-thickness tears and large partial-thickness tears
    - Arthroscopic rotator cuff repair
    - Arthroscopically assisted rotator cuff repair (mini-open technique)
    - Open rotator cuff repair

DISPOSITION
N/A

PROGNOSIS
- Nonsurgical treatment
  - Rotator cuff tears: success rate 33–65%
    - Unfavorable outcome if:
      - Rotator tear >1–2 cm
      - Pretreatment history >1 year
      - Significant functional impairment
    - Few studies used outcome measures or instruments

- Surgical treatment
  - Subacromial decompression for partial-thickness rotator cuff tears
    - Satisfactory result: 75–90% of patients
    - Arthroscopic and open techniques: similar results
    - Arthroscopic: maximal improvement more quickly
    - Patients with worker's compensation claims have less favorable results
  - Rotator cuff repair for full-thickness tears and large partial-thickness tears
    - Satisfactory result in 80–90% of patients
    - Pain relief is predictable.
    - Improvements in function and strength more reliable in younger patients, smaller tears, and patients with recent onset of weakness
- Return to play
  - 6 weeks to 3 months following subacromial decompression for partial-thickness tears (sport-specific)
  - 4–6 months following repair (longer [9–18 months] for the throwing athlete)
  - Criteria: no pain, full range of motion, strength within 90% of contralateral shoulder
- Complications: factors associated with failed repairs
  - Large or massive tears
  - Poor-quality cuff tissue or fatty degeneration of muscle on MRI
  - Inadequate repair
  - Deltoid origin compromise
  - Lateral or radical acromionectomy
  - Insufficient subacromial decompression
  - Excessive subacromial decompression
  - Failure to treat associated AC joint pathology
  - Failure of suture anchors or hardware
  - Failure of graft materials
  - Denervation of deltoid or rotator cuff
  - Infection
  - Deficient or overly aggressive physical therapy

CAVEATS AND PEARLS
- Mobilize retracted tendons: release extra-articular adhesions
- Large and massive tears: release coracohumeral ligament ("interval slide")

- Large and massive tears: repair coracoacromial ligament to prevent "anterosuperior escape"
- Large and massive tears: modify postoperative rehabilitation
- Hydrotherapy useful in later stages of rehabilitation
- Outpatient repair: feasible with interscalene anesthesia
- Partial repair in massive tears better than decompression alone
- Avoid weights early in rehabilitation program
- Think rotator cuff tear in acute dislocation >40 with persistent pain

---

SCAPHOID FRACTURES

ARTHUR RETTIG, MD
RON NOY, MD

HISTORY
- Incidence
  - Most common fracture of the wrist in athletes
  - 70% of carpal fractures
  - 15- to 30-year-old males
- Mechanism of injury
  - Axial force with wrist in dorsiflexion and radial deviation
  - Fall on outstretched hand
  - Jamming/blocking
  - Puncher's scaphoid fracture
- Initial complaints
  - Pain
  - Inability to block (lineman)
  - Decreased range of motion
- Complaints in chronic case
  - Pain
  - With dorsiflexion
- Unable to perform push-up or bench press
  - Increased with cold weather when arthrosis present
- Other pertinent information
  - High index of suspicion
  - Concomitant injuries
    - Scapholunate dissociation
    - Radius fracture – 5%
  - Blood supply

- Distal dorsal ridge
- Proximal pole relatively avascular with fracture
  - Decreased healing
  - Increased rates of nonunion

- Classification
  - Location
    - Waist – 65%
    - Proximal pole – 30%
    - Distal pole – 5%
    - Dorsal ridge avulsion rare
  - Mayo
    - Tuberosity
    - Distal articular
    - Distal third
    - Middle third
    - Proximal pole
  - Russe
    - Horizontal oblique
    - Transverse
    - Vertical oblique
  - Herbert
    - A – Stable acute
    - A1 – Tubercle
    - A2 – Waist, incomplete
    - B – Unstable acute (both corticles involved on x-ray)
    - B1 – Distal oblique
    - B2 – Waist, complete
    - B3 – Proximal pole
    - B4 – Transscaphoid-perilunate fracture-dislocation
    - C – Delayed union
    - D – Established nonunion
    - D1 – Fibrous
    - D2 – Pseudoarthrosis
  - Cooney
    - >1 mm displaced – unstable

PHYSICAL EXAM

- Acute
  - Snuff-box tenderness
  - Decreased range of motion

➤ Swelling
➤ Pain with axial loading of the thumb
■ Chronic
  ➤ Decreased dorsiflexion
  ➤ Weak grip
  ➤ Radial wrist pain

STUDIES
■ Radiographs
  ➤ AP
  ➤ Lateral
  ➤ Dorsiflexed 30° + ulnar deviated 20°
  ➤ Oblique
  ➤ Initial x-rays may be negative
  ➤ Short-arm thumb spica cast
  ➤ Repeat x-rays at 1–2 weeks show periosteal reaction/early callus if fractured
■ MRI
  ➤ Most reliable
  ➤ Most athletes demand early immediate diagnosis
  ➤ Costly
  ➤ Edema around fracture site
  ➤ Shows fracture location well
  ➤ Concomitant injuries
    • Scapholunate ligament ruptures
    • Osteochondral injuries
■ CT
  ➤ False positives if nondisplaced
  ➤ Evaluation of union
■ Bone scan
  ➤ If >48 hours postinjury, no false negatives
  ➤ Nonspecific
  ➤ Invasive

DIFFERENTIAL DIAGNOSIS
■ Scapholunate dissociation
  ➤ Watson clunk test
  ➤ X-ray
  ➤ Terry Thomas sign
  ➤ Scapholunate angle >70°
■ Sprain

- Chondral injury of radioscaphoid articulation
- Contusion of scaphoid (MRI diagnosis)

TREATMENT
- Acute
  - ➤ Nonoperative
    - Indication: nondisplaced
    - Long-arm or Munster thumb spica cast for 4–6 weeks followed by a short-arm thumb spica cast until union
    - Slight radial deviation and volar flexion to relax radioscapho-capitate (RSC) ligament
    - Average time to union 9–12 weeks
    - Longer time to union as fracture site more proximal
    - Longer return to sports
    - 95% union rate
  - ➤ Operative
    - Indications
      - Displaced fractures
      - Nondisplaced fractures in athletes or laborers
      - Relative – proximal pole
    - Open reduction and internal fixation
      - Compression screws (most reliable)
      - K-wires
      - Volar approach for waist and distal fractures
      - Limited transscaphotrapezial
    - Russe
      - Dorsal approach – proximal pole fractures
      - Postoperative short-arm thumb spica
        - Proximal pole 4–6 weeks
        - Waist and distal 1–2 weeks
      - Earlier range of motion
      - Earlier return to sport
      - 4 weeks in playing cast (depends on sport and position)
      - Replace into short-arm thumb spica cast after game
      - Average 5–6 weeks – without cast
- Chronic
  - ➤ Delayed diagnosis 4–6 months postinjury
    - Nonoperative
      - Indications: nondisplaced-stable, 3–6 months to union
    - Operative
      - Indications: displaced, nondisplaced in an athlete

- Open reduction and internal fixation
  - Same approach as acute fractures
  - Usually require bone grafting
- Stable nonunion
  - Russe corticocancellous bone graft with or without internal fixation
- Unstable nonunion
  - Interpositional bone graft and internal fixation
  - Recreation of scaphoid shape
  - Eliminate humpback deformity
- Viability of fracture fragments
  - Punctate bleeding most reliable at time of surgery
  - If not viable, use vascularized bone graft or excise (especially in proximal pole fractures)
- ➤ Arthrosis
  - Salvage procedures: excision and partial fusion, proximal row carpectomy
- ➤ Failed bone graft procedures: repeat graft or salvage procedures – vascularized bone graft

DISPOSITION
N/A

PROGNOSIS
- ■ Nonsurgical treatment
  - ➤ 95% union rate
  - ➤ Long time to union
- ■ Surgical treatment
  - ➤ Acute
    - 95% union rate
    - Earlier return to play
    - Earlier motion
  - ➤ Chronic
    - Higher nonunion rates
    - Follow-up routine
    - Repeat x-rays at 1, 2, 4, 6, 10 weeks and then as necessary
    - Consider CT scan to evaluate for union if painful
- ■ Complications
  - ➤ Nonunion
  - ➤ Malunion
  - ➤ Scaphoid nonunion advanced collapse

➤ Humpback deformity
➤ Posttraumatic arthrosis

CAVEATS AND PEARLS

- Suspect scaphoid fracture in athlete with anatomic snuff-box tenderness
- Cannulated AO threaded washer/compression screw system with limited volar approach for waist fractures does not violate radiocarpus joint
- Herbert compression screw with dorsal approach for proximal pole fractures
- Always discuss risks and benefits of all options in detail with player, family, and coach/athletic trainers
- Placement of screw in central third increases union rate and decreases time to union
- Electrical stimulation controversial for delayed union

SCAPULAR FRACTURES

CARLOS A. GUANCHE, MD

HISTORY

- Direct trauma most frequent (70%)
- Axial load via upper extremity also possible
- Commonly confused with acute rotator cuff tear
- Most commonly motorcycle or motor vehicle accidents
- May occur in football and soccer
- High incidence of associated rib, clavicle, and pulmonary injuries (up to 70%)

PHYSICAL EXAM

- Painful glenohumeral motion
- Occasional scapulothoracic crepitus
- Ecchymoses after 24–48 hours (can be extensive)
- Rotator cuff dysfunction (may mimic acute rotator cuff tear)
- Examine for rib and clavicle fractures (up to 50%)
- Examine for brachial plexus injuries (up to 12%)
- Possible ipsilateral brachial and subclavian artery injury (11%)
- Examine for pulmonary injury (up to 50%)

STUDIES

- Radiographs
  - Scapular AP, scapular lateral and axillary views will show bony injury
  - Chest x-ray to evaluate for possible pneumothorax
- CT scan
  - In cases of glenoid involvement (including neck fractures)
  - Best for evaluation of intra-articular displacement
  - Include entire scapula
  - 3-D reconstructions helpful in management
- MRI
  - Best for evaluation of rotator cuff and possible labral involvement

DIFFERENTIAL DIAGNOSIS

- Rotator cuff tear – re-examine over several days unless MRI confirms no involvement
- Glenohumeral dislocation
- Labral tear
- Brachial plexus injury

TREATMENT

- Acute
  - Establish complete diagnosis
  - Ice posteriorly
  - Sling for comfort
  - Consider CT or MRI following plain films
  - Ensure glenohumeral joint is reduced
- Treatment considerations
  - Age
  - Activity level
  - Scapular neck fractures
    - Make up two thirds of scapular fractures
    - Usually impacted and extra-articular
    - Classification
      - Type I – nonangulated, nondisplaced
      - Type IIa – shortened, displaced >1 cm
      - Type IIb – angulated >40°
  - Glenoid fossa fractures (Goss classification)
    - Type Ia – anterior lip
    - Type Ib – posterior lip

- Type II – transverse, inferior glenoid
- Type III – transverse, superior glenoid
- Type IV – transverse, through body
- Type V – combination of types II and IV
➤ Scapular body fractures (Ada & Miller classification)
  - Type I – acromion, spine, coracoid
  - Type II – neck fracture
  - Type III – glenoid fracture
  - Type IV – body fractures
➤ Superior shoulder suspensory complex (SSSC)
  - Bony and soft tissue ring comprising glenoid, coracoid, cora-coclavicular ligaments, distal clavicle, and acromioclavicular joint
■ Treatment Options
  ➤ Surgical indications
    - Glenoid fossa displacement >5 mm anterior and >10 mm posterior
    - Glenoid neck fracture with >1 cm displacement or 40° of angulation
    - Persistent subluxation
    - Instability of glenohumeral joint
    - Disruption of SSSC
■ Nonoperative treatment
  ➤ Sling 2–4 weeks (depending on glenoid fossa involvement)
  ➤ Early pendulums

DISPOSITION
N/A

PROGNOSIS
■ Nonsurgical treatment
  ➤ Good results if glenoid articular surface is congruent and SSSC not disrupted
  ➤ Return to full activity likely
■ Surgical treatment
  ➤ Good results if glenoid articular surface well reduced
■ Return to play
  ➤ Same for surgical or nonsurgical treatment
  ➤ 8–10 weeks once bony consolidation occurs and range of motion and strength of shoulder girdle approach normal
  ➤ Contact allowed once fracture is consolidated

- Complications
  - Operative: nonunion of fracture, suprascapular nerve damage, posttraumatic arthrosis
  - Nonoperative: posttraumatic arthrosis, suprascapular nerve entrapment in fracture callus

CAVEATS AND PEARLS
- Ensure adequate initial radiographs
- Fully evaluate for pulmonary injuries
- Fully evaluate for brachial plexus injuries
- Evaluate for dislocation and continued disability with this component
- Evaluate for suprascapular nerve entrapment
- Significant impingement may occur if operative fracture is treated nonoperatively
- Surgical approach dictated by glenoid articular surface involvement
  - Anterior lip: anterior deltopectoral approach may require coracoid osteotomy for exposure
  - Posterior lip: posterior approach with deltoid detachment off scapular spine

SCAPULAR WINGING

CARLOS A. GUANCHE, MD

HISTORY
- Most commonly, insidious onset of vague shoulder girdle pain
- Possible direct trauma, traction or penetration injury over spinal accessory nerve distribution (trapezius) or long thoracic nerve distribution (serratus anterior)
- Rarely over dorsal scapular nerve distribution (rhomboid palsy)
- Possible recent surgical biopsy of lymph nodes in posterior cervical triangle (trapezius) or axillary region (serratus anterior)
- Possible pain secondary to impingement or radiculitis from brachial plexus traction
- Possible stiffness in shoulder from secondary adhesive capsulitis
- Possible remote scapular fracture
- Possible noise emanating from scapulothoracic joint
- Possible history of fascioscapulohumeral muscular dystrophy

PHYSICAL EXAM

- Static position of scapula
  - Normal in some situations (including rhomboid palsy)
  - Inferior angle laterally displaced with trapezius palsy
  - Inferior angle medially displaced with serratus anterior palsy
- Muscle atrophy evaluation (possible congenital absence)
  - Serratus anterior, trapezius, rhomboideus major and minor
- Examine scapulothoracic rhythm from posterior both with and without resistance
- Examine at 30°, 90°, and 150° of abduction and measure translation of inferior border from midline
- Compare contralateral (uninvolved) translation
- Examine for palpable crepitus and/or snapping
- Examine distal extremity for neurologic involvement of brachial plexus
- Complete examination of shoulder girdle, including sternoclavicular joint

STUDIES

- Radiographs
  - Scapular AP, scapular lateral and axillary views will show bony prominence (either scapula or rib)
- CT scan
  - Consider in bony abnormality
  - Include both scapulae in study to check for asymmetry
- MRI
  - Consider in muscular atrophy
  - Consider if a tumor is suspected
  - Consider in congenital anomalies of the muscles
- EMG
  - If neurologic abnormalities are present
  - In cases of muscle atrophy

DIFFERENTIAL DIAGNOSIS

- Posttraumatic winging
- Brachial plexus tumor
- Brachial plexus neuritis
- Postsurgical damage (node biopsy)
- Osteochondroma in scapulothoracic articulation
- Fascioscapulohumeral muscular dystrophy
- Deltoid fibrosis (congenital or secondary to multiple IM injections)

TREATMENT

■ Based on classification of winging
  ➤ Primary
   • Neurologic (trapezius, serratus anterior, rhomboideus palsies)
   • Soft tissue abnormalities (contracture, agenesis, avulsion)
   • Bursal (three common bursa; two under superior half, one under inferior angle)
   • Osseous (osteochondroma, tumor, fracture malunion)
  ➤ Secondary
   • Originates from glenohumeral joint abnormalities that disrupt scapulothoracic dynamics
   • Limited glenohumeral motion leads to excessive compensatory use of the periscapular muscles and subsequent fatigue
  ➤ Voluntary
   • Rare; largest series includes four patients
   • Extended rehab
   • Psychiatric consult
■ Initial, acute winging
  ➤ Based on EMG finding
  ➤ Rehab with serial EMGs is alternative (6 months to 1 year)
  ➤ In nerve transection, cable graft may be considered
  ➤ Neurolysis may be considered with results superior if performed within 6 months of injury
■ Operative treatment
  ➤ Usually involves either fusion (static) or transfer (dynamic) procedures
   • Static: scapulothoracic arthrodesis or stabilization using fascial slings
   • Dynamic: all involve muscle transfers
     • Trapezius palsy
       • Eden-Lange procedure: transfer levator scapulae and rhomboids laterally
       • 87% good/excellent results
     • Serratus anterior palsy
       • Transfer of sternocostal head of pectoralis major with fascia lata extension
       • 70–90% success rate
  ➤ Contraindication for transfer or fusion: ability to participate in activities without significant disability

➤ Extended rehab with activity modification is an option in high-level athletes
➤ Chronic bursitis can be treated with arthroscopic debridement
➤ Bony prominence may be resected open or arthroscopic

DISPOSITION
N/A

PROGNOSIS
■ Nonsurgical treatment
  ➤ In nonthrowing athletes, excellent prognosis
  ➤ Return to full activity based on functional ability
■ Surgical treatment
  ➤ Depends on etiology
    • Congenital: good prognosis; patients compensate well
    • Postsurgical nerve injury: based on nerve defect, 70-90% success rate with transfers for daily activities
      • No series of transfers on athletes
  ➤ Transfers limited for overhead activity and significant lifting for 3 months
■ Return to play
  ➤ Same for surgical or nonsurgical treatment
  ➤ 8–10 weeks once bony consolidation occurs and range of motion and strength of shoulder girdle approach normal
  ➤ Contact allowed once fracture is consolidated
■ Complications
  ➤ Nonoperative: shoulder impingement secondary to overall shoulder girdle mechanical malalignment
  ➤ Operative:
    • Fusion: nonunion, recurrent winging, painful pseudoarthrosis, pneumothorax
    • Transfers: failure of transfer, fibrosis, recurrence of winging
    • Arthroscopic debridement: continued pain, pneumothorax, nerve injury

CAVEATS AND PEARLS
■ Secondary winging due to glenohumeral abnormalities is most common
■ Severe pain and acute winging may be due to brachial plexus neuritis or Parsonage-Turner syndrome
■ Lateral position of inferior scapula at rest indicates trapezius palsy

- Medial position of inferior scapula at rest indicates serratus anterior palsy
- Minimal winging at rest indicates bony tumor in articulation or rhomboid weakness
- Congenital absence of serratus anterior, trapezius, and rhomboids has been reported; typically asymptomatic
- Remote obstetric palsy can lead to well-compensated winging
- Fascioscapulohumeral muscular dystrophy presents in the 30s or early 40s
- May have associated problems with facial expression, especially ability to whistle
- Autosomal dominant inheritance
- Usually bilateral winging

SESAMOID PROBLEMS

THOMAS O. CLANTON, MD

HISTORY
- Primary complaint is pain
- Pain localized beneath first metatarsal head aggravated by weight-bearing
- Stair climbing and sports participation provoke symptoms
- Often no specific precipitating event except in acute fractures

PHYSICAL EXAM
- Tenderness to direct palpation under the metatarsal head
- Tenderness may localize to specific sesamoid
- Restriction of motion secondary to pain
- Nonspecific findings: swelling, warmth, erythema, decreased plantarflexion strength, increased pain with dorsiflexion, supinated gait

STUDIES
- **Radiographs**
  - Standing AP and lateral views of the foot are routine
  - Additional views can be helpful
    - Oblique views (medial and lateral) useful for fractures and arthrosis
    - Tangential (coronal plane) sesamoid views useful for focal arthrosis or sagittal plane (axial) fractures

- **Bone scan**
  - Helpful to localize pathology but high rate of false positives
  - Often shows increased uptake before x-ray changes
- **CT scan**
  - Helpful for delineating extent of metatarsosesamoid arthrosis, defining fracture pattern
- **MRI**
  - May help diagnose sesamoid stress fracture, avascular necrosis, and acute infection

DIFFERENTIAL DIAGNOSIS
- **Sesamoiditis**
  - Often history of trauma or overuse
  - Risk factors: cavus foot or plantarflexed first metatarsal
  - Characterized by pain and tenderness localized to sesamoid – usually tibial (75%)
  - Plantar swelling may be present
  - Diagnosis of exclusion: rule out other causes of sesamoid pain
  - Nonoperative treatment: relieve stress on the sesamoid
    - Metatarsal pads placed proximal to the sesamoids
    - Soft arch support
    - Lower heel height
    - Stiffen sole of the shoe, add rocker sole or metatarsal bar
    - Activity modification
    - Anti-inflammatory medication
  - Surgery: only after failure of prolonged conservative treatment ~6 months
    - Excision of involved sesamoid
- **Stress fractures**
  - Usually the tibial sesamoid
  - History of activity-related pain, usually runners
  - Tenderness with palpation and with first metatarsophalangeal hyperdorsiflexion
  - Radiographs positive 3–6 weeks after symptom onset
  - MRI or bone scan helpful for diagnosis
  - Nonoperative treatment
    - Short-leg walking cast for 6 weeks
    - Activity modification
    - Orthosis or metatarsal pad
  - Surgical treatment

- Only after conservative treatment is exhausted >6 months
- Sesamoid excision permits a return to activity in 6–8 weeks
- Alternative to excision: curettage and autogenous bone grafting: heals by 12 weeks and retains flexor strength

■ **Acute fractures**
➤ Mechanism of injury: fall from a height, crush injury, forced great toe dorsiflexion and abduction
➤ Tibial sesamoid more commonly fractured
➤ Usually transverse
➤ Distinguish from partite sesamoid (see "Caveats and Pearls")
  - May require bone scan to differentiate
  - Remember that bipartite sesamoids are easier to fracture
➤ Nonoperative treatment
  - Short-leg walking cast or walking boot for 6–8 weeks
  - Shoe modifications: stiff sole shoe, rocker bottom, metatarsal pad
➤ Surgical treatment
  - Excision vs. autogenous bone grafting
  - Fractures can occur with first metatarsophalangeal dislocations – check metatarsophalangeal joint stability

■ **Osteochondrosis**
➤ Unknown etiology
➤ Characterized by painful fragmentation of sesamoid
➤ Most common in active, young adult females
➤ Symptoms present for 6–12 months before radiographic changes
➤ Radiographic findings
  - Fragmentation
  - Trabecular irregularity
  - Cysts, sclerosis
  - Flattening and hypertrophy
➤ Pathologic findings
  - Focal bone necrosis
  - New bone formation
  - Chondroid metaplasia
  - Irregular osteosclerosis
  - Cartilage degeneration
➤ Treatment
  - Similar to treatment for sesamoiditis
  - Dorsiflexion osteotomy at the base of first metatarsal may be considered for plantarflexed first ray

■ **Arthritis**
➤ Includes degenerative, rheumatoid, seronegative, and crystalline arthropathies
➤ Clinical presentation
  • Tenderness under affected sesamoid
  • Synovitis
  • Decreased first metatarsophalangeal motion
➤ Treatment
  • Nonoperative treatment similar to sesamoiditis
  • Surgery after failure of nonoperative treatment
    • If disease is isolated to one sesamoid, then excise
    • If both sesamoids involved, fuse first metaphalangeal (±excision of sesamoids)

TREATMENT
■ See "Differential Diagnosis" under specific diagnoses

DISPOSITION
N/A

PROGNOSIS
■ Potential complications
  ➤ Cock-up deformity, especially after excision of both sesamoids
  ➤ Hallux varus after fibular sesamoidectomy
  ➤ Hallux valgus after tibial sesamoidectomy
  ➤ Weakness in push-off, active plantarflexion

CAVEATS AND PEARLS
■ Key to diagnosis: pain localized beneath first metatarsal head
■ Initial treatment almost always nonsurgical except wide diastasis or severe comminution
■ Sesamoid excision usually permits return to activity in 6–8 weeks
■ Sesamoid curettage and autogenous bone grafting heals by 12 weeks and retains flexor strength (not yet universally accepted)
■ Sesamoids encased in plantar plate and flexor hallux brevis tendon
■ Bipartite sesamoids occur in 5–30% general population
■ 90% of partite sesamoids are tibial; 25% incidence of bilaterality
■ Form from enchondral ossification, complete by 11th year (tibial first, then fibular)
■ Tibial sesamoid may be multipartite, fibular rarely so
■ Functions of sesamoids

➤ Protect the flexor hallucis longus tendon and first metatarsal head
➤ Distribute load transmission to the medial forefoot
➤ Points of insertion for the intrinsic muscles and tendons
➤ Increase moment arm of intrinsics to increase the strength of flexor hallucis brevis/longus

SHIN SPLINTS

JEFFREY A. GUY, MD
REVISED BY CHARLES NOFSINGER, MD

HISTORY

■ *Definition:* ache, sharp pain, or pressure in the medial lower leg experienced during sporting activity, usually relieved at rest
■ Risk factors:
➤ High-impact sports on hard surfaces such as aerobics, basketball, volleyball
➤ Tight or weak gastrocnemius muscles
➤ Worn shoes
➤ Recent shoe changes
➤ High arches
■ More appropriately called "medial tibial periostitis"
■ No history of trauma
■ Common in runners or any athletes with high demands placed on their lower extremities, especially with high-impact or jumping activities
■ Etiology – Usually inflammatory

PHYSICAL EXAM

■ Pain over medial border of tibia
■ Pain worse with resisted plantarflexion
■ May have swelling over medial border or tibia

STUDIES

■ Check compartment pressures to rule out chronic compartment syndrome if diagnosis in doubt.
■ Bone scan to rule out stress fracture
■ Bone scan may have diffuse uptake consistent with periostitis.

DIFFERENTIAL DIAGNOSIS

■ Stress fracture

- Tendinitis
- Nerve entrapment
- Chronic compartment syndrome

TREATMENT
- Rest, ice, compression, elevation
- Activity modification
- Orthotics
- Anti-inflammatory medication
- Change of playing surface
- Rarely surgical debridement necessary
- Stress fracture responds well to tibial nailing
- Chronic compartment syndrome treated with fasciotomies

DISPOSITION
N/A

PROGNOSIS
- Good if recognized and treated early
- Chronic cases may take up to 6 months or surgical intervention to resolve.

CAVEATS AND PEARLS
- Use pain as a guide for rehabilitation. If it hurts, don't do it.

SHOULDER IMPINGEMENT

JOHN URIBE, MD
REVISED BY CHARLES NOFSINGER, MD

HISTORY
- Acute – traumatic
- Chronic – age-related
  - ➤ Young (<40): sports, work
  - ➤ Older: insidious
- Mechanism
  - ➤ Compression of rotator cuff against acromion from:
    - Direct blow on shoulder
    - Fall on flexed elbow
  - ➤ Repetitive microtrauma fatigue
    - Rotator cuff tendinosis, subacromial bursitis

> Degenerative irritation of cuff/bursae by:
  - Anterolateral subacromial osteophyte
  - Thickened coracoacromial (C-A) ligament
  - Type III acromion
- Initial complaints
  > Pain with activities shoulder height and above
  > Pain when sleeping on affected side
  > Pain localized to lateral aspect of shoulder

PHYSICAL EXAM

- Evaluate active and passive range of motion
- Rule out thoracic scoliosis, winging scapula
- Impingement sign (Neer, Hawkins) – pain with internal rotation, abduction against fixed acromion
- Painful forward flexion arc (60°–120°)
- Greater tuberosity tender to palpation (arm extended)
- Pain with terminal internal rotation
- Decreased internal rotation common
- About 60% of patients have decreased supraspinatus strength
- Crossover test may be positive
- Apprehension test may be positive but relocation test negative

STUDIES

- Radiographs
  > True AP, axillary, caudal tilt
    - Rule out glenohumeral (GH) degenerative joint disease; calcific tendinitis, high-riding humeral head (rotator cuff tear), acromioclavicular (AC) degenerative joint disease, os acromiale, tumors
  > Outlet view
    - Type III acromion
    - Anterolateral acromial osteophyte
- Impingement test
  > Local anesthetic into subacromial space
  > Positive test – immediate relief of symptoms
- MRI
  > Only for refractory cases
  > Supraspinatus tendinosis, edema/thickening subacromial bursae
  > Osteophyte formation on acromion or undersurface AC joint
  > Rule out partial- or full-thickness rotator cuff tears

DIFFERENTIAL DIAGNOSIS
- Rotator cuff tears (partial- and full-thickness)
- Calcific tendinitis
- AC joint arthrosis
- Instability GH joint
- SLAP lesions (superior labral tears)
- Bicipital tendinitis
- Early adhesive capsulitis
- Tumors

TREATMENT
- **Nonoperative**
  - Minimize use of arm at shoulder height or above for 3–6 weeks
  - Stop inciting activities (overhead sports, etc.) 3–6 weeks
  - Rotator cuff strengthening program
  - Strengthen scapular stabilizers
  - Long-acting anti-inflammatory 3–6 weeks
  - Subacromial injection with steroid and local anesthetic
- **Surgical**
  - Open (Neer) subacromial decompression
    - Quick, decreased cost (no special equipment)
    - Requires resection of bone from acromion and detachment of C-A ligament
    - Limited exposure – may miss concurrent pathology
    - Possible deltoid detachment
  - Arthroscopic subacromial decompression
    - Evaluate GH joint and entire subacromial space
    - Rule out instability, rotator cuff tears, SLAP lesions, biceps degeneration
    - Visual monitoring of pathology allows for selective treatment
    - Subacromial bursectomy sufficient in majority
    - Bursal surface of cuff may be inflamed or roughened
    - Resect C-A ligament when frayed or inflamed
    - Bony decompression when:
      - Osteophyte present
      - Type III acromion
      - Unstable os acromiale
    - Resect distal clavicle if AC joint involved
- **Postoperative management**
  - Sling for comfort

➤ Begin full active ROM – avoid pure abduction and forward flexion initially – overhead exercise in scapular plane
➤ Resume nonoperative protocol

DISPOSITION
N/A

PROGNOSIS
■ Nonoperative
➤ >70% respond to treatment
➤ Consider surgical intervention when:
• Minimal or no improvement after 12 weeks treatment
• Symptoms recur after resuming activities ×2
■ Operative
➤ Restricted overhead activities 3–6 weeks
➤ Unrestricted (sports, etc.) 12 weeks

CAVEATS AND PEARLS
■ Impingement test negative, surgical outcome poor
■ To differentiate impingement from AC joint arthrosis, selectively infiltrate subacromial space first
■ Young patients rarely require more than a subacromial bursectomy
■ Impingement + ligamentous laxity usually – symptomatic instability
■ Releasing C-A ligament not benign in patient who may need total shoulder
■ Radiofrequency device very useful for:
➤ Exposing bony undersurface of acromion
➤ Cauterization
➤ Releasing C-A ligament
■ Main reason for treatment failure is missed concurrent condition (AC degenerative joint disease, SLAP lesion, instability)

SINDING-LARSEN SYNDROME

JACK ANDRISH, MD
JAMES S. WILLIAMS, MD

HISTORY
■ Age: skeletally immature, usually 8–12

- Incidence: males > females
- Insidious onset, usually presents as anterior knee pad syndrome
- Etiology: repetitive running and jumping (eccentric loading)

PHYSICAL EXAM
- Tender inferior pole of patella ± soft tissue swelling
- Tight hamstrings and tight quadriceps
- Pain with knee flexion

STUDIES
- Plain radiographs: may be normal, but classically described fleck of calcification anterior to inferior pole of patella

DIFFERENTIAL DIAGNOSIS
- Patellofemoral stress syndrome
- Jumper's knee (skeletally mature counterpart)
- Internal derangement – Plica syndrome, osteochondritis dissecans, meniscus tear
- Patellar sleeve fracture (acute)
- Bipartite patella

TREATMENT
- Similar to Osgood-Schlatter disease
- Cryotherapy, stretching program for hamstrings and quadriceps, activity as tolerated (period of restricted running if pain causes limp or loss of "fun factor")
- Consider NSAIDs

DISPOSITION
N/A

PROGNOSIS
- Excellent; self-limited condition, responds well to treatment

CAVEATS AND PEARLS
- Reassure the family that this is a self-limited condition and will not lead to harm within the knee.
- Resolution may take 12–18 months.

SLAP LESIONS (SUPERIOR LABRAL LESIONS ANTERIOR TO POSTERIOR)

JOHN URIBE, MD
REVISED BY CHARLES NOFSINGER, MD

HISTORY

- Acute trauma – usually due either to compressive force on glenohumeral (GH) joint or sudden traction injury to arm
- May have insidious onset
- Mechanism
  - ➤ GH traction (66%)
    - Anterior traction
      - Follow-through phase of throwing
      - Water skiing
  - ➤ Superior traction
    - Holding on while falling from height
  - ➤ Inferior traction
    - Heavy dead lift
  - ➤ Compression
    - Fall on abducted arm, lateral blow
  - ➤ Repetitive trauma (66%)
    - Overhead sports
    - Work (swinging heavy hammer, etc.)
    - Decreased ability of GH joint with SLAP to resist external rotation during shoulder abduction external rotation
- Symptoms
  - ➤ Vague deep shoulder pain
  - ➤ Pain increases with overhead activity, especially throwing
  - ➤ Occasional symptoms of catching, popping, snapping
  - ➤ "Dead arm" feeling in throwers

PHYSICAL EXAM

- No physical finding specific for SLAP lesion
- Overlap of physical signs from associated pathology common
- Impingement sign usually positive; impingement test (infiltration) negative
- Apprehension test positive with SLAP + Bankart lesion
- Relocation test positive with posterior SLAP
- Internal rotation usually decreased

- Superior load test; downward pressure on acromion with upward pressure on elbow produces pain
- Downward pressure on cross-chest internally rotated extended forearm pushing upward and outward reproduces symptoms (O'Brien's)
- Tests that increase tension of biceps may produce symptoms (Speeds, Yergason)
- Compression rotation GH joint – trap torn labrum
  - Pain
  - Click, pop, catch

STUDIES
- Radiographs
  - True AP, axillary, outlet – usually normal
  - CT arthrogram – poor specificity
- MRI
  - Accuracy depends on:
    - Field strength of magnet
    - Shoulder coil
    - Experience of reader
  - MR arthrography (gadolinium, saline) enhances labral separation, improves staging
  - >90% sensitive, 42% specific
- Arthroscopy
  - Definitive source for diagnosis and classification
  - Entity and management arthroscopically based

DIFFERENTIAL DIAGNOSIS
- Partial rotator cuff tear (internal impingement)
  - >25% SLAP lesions have associated partial cuff tears
- Rotator cuff tear
- Rotator cuff tendinitis
- Bicipital tendinitis
- Impingement syndrome
- Anterior/multidirectional instability
- SLAP lesions can be associated with all of above (<30% isolated)

TREATMENT
- Nonoperative
  - Improve GH stability with rotator cuff and shoulder stabilizer strengthening

> Decrease inflammation
  - Anti-inflammatories
  - Avoid inciting activities, "active" rest
- Operative
  > Depends on arthroscopic appearance (Snyder)
  > Type I – fraying of superior labrum; biceps anchor well attached to glenoid
    - Debride to stable rim if significant tear
    - Rule out associated instability
  > Type II (~50%) – detached superior labrum and biceps anchor
    - Abrade glenoid, reattach with suture anchors
  > Type III – bucket handle tear of superior labrum, biceps anchor firmly attached
    - Debride bucket handle tear
  > Type IV – bucket handle tear with extension into biceps
    - Dependent on age and activity level
    - Repair with multiple sutures in young active patients if >50% biceps torn
    - Debride complex when <50% involved
    - Consider tenodesis biceps in sedentary patients with tendinitis symptoms + >50% tear
  > SLAP lesion may extend more anterior (Bankart), into middle GH ligament, or have unstable flap
    - Bankart reconstruction + SLAP repair
    - SLAP repair + repair middle GH ligament
    - Debride flap and repair SLAP
  > Treat associated pathology
- **Rehabilitation**
  > Sling with arm in neutral position for 3 weeks
  > Begin internal rotation and external rotation isometric exercises, gentle active range of motion
  > At 6 weeks progress range of motion, begin resistance strengthening of shoulder stabilizer, cuff, and biceps, emphasize recovery of internal rotation
  > Pitchers need throwing program, return 4–6 months
  > Full activity at 3–4 months
  > May depend on associated pathologic condition

DISPOSITION
N/A

PROGNOSIS

- Nonoperative treatments usually unsuccessful
- Surgical repair >80% return to overhead sports
- Debridement type II without repair: mixed results

CAVEATS AND PEARLS

- 4–12% of shoulder arthroscopies have significant superior labral lesions
- Normal anatomic variants confused with SLAP
  - ➤ Sublabral foramen/recess
  - ➤ Absence of anterosuperior labrum with cordlike middle GH (Buford complex)
- Superior labral separation from glenoid common in older individuals (>55), not pathologic
- Intact biceps anchor dynamically decreases tension on inferior GH ligament

---

SNAPPING HIP

DAVID DREZ, JR., MD
REVISED BY CHARLES NOFSINGER, MD

HISTORY

- Causes for snapping hip
  - ➤ External cause – iliotibial track sliding over greater trochanter
  - ➤ Internal causes – iliopsoas tendon snapping over:
    - Femoral head – most common cause
    - Iliopectineal eminence
    - Exostosis of lesser tuberosity
  - ➤ Intra-articular causes
    - Acetabular labral tear
    - Loose bodies and fracture fragments
    - Hypertrophied ligamentum teres
    - Synovitis
    - Synovial chondromatosis
    - Chondral lesions
- Symptoms
  - ➤ General symptoms
    - Audible snapping, usually with flexion and extension of hip during exercise or activities of daily living

- Often accompanied by pain
- Patient can frequently demonstrate snapping
➤ External snapping symptoms
  - Pain over greater trochanter
  - Occasional radiation of pain to knees
  - May say hip is dislocating
➤ Internal snapping symptoms
  - Discomfort on front of hip (groin)
  - Snapping felt deep in groin
➤ Intra-articular snapping
  - Usually complain of clicking rather than snapping
  - Pain is primary complaint – radiation toward gluteus is common
  - May have history of trauma
  - Sensations of giving way and catching are common

PHYSICAL EXAM
■ External snapping
  ➤ Localized tenderness over greater trochanter
  ➤ Place patient on side with affected hip up
    - Patient actively flexes hip
    - Examiner palpates area of greater trochanter – snapping felt
    - Block snapping by applying pressure at level of greater trochanter
  ➤ Above can also be done with patient standing
■ Internal snapping
  ➤ Frequently reproduces snapping by having patient lie supine and flex and extend hip
    - Sometimes helps to flex and then abduct hip followed by extension and abduction
    - Can block snapping by applying finger pressure over iliopsoas tendon at level of femoral head
  ➤ Elicit pain by flexion of hip against resistance
■ Intra-articular snapping
  ➤ Restricted motion, esp. internal rotation
  ➤ Limp
  ➤ Causes include labral tears, loose bodies, synovial folds

STUDIES
■ Plain radiographs of hip and pelvis – always take to exclude other causes

- CT arthrogram – loose body identification
- MRI with and without gadolinium – labral tear identification
- Ultrasonography – questionable value
- Iliopsoas bursography
  - ➤ Valuable to diagnose snapping due to iliopsoas

DIFFERENTIAL DIAGNOSIS

- Habitual hip dislocation, esp. teenagers
- Slipping of long head of biceps over ischial tuberosity
- Hip arthritis
- Tumors
- Referred pain from lumbar spine

TREATMENT

- Nonoperative
  - ➤ Rest and avoidance of activities that produce snapping and pain
  - ➤ Stretching program of involved muscles
  - ➤ Short course of nonsteroidal anti-inflammatories
  - ➤ Steroid injection
- Surgical treatment
  - ➤ External type
    - Surgery rarely necessary
    - If fails to improve
      - Excise greater trochanteric bursa
      - Z-plasty of iliotibial band
  - ➤ Internal type
    - Surgery rarely necessary
    - If fails to respond
      - Lengthening of posterolateral tendinous portion of iliopsoas tendon
    - Possible arthroscopy of iliopsoas bursa and release
  - ➤ Intra-articular type
    - Arthroscopic procedure
    - Arthrotomy may be needed

DISPOSITION
N/A

PROGNOSIS

- Most cases of external and internal snapping respond to nonoperative treatment over 6–12 months.

- Many patients have benign, asymptomatic snapping and need no treatment.
- If surgery required, results are good if no significant intra-articular pathology is present.

CAVEATS AND PEARLS
- Many cases of snapping hip are asymptomatic.
- If symptomatic snapping is present, must determine cause.
- Most cases of external and internal snapping respond to nonoperative treatment.

SNAPPING SCAPULA

CARLOS A. GUANCHE, MD

HISTORY
- Audible noise emanating from scapulothoracic joint
- May or may not be associated with pain
- Occasional history of direct trauma
- More common in high-level overhead athletes
- Diminished range of shoulder motion
- Winging scapula in up to 50%

PHYSICAL EXAM
- Static position of scapula
  - Normal in some situations (including rhomboid palsy)
  - Displacement of inferior angle compared to contralateral side
- Muscle atrophy evaluation (possible congenital absence)
  - Serratus anterior, trapezius, rhomboideus major and minor
- Examine scapulothoracic rhythm from posterior both with and without resistance
- Examine at 30°, 90°, and 150° of abduction and measure translation of inferior border from midline
- Compare contralateral (uninvolved) translation
- Examine for palpable crepitus and/or snapping
- Superior, medial angle pain most common
- Throwers may have pain at inferior angle
- Complete examination of shoulder girdle, including sternoclavicular joint

STUDIES
- Radiographs
  - Scapular AP, scapular lateral and axillary views will show bony prominence (either scapular or rib)
  - Usually normal, but need to rule out tumor
- CT scan
  - Consider in cases of bony abnormality (best for osteochondroma)
  - Consider in positional abnormalities
  - Include both scapulae in study to check for asymmetry
- MRI
  - Soft tissue crepitus best evaluated with this modality
  - Evaluate entire scapulothoracic articulation
  - Best for evaluation of chronic bursitis
  - Consider glenohumeral MRI if scapulothoracic joint is normal

DIFFERENTIAL DIAGNOSIS
- Scapulothoracic bursitis
- Bone
  - Osteochondroma (rib or scapula)
  - Rib fracture
  - Scapular fracture
  - Hooked superomedial angle of scapula
  - Luschka's tubercle
  - Reactive bone from chronic avulsion of muscle or overuse
- Snapping secondary to glenohumeral abnormality

TREATMENT
- Acute
  - Relative rest, anti-inflammatory medications
  - Periscapular strengthening exercises
  - Consider scapulothoracic corticosteroid injection
    - Patient supine
    - Inject from medial border of clavicle
    - Patient's arm internally rotated on back to maximize opening of scapulothoracic space
- Chronic
  - Repeat injections if some improvement occurs with initial injection (6 weeks apart)
  - Biomechanical analysis of motion

- Especially in overhead throwing sports
- Consider video analysis
➤ Consider CT or MRI in refractory cases
■ Surgical intervention
➤ Arthroscopic debridement
- Two portals, both below level of scapular spine to avoid spinal accessory nerve
- Three areas to consider where bursae are commonly encountered
  - Infraserratus bursa: between serratus anterior and chest wall
  - Supraserratus bursa: between serratus anterior and subscapularis
    - There may be a bony prominence superomedially that may require resection
  - Inferior angle bursa between serratus anterior and chest wall
    - May also require inferior angle excision along with bursectomy
➤ Open debridement
- Superior half or inferior half, depending on pain or evident pathology
- Release rhomboids and/or levator scapulae off and reattach through drill holes

DISPOSITION
N/A

PROGNOSIS
■ Nonsurgical treatment
➤ Good/excellent results in most situations
➤ Strengthening of periscapular muscles continued indefinitely
■ Surgical treatment
➤ 75% good/excellent results with open or arthroscopic treatment
➤ No large series on arthroscopic treatment yet available
■ Return to play
➤ Nonoperative
- When symptoms of crepitus and consequent pain resolve
- Crepitus by itself is no contraindication to participation
➤ Operative

- Arthroscopic: when strength and motion of glenohumeral girdle appear normal
  - Varies by extent of debridement
    - Simple bursectomy: 10 days to 2 weeks
    - Bony resection: 2–3 weeks
  - Open: varies by extent of periscapular muscle release
    - 6–8 weeks in most situations requiring reattachment of muscles
- Complications
  - ➤ Nonoperative: shoulder impingement secondary to overall shoulder girdle mechanical malalignment
  - ➤ Operative
    - Scapulothoracic and glenohumeral stiffness
    - Nerve injury with surgical approaches
    - Pneumothorax (rare)

CAVEATS AND PEARLS
- Location of bursitis is generally sport-specific
  - ➤ Volleyball, swimming: superomedial
  - ➤ Throwers: inferomedial
- Bony crepitus rare
- Avoid arthroscopic portals superior to scapular spine to avoid spinal accessory nerve injury
- Evaluate both scapulae if CT or MRI is obtained to assess for bony impingement
- Acute trauma often brings attention to previously unnoticed snapping
  - ➤ Evaluate contralateral scapula before initiating treatment
- Osteochondromas occur in 1% of the population; malignant degeneration rare
- Exostoses are generally diagnosed before age 20
  - ➤ Most are on the ribs, but can occur on the spine (Sprengel's deformity) and scapula (Luschka's tubercle)

SPINAL CORD INJURIES

HOWARD S. AN, MD PhD

HISTORY
- Average age: male in 30s
- Bimodal distribution: 15–24 years and >55 years

- Sports: 6–13% of cases
- Mechanism examples
  - Diving into shallow pool/water
  - Football – axial load
  - Fall
- Injury
  - Inability to move extremities
  - Possibly concomitant head injury

PHYSICAL EXAM
- On field
  - Do not remove helmet
  - Remove mask rather than helmet
  - Removal of helmet puts neck into hyperextension
  - ABCs of resuscitation
  - Stabilize neck
- Neurologic evaluation
  - Complete injury
    - No motor or sensory function below the zone of injury (C6 quadriplegia means at least 3/5 muscle strength of wrist dorsiflexion)
  - Incomplete injury
    - Partial preservation of motor or sensory function below the zone of injury
  - Anterior cord syndrome
    - Damage to anterior two thirds of cord
    - Sparing of posterior third
    - Damage to pyramidal tracts
    - Loss of motor function at level of injury
    - Preservation of vibration and position sense
  - Central cord syndrome – most common
    - Motor weakness/paralysis upper extremity
    - Relative sparing of lower extremities
    - Common in ankylosing spondylitis
  - Brown-Sequard syndrome rare
    - Damage to half spinal cord
    - Ipsilateral motor weakness
    - Ipsilateral loss of proprioception
    - Contralateral loss of pain, temperature, light touch
  - Posterior cord syndrome – least common
    - Loss of vibratory sense, proprioception

➤ Mixed syndrome
➤ Spinal shock
  • Hypotension without tachycardia (motor, sensory and reflexes are absent but cannot determine complete injury until bulbocavernosus or other reflexes return, usually within 24 hours)
➤ Autonomic dysreflexia
  • May occur in spinal cord injury above the sympathetic splanchnic visceral outflow (above T6)
  • Headache (paroxysmal hypertension)
  • Sweating
  • Nasal congestion and "goose bumps" activated by noxious stimuli – pain, thermal, or urinary distention

STUDIES
■ Radiographs
  ➤ Variation among centers of 3 vs. 5 film series
  ➤ AP, lateral, obliques, open mouth
  ➤ Spinous process alignment, and open mouth view for C1 and C2
  ➤ Must see C7-T1 (obtain swimmer's view if necessary)
    • 10% cervical fractures at C7
  ➤ Soft tissue anterior to the cervical spine measures about 10 mm at C1, 4-5 mm at C2-4, and up to 15 mm at C4-C7
  ➤ Loss of lordosis may be an important sign
  ➤ Vertebral alignment: >3.5 mm displacement and >11 degrees angulation are significant for instability
  ➤ Spinal canal diameter 17 mm (normal), <14 mm (stenosis)
  ➤ Spinal canal/vertebral body ratio <0.8 abnormal
  ➤ Obliques: intervertebral foramen/pedicles
  ➤ Flexion/extension views: ligamentous injuries (usually 3 weeks later)
■ CT scan
  ➤ Best modality for bony lesions
  ➤ Reconstructive images shows details in sagittal, coronal or three dimensions
■ MRI
  ➤ Prognosis after spinal cord injury
  ➤ Distinguish between cord edema vs. hemorrhage
  ➤ Soft tissue injuries such as herniated disk or ligamentous injury can be diagnosed
  ➤ Controversial timing of MRI

➤ Advantage – pre-reduction MRI can rule out herniated nucleus pulposus

DIFFERENTIAL DIAGNOSIS
■ Cord injury: complete vs. incomplete
■ Transient quadriplegia
■ Associated cervical fracture
■ Possible multiple-level fractures
■ Brachial plexus injury
■ Head injury

TREATMENT
■ Evaluation (as in "Physical Exam" section)
■ Resuscitation
➤ Nasal intubation safer than jaw thrust
■ Immobilization
➤ Apply hard cervical collar
➤ Keep helmet in place
■ Transport
➤ <50 miles – ambulance
➤ 50–150 miles – helicopter
➤ >150 miles – fixed-wing airplane
■ Hospital management
➤ Methylprednisolone 30 mg/kg over 15 minutes, then repeat 5.4 mg/kg per hour for 24 hours
➤ Initiate within 8 hours after injury
■ Surgical treatment
➤ Controversial for complete injury with cord compression without fracture
➤ High-dose corticosteroids administered early within 8 hours of injury to improve prognosis (see dosage above)
➤ Spinal cord recovery is better if bony impingement is removed for incomplete types
➤ Decompression may improve nerve root recovery even for complete injuries

DISPOSITION
N/A

PROGNOSIS
■ Complete

> Usually remains complete but one- or two-root recovery is expected, particularly in cervical-level injuries
- Incomplete
  > Potential for significant recovery, particularly in Brown-Sequard
    - Posterior cord – functional recovery fair
    - Central cord – functional recovery fair to poor
    - Brown-Sequard – prognosis for ambulation excellent
    - Anterior cord – functional recovery dependent on level and degree of deficit

CAVEATS AND PEARLS
- Suspect neck injury in unconscious athlete until proven otherwise
- Document level of injury
- Determine whether complete or incomplete injury
- High-dose methylprednisolone indicated
- Spinal shock is defined as hypotension without tachycardia
- Spinal shock may last 24 hours
- Cannot prognosticate recovery until spinal shock resolves
- Missed lesions common in noncontiguous injuries; intoxicated, comatose patients; and multiple trauma victims
- Keep helmet on athlete – remove face mask!

SPINAL STENOSIS

GUNNAR ANDERSSON, MD, PhD

HISTORY
- **Definition:** Narrowing of the spinal canal and/or spinal foramina (nerve canals)
- Can be classified by etiology, location, and symptoms
  > Etiology: congenital, traumatic, degenerative
    - Degenerative most common
    - Caused by degenerative disk bulging, facet joint osteoarthritis, and bundled, thickened ligamentum flavum
    - Symptoms gradual or sudden
    - Not work-related, but strongly age-related
    - Sometimes caused by degenerative spondylolisthesis
    - Degenerative spondylolisthesis usually at L4/5; six times more common in women
  > Location: central and/or lateral
    - Central means spinal canal is narrowed

- Lateral means lateral recess or nerve canal is narrowed
- Central and lateral stenosis may both be present

➤ Symptoms: radiculopathy, atypical leg symptoms, neurogenic claudication

- Radiculopathy and atypical leg symptoms most common with lateral stenosis
- Neurogenic claudication most common with central stenosis
- Radiculopathy: pain in the distribution of one or several nerve roots
- Atypical leg symptoms can be pain, achiness, numbness, tingling, weakness, heaviness, etc.
- Neurogenic claudication: leg symptoms with walking that improve when stopping, bending, or sitting
  - Can occur when standing
  - Bending often gives symptom relief because the spinal canal and foramina become larger
  - Walking usually painful, biking less so (canal widens)
  - Grocery cart pushing relieves pain (canal widens)
  - Sitting often relieves pain
  - Multilevel stenosis more likely to cause symptoms than single level
  - Rarely: chronic cauda equina syndrome with bowel and/or bladder dysfunction, saddle anesthesia, and weak or absent reflexes

PHYSICAL EXAM

- Clinical exam is often quite normal
- Usually flattened lordosis, mildly decreased spinal range of motion
- Usually negative straight-leg raise, normal reflexes, motor and sensory function; reflexes often weak or absent in elderly patients
- With radiculopathy (lat. stenosis) straight-leg raise and neurologic exam can be abnormal, corresponding to compressed nerve root
- Always examine hip joints
- Always examine peripheral pulses

STUDIES

- Radiographs unspecific; usually degenerative changes
- Note degenerative spondylolisthesis
- In congenital spinal stenosis, often short pedicles
- MRI study of choice
- CT, myelography, myelo-CT alternatives

- Axial images particularly helpful
- Myelograms sometimes show hourglass deformity
- Spinal deformity such as scoliosis, olisthesis makes scans more difficult to interpret
- Electrodiagnostics are of limited value, but peripheral neuropathy can masquerade
- Vascular studies if vascular claudication suspected
- Provocative tests (e.g., walking) may initiate symptoms
- Flexion/extension views if instability considered

DIFFERENTIAL DIAGNOSIS
- Spinal stenosis patients with radiculopathy
  - Lumbar disk herniation: analyze imaging
  - A small herniation is more symptomatic if pre-existing stenosis
  - Tumors, infections, fractures, etc.: rare
  - Herpes zoster
  - Aortic aneurysm
- Spinal stenosis patients with atypical leg pain
  - Hip osteoarthritis: always examine hip range of motion
  - Myelopathy: often increased reflexes, upper extremity symptoms
- Spinal stenosis patients with neurogenic claudication
  - Vascular claudication: peripheral vascular studies
  - Peripheral neuropathy: patient history/electrodiagnostics

TREATMENT
- Acute
  - Pain medication (rarely narcotics)
  - NSAIDs
  - Activity modification
  - Information
  - Epidural injections (steroid): variable response
  - Corset if spondylolisthesis/instability
  - Physical therapy (conditioning, strengthening, stabilization)
  - Modalities have no effect but may "feel good"
  - Surgical consideration if nonoperative treatment fails
- Chronic
  - NSAIDs
  - Education: benign disorder, activity modification
  - Corset if spondylolisthesis/instability
  - Walking aid if functional difficulty

➤ Epidural steroid injections: not too frequently, not too many
➤ Surgery if severe pain, progressive neurologic changes, unacceptable quality of life, poor treatment response
  • Surgery is always decompression (laminectomy, foraminotomy, etc.)
  • Fusion if degenerative spondylolisthesis, and preserved disk, and back pain

DISPOSITION
N/A

PROGNOSIS
■ Untreated spinal stenosis has variable prognosis; some better, some worse, some unchanged
■ Nonoperative treatment provides acceptable results for many years
■ Symptoms usually variable (sometimes better, sometimes worse)
■ Permanent neurologic dysfunction rare
■ Epidural injections have unpredictable results
■ Surgery provides improvement in 90+%, excellent results in 70+%
■ Results deteriorate long term (10 years +)

CAVEATS AND PEARLS
■ Old person's sciatica
■ Improved with flexion
■ Grocery cart sign: can walk better when leaning on (pushing) grocery cart
■ Spinal stenosis and hip osteoarthritis can be similar: groin pain uncommon with spinal stenosis, common with hip osteoarthritis
■ Do not exceed three epidural injections in 6 months

STERNAL CONTUSIONS

CARLOS A. GUANCHE, MD

HISTORY
■ Direct trauma to chest
■ Most commonly vehicle accident
■ Occasionally in football, soccer, rugby
■ Hockey: direct puck injury
■ Possible cardiac symptoms secondary to blunt injury
■ Dyspnea present in up to 20%

- Palpitations may be noted if dysrhythmia occurs
- Possible head or neck pain/symptoms

PHYSICAL EXAM
- Pain over anterior, mid chest
- Skin usually intact, abrasion possible
- Evaluate for possible aortic root injury by checking for extremity pulse symmetry
- Evaluate for rib fractures, pneumothorax, hemothorax
- Evaluate for signs of pericardial tamponade
- Evaluate for head and/or neck injury

STUDIES

Radiographs
- Chest x-ray to evaluate for possible pneumothorax or other chest injury
- AP and lateral sternal views (technique involves decreasing exposure about 50% to view bony detail better)
- CT scan
- Consider if fracture is questionable on plain films
- May reveal retrosternal hematoma
- Consider if suspicious of other chest injuries

Laboratory
- ECG in suspected cardiac involvement
- Creatine kinase (CK)-mb index if cardiac contusion suspected

Ultrasound
- May use for evaluation of sternal fracture as well as pericardial effusion

Others
- Perform cardiac monitoring as workup proceeds
- Pulse oximetry as workup proceeds
- Echocardiography if symptoms of hemodynamic compromise

DIFFERENTIAL DIAGNOSIS
- Sternal fracture
- Pericardial tamponade
- Aortic dissection
- Rib fracture

TREATMENT
- Establish complete diagnosis

- Local icing
- Hospital admission if cardiac or pulmonary symptoms present (12 hours)
- Relative activity limitation until pain subsides

DISPOSITION

N/A

PROGNOSIS

- Excellent recovery in isolated cases
- Poor prognosis with hemodynamic compromise or pulmonary disruption

Return to play

- Dictated by pain and swelling, usually 7–10 days for significant injury
- Return may be compromised by associated pulmonary or cardiac injuries

Complications

- Cardiac contusion <5%
- Pulmonary contusion <1%
- Aortic disruption <1%
- Diaphragmatic disruption <1%

CAVEATS AND PEARLS

- Mortality rate can be as high as 25% from associated injuries
- Pain may be more diffuse in acute situations, confusing the diagnosis
- Cervical/head injuries occur in up to 50% of contusions
- Normal ossification centers (sternomanubrial and sternoxiphoid) may persist in 10–30% of adults and do not ossify until about 18 years of age
- Cardiac contusion occurs frequently (6–18%)

STERNAL FRACTURES

CARLOS A. GUANCHE, MD

HISTORY

- Direct trauma to chest
- Most commonly vehicle accident
- Occasionally in football, soccer, and rugby
- Hockey: direct puck injury

- Possible cardiac symptoms secondary to blunt injury
- Dyspnea present in up to 50%
- Palpitations may be noted if dysrhythmia occurs
- Possible head or neck pain/symptoms in up to 25%
- Sternal stress fractures can occur in golfers, weightlifters, baseball players, rowers
- Stress fractures may have more diffuse pain

PHYSICAL EXAM
- Possible crepitus over mid chest
- Pain over anterior, mid chest
- Skin usually intact, abrasion possible
- Evaluate for possible aortic root injury by checking for extremity pulse symmetry
- Evaluate for rib fractures, pneumothorax, hemothorax
- Evaluate for signs of pericardial tamponade
- Evaluate for head and/or neck injury

STUDIES
Radiographs
- Chest x-ray to evaluate for possible pneumothorax or other chest injury
- AP and lateral sternal views technique involves decreasing exposure about 50% to view bony detail better

CT scan
- Consider if displacement visualized on plain films
- May reveal retrosternal hematoma
- Consider if suspicious of other chest injuries

Laboratory
- ECG in all cases
- Creatine kinase (CK)-mb index if cardiac contusion suspected

Ultrasound
- May use for evaluation of sternal fracture as well as pericardial effusion

Others
- Perform cardiac monitoring as workup proceeds
- Pulse oximetry as workup proceeds
- Echocardiography if symptoms of hemodynamic compromise

DIFFERENTIAL DIAGNOSIS
- Sternal contusion

- Pericardial tamponade
- Aortic dissection
- Rib fracture

TREATMENT
- Establish complete diagnosis
- Local icing
- Hospital admission if cardiac or pulmonary symptoms present (12 hours)
- Taping or splinting contraindicated secondary to limitation of normal chest expansion
- Consult trauma surgeon early
- Surgical fixation rarely necessary acutely
- Fixation with heavy-gauge wire or nonabsorbable suture if necessary

DISPOSITION
N/A

PROGNOSIS
- Excellent recovery in isolated cases
- Poor prognosis with hemodynamic compromise or pulmonary disruption
- Nonunion is rare, with painful pseudoarthrosis a possibility
- Malunions rare

Return to play
- 6-8 weeks following healing and consolidation of fracture
- Return may be compromised by associated pulmonary or cardiac injuries

Complications
- Cardiac contusion (18–62%)
- Pulmonary contusion (<2%)
- Aortic disruption (<2%)
- Diaphragmatic disruption (<8–8%)

CAVEATS AND PEARLS
- Mortality rate can be as high as 45% from associated injuries
- Cervical/head injuries occur in up to 50% of contusions
- Normal ossification centers (sternomanubrial and sternoxiphoid) may persist in 10–30% of adults and do not ossify until about 18 years of age
- Consult trauma surgeon early

- Insufficiency fractures may occur in patients with osteoporosis, osteopenia, and long-term steroid therapy
- May occur in long-standing severe thoracic kyphosis

STERNOCLAVICULAR JOINT SUBLUXATIONS/DISLOCATIONS

CARLOS A. GUANCHE, MD

HISTORY
- Direct trauma to medial clavicle
- More commonly, indirect force applied to anterolateral or posterolateral shoulder, compressing clavicle
- May be atraumatic (especially in women)
- Chest/shoulder pain may be exacerbated by supine position
- Associated injuries may cause dyspnea, dysphagia, paresthesias

PHYSICAL EXAM
- Acute
  - Local pain and swelling over sternoclavicular (SC) joint
  - Swelling may mask posterior dislocation and seem like anterior
  - Pain over glenohumeral (GH) joint area with shortened and forward-thrust shoulder
  - Significant pain with lateral compression of shoulder
  - View from level of patient's knees for medial clavicular asymmetry
  - Posterior dislocation may be more subtle
  - Examine entire shoulder complex
  - Check bilateral pulses
  - Check for breath sounds
- Chronic
  - Palpable prominence over SC joint
  - Most commonly anterior dislocation
  - Moderate pain with lateral shoulder compression

STUDIES
- Radiographs
  - Serendipity view: tilt 40° from vertical and direct cephalad through the manubrium on a supine patient

➢ Normal clavicles on the same plane
➢ Dislocated clavicle appears anterior or posterior to plane of manubrium
■ CT scan
➢ Often necessary
➢ Include both affected and unaffected SC joints
➢ Also evaluates for soft tissue swelling in mediastinum
➢ Angiography: may be indicated in posterior dislocations with hemodynamic compromise
➢ Esophagoscopy: may be indicated in cases with dysphagia, especially chronic situations

DIFFERENTIAL DIAGNOSIS
■ SC subluxation vs. dislocation
■ Fracture of medial clavicle
■ Fracture of ribs
■ Scapular fracture
■ Sternal fracture or contusion

TREATMENT
■ Acute
■ Subluxation
➢ Local ice and pain control
➢ Sling for comfort
➢ Assess for associated injuries (rare)
■ Dislocations
➢ Closed reduction with conscious sedation
  • Posterior: supine patient, bolster between scapula and spine, apply traction to 90° abducted extremity
  • Anterior: press clavicle posterior and inferior
➢ Failure under sedation leads to general anesthetic
  • Consider grasping clavicle with towel clip through skin
  • Especially important in posterior dislocations
■ Chronic dislocations
➢ Treatment predicated by symptoms and direction
  • Anterior
  • Typically asymptomatic, cosmetic problem
  • Occasional dysfunction at GH joint
  • Consider medial clavicular resection with preservation of costoclavicular ligaments (make osteotomy proximal lateral to distal medial)

- Posterior
  - Commonly symptomatic
  - Attempt closed reduction under general anesthetic
  - Open reduction should be performed with thoracic surgeon
  - Use heavy nonabsorbable suture only (no plates or wire secondary to migration into chest)
  - Typically stable reduction
  - Postreduction, immobilize in figure-of-eight splint for 4 weeks

DISPOSITION
N/A

PROGNOSIS
- Anterior: typically asymptomatic even in unreduced situations
- Posterior: stable after reduction
  - Occasionally symptomatic if unstable

Return to play
- Closed reduction or subluxation: activity as tolerated after normal shoulder girdle strength and motion return (7-10 days)
- May need to immobilize unstable posterior dislocation in figure-of-eight splint for up to 4 weeks
- Open reduction: 12 weeks before completely unrestricted

Complications
- Anterior
  - Minimal risk with exception of cosmetic deformity
  - Occasionally can have chronic pain
  - Medial clavicular instability if aggressive excision performed
- Posterior
  - 25% associated with tracheal, esophageal, or great vessel injury
  - Chronic open reductions at risk for above injuries

CAVEATS AND PEARLS
- Overall incidence higher in males
- Females have increased incidence of atraumatic anterior subluxation associated with general joint laxity
- One of the least dislocated joints (<3%)
- Anterior to posterior 9:1 ratio
- Soft tissue swelling may obscure posterior dislocation – CT if in doubt

- Beware of medial epiphyseal fractures of clavicle in skeletally immature patients
- Assess lateral end of clavicle and entire shoulder girdle following SC dislocation
- Anterior: closed or open reduction usually not successful, but not of functional significance
- No specific treatment indicated for atraumatic anterior dislocations
- In open procedures, the costoclavicular ligament (superior) is critical to preserve

STRESS FRACTURES OF THE ANKLE

GEORGE B. HOLMES, JR., MD

HISTORY
- Mechanism
  - ➤ Repetitive impact trauma
  - ➤ Increase in training (e.g., longer mileage, inadequate rest)
  - ➤ Improper shoe wear or biomechanics
  - ➤ Amenorrhea in underweight female athletes
- Complaints
  - ➤ Pain that limits performance
  - ➤ Swelling may or may not be present.
  - ➤ Gradual increase in intensity of pain over time with continued participation in sports
  - ➤ Localization of pain may be vague.

PHYSICAL EXAM
- A very careful examination will localize pain to the site of the stress fracture.
- Distinguish localization of pain in bone vs. soft tissue.
- Check body mechanics (cavus foot, pes planus, short leg).

STUDIES
- Radiographs
  - ➤ AP, lateral, mortise views of the ankle
  - ➤ AP, lateral, oblique views of the foot
  - ➤ Radiographs may be normal soon after onset of pain.
  - ➤ Look for periosteal changes or callus for long bones.
  - ➤ Cancellous bone (calcaneus) generally will not show callus.

- Bone scan
  - ➤ Most sensitive in diagnosis of stress fracture, especially with normal radiograph
- MRI
  - ➤ Can be helpful (sensitive/specific) for discerning bone edema and stress fractures
- CT scan
  - ➤ Useful in diagnosis of sclerosis and fragmentation in certain stress fractures (navicular fractures and sesamoid fractures)

DIFFERENTIAL DIAGNOSIS
- Tendinitis
- Osteoid osteoma
- Traction periostitis (shin splints)
- Plantar fasciitis

TREATMENT
- Activity modification (all lower extremity stress fractures except navicular fractures, true Jones fractures, sesamoid fractures) for 6–12 weeks
- Cast
  - ➤ Initial treatment is nonweight-bearing for 6 weeks for acute navicular, Jones, and sesamoid stress fractures.
  - ➤ Weight-bearing cast for stress fractures of the navicular bone, metatarsals, heel stress fracture: 6–8 weeks
- Walking brace: 6–8 weeks
- Postoperative wooden shoe (metatarsal stress fractures)
- Internal fixation
- Bone graft (inlay graft)
- Bone stimulation (external vs. internal)

DISPOSITION
N/A

PROGNOSIS
- Good
- Recurrent stress fractures suggest underlying biomechanical abnormality; must modify biomechanics to prevent recurrence

Complications
- Chronic nonunions
  - ➤ Navicular: goes on to sclerosis and fragment if early fracture is not treated with nonweight-bearing cast

➤ Jones: nonunions are frequently associated with noncompliance in early treatment
➤ Fibula: rare but do occur
➤ Sesamoid: nonunions frequent due to poor vascularity and location

CAVEATS AND PEARLS

■ High suspicion in the active athlete with pain that inhibits performance without a specific injury

---

STRESS FRACTURES OF THE FIFTH METATARSAL

SCOTT A. RODEO, MD

HISTORY

■ Athlete reports insidious onset of pain, mild swelling.
■ Pain has usually been present for a number of weeks.
■ Pain initially occurs only later in the run or after a run.
■ May progress to constant pain with any weight-bearing
■ Due to repetitive cyclical loading below the fracture threshold
■ Most common in athletes involved in running and jumping
■ Rapid increase in training mileage or training frequency
■ May be related to change to harder running surface
■ Changes in shoes or foot orthoses, resulting in unaccustomed stresses on the foot
■ Higher incidence in female runners due to lower bone mass
■ Significant decrease in bone mineral density seen in amenorrheic or oligomenorrheic athletes, especially runners
■ May be seen with excessive supination (stiff varus foot), which places stress on lateral foot
■ Injury/abnormality of first ray (such as turf-toe or hallux rigidus) results in greater load transfer to fifth metatarsal.
■ Assess for history of previous stress fractures.

PHYSICAL EXAM

■ Tenderness over fifth metatarsal
■ Mild swelling may be present over dorsum of foot.
■ Assess for abnormalities in hindfoot alignment.
■ Examine for concomitant abnormality in first ray as cause for altered weight-bearing.

STUDIES

- Plain radiographs (AP, lateral, oblique)
  - Look for radiolucent line (may not see initially), periosteal new bone, or endosteal thickening/intramedullary sclerosis.
  - If radiographs negative, repeat in 3 weeks.
- Bone scan more sensitive than plain radiograph
  - Negative (cold) bone scan indicates poor healing potential.
  - Bone scan may also demonstrate subclinical stress fractures elsewhere.
- MRI very sensitive for early diagnosis, but expensive and not routinely recommended
- May consider DEXA (dual-energy x-ray absorptiometry) to assess bone mineral density if clinically indicated (recurrent stress fractures)

DIFFERENTIAL DIAGNOSIS

- "Stress reaction" – Bone pain due to remodeling
- Injury to cuboid-metatarsal joint
- Peroneus brevis tendinitis/tenosynovitis
- Lateral ankle ligament injury

TREATMENT

- Conservative treatment
  - Initial treatment involves activity modification.
  - Avoidance of repetitive impact activities (running, jumping)
  - Nonweight-bearing
  - Removable boot preferred over short-leg cast (allows removal for ROM exercise)
  - Vitamin D and calcium supplementation
  - May consider pulsed electromagnetic field bone stimulator, but currently no data to support
  - Cross-training to maintain fitness (swimming, upper extremity exercise)
  - Follow progress of healing by physical exam (absence of tenderness) and radiographs every 3–4 weeks
- Operative treatment
  - Surgery required for nonunion
  - Many of these fractures require ORIF
  - Intramedullary screw fixation using 4.5-mm malleolar screw; use largest screw diameter possible

> May need to drill medullary canal (if intramedullary sclerosis) and use bone graft

DISPOSITION
N/A

PROGNOSIS
- Return to activity when no tenderness on bone, no pain with weight-bearing, radiographic evidence of healing
- Return to activity following surgery averages 8 weeks
- Return to repetitive impact activities needs to be very gradual.
- Prognosis for healing of these fractures is guarded due to relatively poor blood supply to bone.
- Complications include recurrent fracture, which is more common with use of smaller screw for ORIF.

CAVEATS AND PEARLS
- Consider early ORIF due to poor healing potential.
- Consider use of custom orthotic to prevent recurrence if abnormalities in hindfoot alignment.
- Consider bone tumor in differential (very rare, Ewing's sarcoma reported here).
- Failure of complete healing common, even after surgery
- Refracture can occur if return to sports too early.

SUPRASCAPULAR NERVE ENTRAPMENT INFERIOR

KEITH MEISTER, MD

HISTORY
- Entrapment of suprascapular nerve distal to supraclavicular notch
- Spinoglenoid notch impingement
  > Spinoglenoid ligament
  > Medial edge of notch
  > Spinoglenoid cyst
  > Eccentric contraction of infraspinatus
- Overhand athletics
  > Volleyball, baseball most common
- Most commonly incidental finding of wasting of infraspinatus muscle on routine screening (volleyballers and throwers)

- Acute onset is rare (acute shoulder dislocation)
- Insidious onset of symptoms by far most common
- Posterior shoulder pain
- Weakness of external rotation
- Loss of velocity/location in throwers (rare)

PHYSICAL EXAM
- Acute (rare onset)
- Chronic
  - Infraspinatus wasting
  - Weakness of external rotation
  - Tenderness over posterior rotator cuff and capsule

STUDIES
- Radiographs
  - AP (internal and external rotation) axillary
  - 30° cephalic tilt view (view supraclavicular notch)
- MRI (with or without contrast)
  - Rotator cuff disease
  - Spinoglenoid cysts
- EMG and nerve conduction studies only in symptomatic patient
- EMG
  - After 3–4 weeks in acute patient
  - Immediate in chronic patient
  - May be normal with an obvious clinical deficit of the nerve
- Nerve conduction studies
  - Beginning at Erb's point, should be abnormal to confirm true diagnosis of nerve compression
  - After 3–4 weeks in acute patient
  - Immediate in chronic patient

DIFFERENTIAL DIAGNOSIS
- Intra-articular shoulder pathology
  - Internal impingement
  - Rotator cuff/labral pathology
  - Instability
- Suprascapular nerve entrapment superior
  - Injury to nerve at supraclavicular notch and proximal
- Acute/prolonged burner syndrome
- Brachial neuritis
- Cervical root compression (C5, C6)

TREATMENT
- Routine preventive shoulder exercise program in the asymptomatic overhand athlete
- Acute
  - Conservative follow-up
  - Initiate physical therapy if acute musculoskeletal injury is stable
  - Surgical decompression after failure of 3–6 months of conservative management
- Chronic
  - Rest from inciting activity, supportive measures (NSAIDs, etc.)
  - Initiate shoulder strengthening and stretching program
  - Surgical decompression: minimum of 3 months of rest with clinical complaints, well-established infraspinatus atrophy, and confirmatory nerve conduction studies
- Surgical release
  - Spinoglenoid cyst: arthroscopic vs. open excision
  - Medialization of spinoglenoid notch
  - After surgery, early range of motion and strengthening
- Surgical complications
  - Injury to suprascapular nerve

DISPOSITION
N/A

PROGNOSIS
- Re-evaluate conservative program at 3- to 4-week intervals
- Conservative management: expectations of complete recovery in most
- Open decompression typically successfully
- Relief from decompression is often profound and immediate
- Return to play
  - Initiate overhand activities when strength 80% of unaffected side
  - Overhand athletes: complete interval throwing program
  - Contact sports: absence of symptoms and 90% strength

CAVEATS AND PEARLS
- Be aware of proximal entrapment process, suprascapular nerve entrapment superior
- Presence of asymptomatic atrophy in up to 15% of elite volleyball players

- Profound weakness in throwers may lead to other more complicated processes – rotator cuff disease, instability, labral damage
- Only 30–40% of maximum strength of the infraspinatus is used in throwing; therefore, some loss of external rotation strength may not be clinically relevant

---

SUPRASCAPULAR NERVE ENTRAPMENT SUPERIOR

KEITH MEISTER, MD

HISTORY

- Stretch and/or compression of the nerve proximal to or at the suprascapular notch
- Acute
  - ➤ Direct blow to Erb's point or supraclavicular fossa
  - ➤ Stretch injury with forceful scapular protraction and/or shoulder depression
  - ➤ Fractures of suprascapular notch
- Chronic
  - ➤ Repetitive overhand athletics (volleyball, throwing)
  - ➤ Malunited or ununited clavicle fractures
- Vague shoulder discomfort
- Weakness/pain during overhead activities
- Pain may localize to posterior shoulder
- Chronically complaints of atrophy, decreased performance

PHYSICAL EXAM

- Complete exam of neck and proximal extremity
- Tenderness of supraclavicular fossa, posterior shoulder
- Weakness of shoulder abduction strength
- Weakness of external rotation strength
- Chronic atrophy of infra- vs. supraspinatus fossa is more readily apparent
- Aggravation of symptoms with shoulder adduction
- Lidocaine injection into supraclavicular fossa may acutely resolve pain

STUDIES

- Radiographs
  - ➤ AP (internal and external rotation), axillary
  - ➤ 30° cephalic tilt view (view supraclavicular notch)

- MRI (with or without contrast)
  - Rotator cuff disease
  - Spinoglenoid cysts
- EMG
  - After 3–4 weeks in acute patient
  - Immediate in chronic patient
  - May be normal with an obvious clinical deficit of the nerve
- Nerve conduction studies
  - Beginning at Erb's point, should be abnormal to confirm true diagnosis of nerve compression
  - After 3–4 weeks in acute patient
  - Immediate in chronic patient

DIFFERENTIAL DIAGNOSIS
- Suprascapular nerve entrapment inferior
  - Injury to the nerve distal to the supraclavicular notch, usually at the spinoglenoid notch and distal
- Acute/prolonged burner syndrome
- Rotator cuff disease
- Brachial neuritis
- Cervical root compression (C5, C6)

TREATMENT
- Acute
  - Conservative follow-up
  - Initiate physical therapy if acute musculoskeletal injury is stable
  - Surgical decompression if associated with acute fracture of supraclavicular notch
  - Surgical decompression after failure of 3–6 months of conservative management
- Chronic
  - Surgical decompression with well-established atrophy and confirmatory nerve conduction studies
- Surgical release
  - Release of transverse scapular ligament and widening of bony notch
  - After surgery, early range of motion and strengthening
- Surgical complications
  - Injury to suprascapular nerve
  - Uncontrolled bleeding from suprascapular artery
  - Injury to spinal accessory nerve with dissection of trapezius

DISPOSITION
N/A

PROGNOSIS
- Re-evaluate at 3- to 4-week intervals
- Expectations of complete recovery with a combination of conservative management and open decompression
- Relief from decompression is often profound and immediate
- Return to play
  - Initiate overhand activities when strength 80% of unaffected side
  - Overhand athletes: complete interval throwing program
  - Contact sports: absence of symptoms and 90% strength

CAVEATS AND PEARLS
- Be aware of distal entrapment process, suprascapular nerve entrapment inferior
- Profound weakness in throwers may lead to more complicated processes – rotator cuff disease, instability, labral damage

---

SYNDESMOSIS SPRAINS

CAROL FREY, MD
REVISED BY CHARLES NOFSINGER, MD

HISTORY
- Injury to the syndesmosis occurs in about 5% of all ankle sprains.
- Referred to as "high ankle sprain"
- Mechanism
  - External rotation most significant force
  - Pronation/abduction or pronation/eversion
- Patient reports pain, swelling over injured ligaments.

PHYSICAL EXAM
- Acute swelling anterior that progresses to diffuse swelling and ecchymosis
- Point of maximum tenderness over injured ligaments, particularly the AITFL (anterior inferior tibiofibular ligament)
- Can be tender proximal to ankle over syndesmosis
- Squeeze test

➤ Positive if injured syndesmosis
➤ Compress tibia & fibula at midcalf
➤ Reproduces pain at syndesmosis if positive
■ Squeeze test will also elicit pain if there is a high fibula fracture (Maisonneuve fracture).
■ External rotation test
  ➤ Knee at 90°
  ➤ Ankle in dorsiflexion
  ➤ External rotation at foot
  ➤ Causes marked pain over syndesmosis if positive

STUDIES
■ Radiographs
  ➤ AP, mortise, and lateral x-rays of ankle
  ➤ Go through differential and rule out.
  ➤ Measure syndesmosis 1 cm superior to the ankle joint line on AP and mortise. Should not measure >5 mm.
  ➤ Medial clear space should not be >5 mm.
  ➤ Check for high fibula fractures.
  ➤ Check for avulsion fractures off the tibia.
■ Stress tests
  ➤ Eversion stress test
    • AP
    • Look for diastasis.
■ Arthrogram may show leakage of dye superior to plafond.
■ CT or MRI may show widening of syndesmosis.

DIFFERENTIAL DIAGNOSIS
■ Avulsion fracture of calcaneus, talus, lateral malleolus, base of fifth metatarsal
■ Fracture of lateral process of talus
■ Fracture of proximal fibula
■ Neuropraxia of superficial or deep peroneal nerve
■ Osteochondral fracture of talar dome
■ Peroneal tendon tear or subluxation
■ Subtalar joint sprain

TREATMENT
■ Stable incomplete sprain
  ➤ Nonweight-bearing cast for 4–6 weeks
  ➤ May recover slowly

- Unstable or complete tear
  - Reduce and stabilize syndesmosis with nonlagged transfixion screw through 3 cortices.
  - Emphasize foot in dorsiflexion while placing transfixion screw.
  - Open repair of the AITFL optional, based on degree of damage or instability
  - ORIF of fibular fracture if present
  - Immobilize in a nonweight-bearing cast 4-6 weeks.
  - Full weight-bearing at 6 weeks with screw removal at 12–16 weeks
- Complications
  - Poor reduction of syndesmosis
  - ORIF advised if reduction difficult
  - Overreduction from "lagging" syndesmosis may limit dorsiflexion of ankle.
  - Late screw breakage, usually from failure to remove screw
  - Synostosis

DISPOSITION
N/A

PROGNOSIS
N/A

CAVEATS AND PEARLS
- Failure to recognize is the major pitfall. Must be suspicious!
- Late instability or failure of reduction is usually due to too-early removal of syndesmosis screw.
- Late screw breakage and pain due to failure to remove screw
- Better to break a screw than to have a recurrent spread instability of the syndesmosis.
- Complete or incomplete synostosis of the tibia-fibula may be painful, especially with push-off. Probably results from original injury.
- Must have talus in dorsiflexion at the time of placement of nonlagged screw

TENNIS LEG

JEFFREY GUY, MD

HISTORY

- Medial gastrocnemius-soleus muscle tear
- Mechanism: Usually with maximum extension of knee and dorsiflexion of ankle
- Usually occurs at musculotendinous junction
- Rare but more common in tennis players and other sports activities requiring jumping
- May be associated with prodromal ache or stiffness
- Usually associated with audible snap or pop with sudden acute pain in calf
- Patients usually feel as if they have been struck or kicked in the back of the leg.
- Pain and swelling over next 24 hours

PHYSICAL EXAM

- Marked calf swelling and pain
- Tenderness at musculotendinous junction of medial gastrocnemius
- Pain increased with dorsiflexion of ankle

STUDIES

- Radiographs
  - ➤ Plain radiographs useful only if associated with a traumatic event and/or a fracture is in your differential
- MRI
  - ➤ Study of choice
  - ➤ MRI should identify hemorrhage within the gastrocnemius muscle and the tear without difficulty.
- Ultrasound
  - ➤ Found to be useful in lower extremity tendon injuries, but mostly with the Achilles tendon
  - ➤ May be useful to rule out thrombophlebitis

DIFFERENTIAL DIAGNOSIS

- Thrombophlebitis
- Posterior compartment syndrome

TREATMENT
- Nonoperative
  - ➤ Aggressive early rehab with first 48 hours of ice, compression, and elevation
  - ➤ Crutches as needed
  - ➤ Active assisted ROM and passive stretching
  - ➤ Heel lift
  - ➤ Strengthening exercises as comfort allows, usually by 2 weeks
  - ➤ Gradual return to sports activity, with full return after 90% normal strength has been attained

DISPOSITION
N/A

PROGNOSIS
- Good with proper rehab

CAVEATS AND PEARLS
- Early diagnosis and aggressive rehab essential to full return to sport
- While rare, always consider the diagnosis of compartment syndrome, which may occur in association with an acute rupture.

THORACIC COMPRESSION FRACTURES

JOHN W. NOBLE, JR., MD

HISTORY
- By definition, involves anterior column of thoracic spine
- Requires substantial trauma to occur in the young athlete
- In the absence of significant trauma, be concerned about pathologic fracture
- Older athletes are more likely to sustain a compression fracture due to osteoporosis
- Mechanism of injury is either acute flexion load or axial compression
- Ask about any transient or permanent neurologic symptoms in the lower extremities
- Any compression fractures occurring with trivial trauma should be thoroughly investigated

PHYSICAL EXAM
- Level of injury ascertained by percussion of the spinous process
- Kyphosis may be present with significant compression
- Paraspinal muscle spasm frequently present
- Thorough neurologic examination imperative
- If any question of neurologic deficit exists, check perianal sensation and rectal exam

STUDIES
- Radiographs
  - AP and lateral should be diagnostic of a compression fracture
  - Should not be confused with Scheuermann's kyphosis
  - Percentage of compression of the anterior column should be ascertained
  - >50% compression associated with posterior ligament injury
  - Posterior retropulsion of the vertebral body by definition is indicative of a burst fracture
  - Difficult to exclude burst fractures on the basis of plain radiographs alone
- CT scan
  - Allows visualization of middle column
  - Allows evaluation of spinal canal
  - May determine size of lesion in pathologic fracture
- MRI
  - May be useful for identifying occult compression fractures in the older athlete
  - Frequently helpful in excluding pathologic fracture
  - Allows multiplanar imaging
- Radionuclide scanning
  - May help diagnose occult compression fracture
  - Usually not necessary in the young healthy athlete

DIFFERENTIAL DIAGNOSIS
- Primary tumor
  - Aneurysmal bone cyst
  - Hemangioma
  - Giant cell tumor
  - Eosinophilic granuloma
- Metastatic carcinoma
  - Breast

- ➤ Lung
- ➤ Prostate
- ■ Hematologic disorder
  - ➤ Lymphoma
  - ➤ Leukemia
  - ➤ Multiple myeloma
- ■ Infectious
  - ➤ Mycobacterial
  - ➤ Fungal
  - ➤ Pyogenic osteomyelitis
- ■ Osteomalacia

TREATMENT
- ■ Nonoperative
  - ➤ Minimal compression fractures treated with analgesics and orthosis
  - ➤ Types of orthoses
    - • Jewett hyperextension brace
    - • Molded TLSO
  - ➤ Braced for 6–12 weeks, depending on age and quality of bone
- ■ Operative
  - ➤ **Acute**
    - • Few indications for surgery, except for flexion-distraction injuries with >50% loss of anterior height
  - ➤ **Chronic phase (compression fracture >50%)**
    - • May lead to chronic pain
    - • May lead to late or progressive kyphosis
    - • Some authors advocate internal fixation and fusion, though this is controversial

DISPOSITION
N/A

PROGNOSIS
- ■ **Nonsurgical treatment**
  - ➤ Most compression fractures heal without significant consequence
  - ➤ Late instability or kyphosis may develop
  - ➤ For compression fractures >50% and pathologic fractures, prognosis depends on underlying disease state
  - ➤ Surgical results for high-grade compression fractures mixed

- ◼ **Return to play**
  - ➤ **Nonoperative**
    - The athlete who has been braced may return when evidence of radiographic healing is apparent
    - Should have no pain and normal range of motion prior to return
  - ➤ **Postsurgical**
    - Contact sports are not allowed for patients who have undergone fusion
    - Once fusion is confirmed, the athlete may return to noncontact sport

CAVEATS AND PEARLS
- ◼ High index of suspicion to rule out pathologic fracture with minimal trauma
- ◼ Beware of undiagnosed burst fracture in the older athlete
- ◼ Inquire about bowel and bladder symptoms, particularly in the older athlete
- ◼ History of obvious injury should be apparent in the younger athlete

---

THORACIC DISK DISEASE

JOHN W. NOBLE, JR., MD

HISTORY
- ◼ May be present in athletes, but not usually related to athletic injury
- ◼ Presents with a myriad of symptoms
- ◼ Most frequent in men aged 30 to 50
- ◼ Classic thoracic disk herniation is rare
- ◼ Most frequently involves lower thoracic spine
- ◼ Signs and symptoms related to location of disk herniation
- ◼ Lateral herniation may produce radiating pain, which follows specific dermatome
- ◼ Nonspecific dorsal pain may be present
- ◼ May be a vague history of minor antecedent trauma

PHYSICAL EXAM
- ◼ Lateral thoracic disk herniation
  - ➤ Focal tenderness at level of herniation
  - ➤ Pain or numbness may follow a dermatomal pattern

- Central disk herniation
  - ➤ Large central herniations may cause spinal cord compression
  - ➤ Spasticity of lower extremities
  - ➤ Hyperactive deep tendon reflexes
  - ➤ Positive clonus
  - ➤ Positive Babinski sign
  - ➤ Altered abdominal reflexes
  - ➤ Paraplegia in severe cases

STUDIES
- Radiographs
  - ➤ AP and lateral of thoracic spine
  - ➤ Usually not helpful in diagnosis
  - ➤ Usually normal, or may indicate spondylitic changes
- MRI
  - ➤ Highly accurate in diagnosing thoracic disk disease
  - ➤ Allows visualization of neural elements
  - ➤ Asymptomatic thoracic disk bulges/herniations frequent
- CT myelogram
  - ➤ Usually not necessary for diagnosis
  - ➤ May be helpful to determine extent of bony compression
  - ➤ May clarify amount of neural compression

DIFFERENTIAL DIAGNOSIS
- Intrathoracic
  - ➤ Angina pectoris
  - ➤ Myocardial infarction
  - ➤ Pericarditis
  - ➤ Aortic aneurysm
  - ➤ Pneumonia
  - ➤ Pleurisy
  - ➤ Pneumothorax
  - ➤ Mediastinal tumors
- Intra-abdominal
  - ➤ Hepatitis
  - ➤ Cholecystitis
  - ➤ Peptic ulcer disease
- Retroperitoneal
  - ➤ Pyelonephritis
  - ➤ Renal colic
  - ➤ Pancreatitis

- Miscellaneous
  - Herpes zoster (shingles)
  - Rib fracture/neoplasm

TREATMENT
- **Acute**
  - Anti-inflammatory medications
  - Physical therapy
  - Bracing
  - Direct injections
  - Selective nerve root block if pain persists
- **With neurologic findings**
  - Surgery indicated for cord compression symptoms
  - Laminectomy contraindicated
  - Transthoracic approach for central disk herniations
  - Transpedicular-transfacetal approach lateral
  - Alternatively, costotransversectomy
  - Video-assisted thoracoscopic diskectomy increasingly used

DISPOSITION
N/A

PROGNOSIS
- **Nonsurgical treatment**
  - Frequently improve with nonoperative management
  - May have persistent localized pain
- **Surgical treatment**
  - Necessary for significant neurologic impairment
  - Radicular symptoms generally improve with surgery
  - Neurologic deficit dependent on degree of herniation
  - Localized pain may persist
- **Return to play**
  - **Nonoperative**
    - May return to participation when asymptomatic
    - Must not have any evidence of cord compression
  - **Postsurgical**
    - Return to sports for posterolateral diskectomy without fusion
    - No contact sports for diskectomy and fusion
    - Once fusion achieved, may return to noncontact sports
- **Complications**
  - Persistent pain
  - Neurologic injury

➤ Empyema
➤ Chronic pain syndrome
➤ Postthoracotomy syndrome

CAVEATS AND PEARLS

- Blood supply to thoracic cord tenuous
- Cord to spinal canal ratio highest in thoracic spine
- Little room for extradural mass
- There is little motion in upper thoracic spine due to constraint of rib cage
- Thoracic disk herniations are frequently misdiagnosed
- Neurologic symptoms may be subtle
- Urinary retention/incontinence may be present with central herniation

---

THORACIC OUTLET SYNDROME

GORDON W. NUBER, MD
REVISED BY CHARLES NOFSINGER, MD

HISTORY

- Constant or intermittent neurovascular compression about the shoulder
- Arm fatigue during the act of throwing over short time span
- Forearm pain like ulnar neuropathy
- Heaviness of throwing arm
- Dull pain from supraclavicular shoulder regions radiates down arm
- Paresthesias inner aspect arm, forearm, ulnar border of hand
- Poorly tolerate arm position of abduction and external rotation (pitching)
- History of trauma to shoulder
- Pain and paresthesias carrying heavy object or wearing arm sling (backpack)
- Blanching, coldness of fingers

PHYSICAL EXAM

- Chronic – loss of pinprick and light touch along C8-T1 dermatomes
- Ulnar sensory changes
- Median nerve motor deficit
- Ischemia of digits

- Adson test abnormal
  - ➤ Pulse lost with full inspiration and head turning toward side
- Wright test abnormal
  - ➤ Radial pulse obliterates with arm abducted and externally rotated
- Roos test abnormal
  - ➤ Slowly open and close hands in overhead position – recreates symptoms
- Exaggerated military maneuver abnormal
  - ➤ Shoulders thrust back, deep inspiration
- All tests look not only for obliteration of pulse but also duplication of symptoms

STUDIES

- X-ray: cervical-thoracic spine to detect anomalous ribs
- Noninvasive vascular tests
  - ➤ Doppler flowmeter
  - ➤ B-mode duplex scan – ultrasound
  - ➤ Photoplethysmography
  - ➤ Nerve conduction velocity tests
- Invasive radiology
  - ➤ Anteriogram – image entire upper extremity in functional position that recreates symptoms
  - ➤ Venogram to look for vein thrombosis

DIFFERENTIAL DIAGNOSIS

- Quadrilateral space syndrome
  - ➤ Posterior humeral circumflex artery occlusion
- Axillary vein thrombosis (effort thrombosis)
- Peripheral nerve lesions
  - ➤ Suprascapular nerve – traction or compression injury (supraganglionic cyst from labral tear)
  - ➤ Long thoracic nerve injury (scapular winging)
  - ➤ Axillary nerve injury – shoulder instability, surgical injury

TREATMENT

- Thoracic outlet syndrome
  - ➤ Conservative
    - If no evidence of aneurysm, emboli, or arterial occlusion
    - Physical therapy to strengthen shoulder girdle musculature
    - Avoid postures and positions that lead to aggravation
    - Avoid shoulder straps or external compression

➤ Surgical
  - Vascular surgeon
  - Aneurysm – resect, bypass graft
  - Cervical rib resection
  - Decompression of scalene muscle or pectoralis minor if compression
  - Embolectomy
- Quadrilateral space syndromes
  ➤ Surgical decompression of quadrangular space through a posterior scapular approach
  ➤ Resection of aneurysm – posterior humeral circumflex artery
- Axillary vein thrombosis
  ➤ Thrombolytic therapy
  ➤ Decompress costoclavicular space – first rib resection
- Suprascapular nerve lesion
  ➤ Exercise program with follow-up nerve condition velocity
  ➤ Surgical decompression
  ➤ If supraganglionic cyst – Decompression arthroscopically, treat labrum tear if present

DISPOSITION
N/A

PROGNOSIS
- Nonsurgical treatment
  ➤ Low probability of resolution unless willing to give up overhead activity
- Surgical treatment
  ➤ If defined lesion or site of neurovascular compression, high likelihood of resolution
- Return to play 6–8 weeks after decompression
- Complications of surgical treatment
  ➤ Infection
  ➤ Persistence of symptoms
  ➤ Pulmonary embolism

CAVEATS AND PEARLS
- Diagnosis depends on high index of clinical suspicion along with thorough examination that includes neurovascular exam
- Arteriogram must be performed in functional position (abduction and external rotation) from shoulder to digits

- All surgical procedures involving vascular pathology should be undertaken by competent vascular surgeon
- Return to play: high probability if defined lesion or compression corrected at time of surgery

---

TIBIA STRESS FRACTURES

JEFFREY GUY, MD

HISTORY
- *Most common*: Overuse injuries usually related to sporting activities requiring repetitive and/or high-impact activity, such as long-distance runners, gymnasts, and dancers
- *Less common*: Overuse or normal physical activity in athletes with poor-quality bone
- Disruption of bone equilibrium: Bone destruction or breakdown exceeds bone formation and repair
- *Risk factors*: High-impact activities, tight muscles and tendons, flat feet, high arches, leg length discrepancy, poor nutrition/eating disorders, and menstrual irregularities
- Most common in proximal two thirds of tibia
- Symptoms usually have a gradual onset, but may also develop with a sudden increase in duration, frequency, or intensity of training
- Pain especially intense with activity, usually relieved with rest
- May progress to complete fracture if not recognized and treated

PHYSICAL EXAM
- May be normal as the patient may be asymptomatic during periods of inactivity
- When symptomatic, pain can be described as dull or sharp depending on progression of fracture.
- Pain is localized over anterior and proximal shaft and may be sensitive to percussion or tapping proximal or distal to involved area.

STUDIES
- Plain radiographs
  - May appear normal acutely
  - Radiodense lines are a sign of attempted healing.
  - "Dreaded black line" (horizontal line in tibial cortex) – seen with chronic injuries

- Bone scan
  - More effective than plain films at identifying an area of increased bone activity
  - May also identify pathologic lesions not apparent on plain film such as osteoid osteoma
- MRI
  - Also effective at identifying stress fractures; more useful when diagnosis is in question
  - May demonstrate bone edema and fracture lines associated with a stress fracture, but also will identify pathologic lesions and soft tissue masses
- CT scan
  - Best test to further characterize bony detail of area involved
  - Helpful in surgical planning

DIFFERENTIAL DIAGNOSIS
- Tibial periostitis
- Chronic compartment syndrome
- Bone tumors

TREATMENT
- Acute
  - Immediate cessation of activity and employ rest, ice, compression, and elevation regimen
  - Modified weight-bearing until painless ambulation achieved
  - Six weeks of modified activity (varies with extent of symptoms)
  - Anti-inflammatory medication as needed
  - Identify and modify training regimen or other etiology thought to contribute to stress fracture
  - Encourage nonweight-bearing cardiovascular activity such as swimming and stationary bike
  - Physical therapy emphasizing stretching regimen
  - Progressive and controlled return to activity
- Chronic nonoperative
  - Permanent cessation of activity
  - Bone stimulator
- Chronic operative
  - Intramedullary reamed rod placement preferred
  - Internal fixation with plate and bone graft

Treatment considerations
- Age

- Training regimen
- Nutrition
- Chronicity

DISPOSITION
N/A

PROGNOSIS
- Good if etiology identified and modified
- "Dreaded black line" on plain radiographs – Poor prognosis with conservative therapy, higher incidence of nonunion

CAVEATS AND PEARLS
- Beware of pathologic bone! Stress fractures can result from normal physical activity in patients with poor bone quality such as osteomalacia.
- Stress fracture can be initial presentation of eating disorder in young women.
- Close follow-up is essential to a safe return to sport.

TIBIAL EMINENCE FRACTURES

ROBERT E. HUNTER, MD

HISTORY
- Stop/start, cut, pivot, jump, twist sports
- Deceleration, valgus/external rotation, varus/internal rotation, hyperflexion
- Acute pain
- Unable to continue activity
- Acute swelling/hemarthrosis
- Complaints of "giving way"
- Children > adults (60:40%)

PHYSICAL EXAM
- Inspection
  - ➢ Moderate to tense effusion
- Palpation
  - ➢ Often associated medial collateral ligament (MCL) pain (prox > mid > distal)
  - ➢ ROM
    - Extension restricted 5–20°

- Stability
  - Generally unstable with + Lachman and + pivot shift
  - Can be stable if fracture nondisplaced
  - MCL laxity often present 30°>0°

STUDIES
- AP/lateral x-ray
  - Displacement
  - None to minimal (<1.0 mm) – Type I
  - Tipped with anterior fragment displaced (fish-mouth) – Type II
  - Completely displaced – Type III
  - Eminence fracture can extend into the weight-bearing surface of plateau
- MRI
  - Confirms x-ray
  - Useful for diagnosis of associated meniscal damage

DIFFERENTIAL DIAGNOSIS
- Hemarthrosis
  - Anterior cruciate ligament (ACL) rupture
  - Patella fracture
  - Peripheral meniscus tear
  - Tibial plateau fracture
  - Patellar dislocation
- "Instability"
  - Quad tendon rupture
  - Patellar tendon rupture
  - ACL tear
  - MCL rupture

TREATMENT
- Nonoperative
  - Nondisplaced and stable
    - Brace in extension – 4 weeks
    - Passive ROM ±
    - Prone knee flexion/extension
    - Weight-bearing as tolerated
    - Full function at 12 weeks
- Operative
  - Displaced
    - Unstable (+ Lachman)
    - Arthroscopic techniques work for virtually all fractures

- Clean, reduce, pin, fixation
- Fixation options
  - Cannulated screws
    - Large fragment
    - Adult
  - Nonabsorbable suture
- Comminuted
  - ➤ Open growth plates
    - Brace in extension – 4 weeks
    - Passive ROM or
    - Prone knee flexion/extension with good leg assist
    - Weight-bearing as tolerated
    - Full function at 12 weeks

DISPOSITION
N/A

PROGNOSIS
- Dependent on reduction, fixation, and ROM
- Anatomic reduction and stable fixation predict good outcome.
- Full extension is critical to good outcome; therefore, brace in extension.
- ACL damage can accompany avulsion, resulting in residual laxity, even if reduction is anatomic.

CAVEATS AND PEARLS
- Both fracture displacement and pathologic laxity suggest the need for surgical repair.
- A fracture that looks anatomically aligned but that presents with pathologic laxity is moving; fix it.
- Try to avoid screw fixation in children with open growth plates.
- #5 Ethibond passed over the fracture and tied over the anterior/medial tibial cortex gives very solid fixation.
- >50% of displaced avulsion fractures have interposition of a meniscus or intermeniscal ligament.
- Interposed soft tissue must be removed to allow for full fracture reduction.
- An ACL tibial guide works well for drilling holes and passing suture.

TIBIAL PLATEAU FRACTURES

ROBERT E. HUNTER, MD

HISTORY

- Valgus/axial load
- Pedestrian vs. auto
- Sports
- Fall
- Acute, severe pain
- Unable to bear weight
- Acute swelling
- Frequent associated ligamentous damage
  - Medial collateral (MCL) > Anterior cruciate (ACL) > Posterior cruciate (PCL)
- Frequent associated meniscal damage
  - Lateral > Medial

PHYSICAL EXAM

- Inspection
  - Tense effusion/hemarthrosis
  - Often lateral contusion/abrasion
  - May have deformity (valgus)
- Palpation
  - MCL pain – Proximal > mid > distal
  - Lateral tibial plateau pain
- ROM restricted
- Stability
  - Often MCL laxity: 30°>0°
  - Occasionally ACL laxity: + Lachman
  - False pivot due to depressed lateral plateau

STUDIES

- Radiographs
  - AP/lateral/obliques
  - Look for change of bone density lateral tibia
  - Look for break in cortex (lateral view > AP)
  - Look for lateral plateau wider than lateral femoral condyle on AP view
  - Underestimates amount of displacement
  - Subtle fractures can be missed

- MRI
  - Very sensitive
  - Evaluate for displacement, comminution
  - Lateral meniscus frequently torn
  - Very helpful in surgical planning
- CT
  - Not as helpful as MRI
  - Good for fracture evaluation

DIFFERENTIAL DIAGNOSIS

- Hemarthrosis
  - ACL, patellar fracture, peripheral meniscus tear, tibial spine avulsion
- "Instability"
  - Quad tendon rupture, patellar tendon rupture, ACL tear, tibial spine avulsion, MCL rupture
- Deformity
  - Patellar dislocation, tibial fracture, distal femur fracture

TREATMENT

- Nonoperative
  - Stable fracture pattern
  - Nondisplaced (<2.0 mm)
  - Normal menisci
  - Poor surgical candidates
  - Hinged brace – Full ROM
  - Crutches – Nonweight-bearing up to 6 weeks
  - Physical therapy for quad strength/control
- Operative
  - Unstable fracture pattern (vertical split)
  - Displacement (>2.0 mm)
  - Displaced meniscus
  - Torn meniscus
- Operative options
  - Scope/percutaneous fixation
  - Scope/percutaneous reduction + bone grafting/percutaneous fixation
  - Open reduction/internal fixation +/− bone grafting
    - Screws
    - Plates
  - External fixation

DISPOSITION
N/A

PROGNOSIS
- Dependent on
  - ➤ Bony alignment
  - ➤ Ligamentous stability
  - ➤ Quality of cartilage (articular and meniscal)
- Bony healing predictable
  - ➤ Subsidence can occur in osteoporotic bone
- High-impact sports/activities (running) not recommended
- Painful metal often requires removal

CAVEATS AND PEARLS
- Acute, tense effusion is generally a fracture.
- MRI will show many plateau fractures not visible with plain x-ray.
- Acute effusion, normal patellofemoral exam, normal stability, full extension: think plateau fracture.
- Pivot shift maneuver can feel positive due to displacement of lateral plateau.
- Fracture that starts in the interspinous region of the tibia and exits medially can be associated with severe nerve/artery damage.
- Always do a complete neurovascular exam of lower leg before treatment.
- Scope management, when possible, has less morbidity and allows for better reduction and faster recovery with fewer complications than open techniques.
- Never sacrifice a meniscus for visualization or reduction.
- Minimize exposure to avoid soft tissue stripping and avascular bone.
- Two small incisions (medial and lateral) are better than one large central incision.
- Aggressively restore ROM but delay weight-bearing (full weight-bearing at 6–12 weeks).

TIBIAL TUBERCLE AVULSION

MATTHEW SHAPIRO, MD

HISTORY
- Occurs at proximal tibial physis, in region of insertion of patellar tendon
- Questionably associated with Osgood-Schlatter disease
- Occurs as stress-related failure deep to the ossified portion of the tibial tubercle
- Transitional fracture: occurs in adolescents in whom the posterior portion of the proximal tibial physis is already closed

PHYSICAL EXAM
- Pain, swelling, deformity at tibial tubercle
- Pain or inability to extend knee
- Type III injuries associated with traumatic hemarthrosis

STUDIES
- Classified by x-ray according to Ogden
  - Type I: fracture line through ossified portion of tibial tubercle
  - Type II: fracture line exits anteriorly, at level of proximal tibial physis
  - Type III: fracture line vertical, exiting intra-articularly (Salter-Harris type III fracture)

DIFFERENTIAL DIAGNOSIS
- Type I fractures may simulate Osgood-Schlatter disease.
- Rule out sleeve-type fracture of patella.

TREATMENT
- Nondisplaced Type I fractures may be treated in a cylinder cast for 4–6 weeks.
- Displaced fractures require open reduction/internal fixation followed by 4–6 weeks immobilization.

DISPOSITION
N/A

PROGNOSIS
- Expect full recovery with above treatment.

CAVEATS AND PEARLS

- Since these are transitional fractures, there is no concern about placing hardware across the physis (it is already closing).

TRANSIENT QUADRIPLEGIA

JOHN D. KELLY, IV, MD
REVISED BY CHARLES NOFSINGER, MD

HISTORY

- Collision injury
- Mechanism: hyperextension, axial load, or rarely hyperflexion to cervical spine
- Bilateral burning paresthesia with varying degrees of bilateral extremity weakness or paralysis
- Neurologic symptoms may involve both arms, both legs, or all four extremities
- Complete recovery usually 10–15 minutes, although some require up to 48 hours to resolve
- Neck pain may or may not be present

PHYSICAL EXAM

- Neck range of motion usually normal or near-normal
- Acutely may have sensory loss in both hands and/or both feet
- Acute loss of bilateral upper extremity and/or lower extremity motor strength
- "Long tract" signs may or may not be present acutely

STUDIES

- Cervical spine x-rays
  - Lateral cervical spine all cases
  - Include flexion/extension if neck pain present
  - Torg ratio <.80 on lateral cervical spine x-rays indicates canal stenosis
    - Canal size divided by vertebral body width
    - Poor positive prediction
  - Absolute stenosis defined as AP canal diameter <10 mm
- MRI to rule out "nonbony" compression
  - Large central disk
  - Measures "functional reserve" of cord and cord edema

➤ For all deficits lasting >15–20 minutes – definite indication for MRI
■ Lateral flexion/extension radiographs if no bony or soft tissue cord compressive lesion seen
➤ Rule out instability as cause of cord compression

DIFFERENTIAL DIAGNOSIS
■ Rule out cervical burst fracture, large central herniated nucleus pulposus, or instability
➤ All the above may cause transient quadriplegia
➤ Lateral flexion/extension and MRI effectively rule out above

TREATMENT
■ Must use spine board precautions
➤ Immobilize on spine board, sand bag to neck/head
➤ Do not remove helmet
➤ Remove face mask if airway compromised
➤ Safe transport to medical facility where radiographs can be safely obtained

DISPOSITION
N/A

PROGNOSIS
■ Generally favorable if secondary to isolated canal stenosis
■ No strong evidence that cord neuropraxia predisposes to permanent neurologic injury (controversial)
■ If associated disk herniation, instability, or chronic degenerative changes, athlete best advised to avoid contact sports
■ Cord edema on MRI relative contraindication to continue contact sports

CAVEATS AND PEARLS
■ Neurosurgery literature suggests higher risk of neural injury with narrow canal size
■ In work-up, consider three mechanisms of cord compression
➤ Bony (stenosis with or without degenerative changes)
➤ Soft tissue herniated nucleus pulposus
➤ Dynamic (instability)
■ MRI can demonstrate dural vs. cord compression and indicate "functional reserve" of cord
■ Prevention: neck, trapezial strengthening; avoidance of "spearing"

TRAUMATIC ANTERIOR SHOULDER INSTABILITY

BRIAN J. COLE, MD
ROBERT A. SELLARDS, MD

HISTORY

- Most common form of shoulder instability – 1.7% in general population
- Mechanism – forceful abduction, external rotation
- Associated findings
  - Bankart 85%: anterior inferior labrum torn from glenoid
  - Hill-Sachs: posterolateral humeral head and cartilage injury
  - Capsular laxity
- Axillary nerve 5–35%: sensory over deltoid, spontaneous resolution
- Recurrence: <20 years old, >90% recurrence; >40 years old, <10% recurrence
- Acute dislocation findings (pre-reduction)
  - Loss of deltoid contour
  - Pain
  - Difficult and painful internal rotation
- Chronic recurrent anterior instability findings
  - Discomfort with abduction and external rotation
  - Rare spontaneous dislocation or subluxation

PHYSICAL EXAM

- Observe for atrophy and abnormal scapular rhythm with forward elevation
- Neurovascular evaluation with emphasis on axillary nerve
- Range of motion with side-to-side comparison
- Rotator cuff testing for weakness (especially in patient >40 years old)
- Apprehension sign: grimacing and feeling as if shoulder will dislocate
- Abduction and external rotation to 90°
- Relocation test
- Apprehension resolved with posterior pressure on proximal humerus

STUDIES

- Radiographs

- ➤ Trauma series: true AP, scapular "Y" and axillary views
- ➤ West Point view – evaluate anterior glenoid
- ➤ Stryker notch view – Hill-Sachs lesion
- ■ MRI
  - ➤ Detects labral lesions
  - ➤ Detects associated pathology
    - • Rotator cuff
    - • Superior labrum
    - • Cartilage
- ■ CT arthrogram (rarely needed)
  - ➤ Revision surgery
  - ➤ Detects glenoid version abnormalities
  - ➤ Defines capsule integrity
  - ➤ Defines labral pathology
- ■ Exam under anesthesia
- ■ Determine principal direction of instability
- ■ Grading (based on translation of humeral head)
  - ➤ 0: normal
  - ➤ 1: to glenoid rim
  - ➤ 2: over glenoid rim with spontaneous reduction
  - ➤ 3: locking over glenoid rim
  - ➤ Abnormal: anterior translation of grade 2 or greater on affected side
  - ➤ Abnormal: posterior translation of grade 3
  - ➤ Normal: bilateral posterior translation of grade 2 or less
- ■ Define secondary direction of instability
- ■ Rotator interval: sulcus sign with inferior traction (space increases between lateral acromion and top of humeral head) in adduction that persists in external rotation
- ■ Test in various arm positions

DIFFERENTIAL DIAGNOSIS
- ■ Other instability patterns (i.e., posterior, bidirectional, multidirectional)
- ■ Superior labral anterior to posterior tears (SLAP lesions)
- ■ Rotator cuff tear

TREATMENT
- ■ Acute dislocation
  - ➤ Reduction maneuver: IV sedation or intra-articular lidocaine
  - ➤ Prone, arm over edge of bed with weight hanging from wrist

➤ Supine, gentle traction-countertraction
➤ Pre- and post-reduction neurovascular and rotator cuff examination
➤ Verify with post-reduction radiographs
➤ Initial treatment
  • Sling immobilization 3–6 weeks (young) or 2–4 weeks (old)
  • Weeks 0–6: gentle, limited range of motion, external rotation to 0°
  • Weeks 6+: restore dynamic stability and range of motion
➤ Activity modification prn
■ Surgical indications
  ➤ Pain, disability with recurrent instability
  ➤ Athlete who is unable to compete
■ Surgical technique: open
  ➤ Limited deltopectoral approach (i.e., coracoid to axillary fold)
  ➤ Subscapularis split vs. lateral incision and separation from capsule
  ➤ Medial-based capsulotomy: isolated Bankart
  ➤ Lateral-based capsulotomy: surgeon preference and need for capsulorrhaphy
  ➤ Repair anterior capsulolabral structures
  ➤ Suture anchors vs. drill holes
  ➤ Capsular shift prn
■ Surgical technique: arthroscopic
  ➤ Advantages: pathology identification, morbidity, motion loss
  ➤ Disadvantages: technical, learning curve
  ➤ Technique
    • One posterior, two anterior portals
    • Suture anchors, single-point fixation device (i.e., Suretac), knotless anchors
    • Repair Bankart lesion anatomically
    • Identify and address all pathology
    • Capsular plication vs. thermal shrinkage where needed
■ Rehabilitation
  ➤ Weeks 2–4: sling
  ➤ Weeks 4–6: early protected range of motion, limited external rotation, no stretching
  ➤ Weeks 6–8: active assisted range of motion
  ➤ Weeks 8+: active range of motion
  ➤ Weeks 12+: pre-injury conditioning
  ➤ Months 6+: sports

■ Results
  ➤ Arthroscopic: contemporary techniques with recurrence rates <10%
  ➤ Open: recurrence rates <10%, surgical morbidity may decrease return to sport

DISPOSITION
N/A

PROGNOSIS
■ Complications
  ➤ Recurrence
  ➤ Stiffness
  ➤ Neurologic injury (axillary nerve)

CAVEATS AND PEARLS
■ Axillary view to determine direction of dislocation
■ Neurologic examination before and after reduction
■ Verify reduction radiographically
■ High recurrence rate in younger patients (90% <20 years old)
■ Shorter-term immobilization in older patients due to risk of stiffness
■ Beware of cuff tears in older patients (>40 years old)
■ Address labral pathology and avoid medializing repair
■ Identify and treat all associated pathology at time of exam under anesthesia and arthroscopy or open reconstruction

---

TRAUMATIC AXILLARY NERVE INJURY

KEITH MEISTER, MD

HISTORY
■ Acute mechanisms
  ➤ Glenohumeral dislocations
  ➤ Fracture/dislocations of proximal humerus
  ➤ Reduction of acute dislocation
  ➤ Intraoperative traction or nerve severing
  ➤ Brachial plexus injury (i.e., burner syndrome)
■ Chronic mechanisms
  ➤ Brachial neuritis

- Acutely decreased sensation of lateral deltoid
- Inability to abduct shoulder

PHYSICAL EXAM
- Complete evaluation of head and neck
- Acute
  - Isolated decreased sensation in lateral deltoid
  - Isolated complete or incomplete paralysis of deltoid
- Chronic
  - Complete or partial wasting of deltoid
  - Isolated posterior third wasting with decreased sensation over lateral deltoid; involves medial branch only
  - Isolated anterior/lateral third wasting involves lateral branch only
  - Inability to abduct shoulder

STUDIES
- Radiographs
  - AP (internal and external rotation), axillary or scapular Y views
- MRI
  - With or without contrast may be indicated in case of recurrent instability
- EMG and nerve conduction studies if no return by 3–4 weeks

DIFFERENTIAL DIAGNOSIS
- Brachial neuritis
- Acute burner syndrome
- Prolonged burner syndrome (>72 hours)
- Quadrangular space syndrome
  - Compression neuropathy of the axillary nerve and branch to the teres minor as it passes through the interval between the muscle bellies of the teres muscles

TREATMENT
- Acute
  - Reduction of fracture or dislocation
  - Re-evaluation of neurologic status following reduction maneuver
  - Initiation of range of motion and strengthening after appropriate treatment of musculoskeletal trauma
  - NSAIDs, sling for comfort, supportive measures

- Chronic
  - ➤ Surgical exploration/neurolysis/grafting of nerve after closed trauma if no sign of recovery after 3–4 months
  - ➤ Dysfunction of anterior deltoid may be treated with rotational transfer of posterior deltoid
  - ➤ Muscle transfers of the long head of the biceps and clavicular head of the pectoralis major
  - ➤ Trapezius muscle transfers not recommended
  - ➤ Scapulothoracic arthrodesis for complete, unrecovered paralysis

DISPOSITION
N/A

PROGNOSIS
- True incidence of acute axillary nerve injury unknown
- Most injuries go undiscovered and recover without sequelae
- If incomplete return in first 72 hours, then re-evaluation every 2–3 weeks
- Results of axillary nerve exploration/neurolysis/grafting at 1 year
  - ➤ Grade 4 muscle function in 60%
  - ➤ Grade 3 muscle function in 70%
- Return to play
  - ➤ Full shoulder range of motion
  - ➤ Normal sensation
  - ➤ 90% recovery of strength

CAVEATS AND PEARLS
- Beware of acute shoulder instability vs. acute burner syndrome
- Document complete and thorough neurologic exam prior to attempt at reduction of suspected fracture or dislocation
- Document repeat neurologic examination following each reduction attempt
- Perpendicular radiographic views of glenohumeral joint in the event of a shoulder dislocation
- Individual with history of recurrent dislocations may reduce without radiographs
- Suggest radiograph prior to reduction in suspected first-time dislocation, particularly if initial reduction attempt does not produce easy reduction of deformity
- Cervical-spine radiographs in the event of multiple burners, with possible need for MRI

TRAUMATIC BOUTONNIERE INJURIES OF THE DIGITS

GERARD GABEL, MD

HISTORY
- Sports > work injury
- Mechanism: axial load, eccentric flexion of proximal interphalangeal (PIP) joint
- Acute: central slip avulsion from middle phalanx
- Chronic: central slip avulsion, fixed lateral band subluxation
- Looks identical to typical "jammed finger" on presentation
- Painful, swollen digit, centered around PIP joint
- Patient may or may not note inability to actively extend PIP joint
- May have sustained volar PIP joint dislocation; ask if someone had to "pop joint into place"
- Most commonly identified subacutely or late due to delay in diagnosis of central slip component
- Chronic: typical PIP flexion/distal interphalangeal (DIP) hyperextension posture; must differentiate boutonniere from more common isolated flexion contracture
- Common sports: football, basketball, baseball

PHYSICAL EXAM
- Acute
  - ➤ Swollen PIP joint
  - ➤ PIP rests in varying degrees of flexion
  - ➤ Weak PIP extension
  - ➤ Tenderness over dorsal, proximal aspect of middle phalanx
  - ➤ Must differentiate PIP sprain (early active range of motion) from boutonniere (delayed active range of motion)
    - Digital block testing
    - 10 cc – Half 5% Marcaine, half 2% Xylocaine, no epinephrine
    - Block digital nerves at web space or neck level
    - Test PIP extension strength of injured and contralateral digit
    - May have deficiency of DIP flexion if subacute or chronic
- Must differentiate from isolated flexion contracture if chronic
  - ➤ Isolated contracture: no deficiency of PIP extension strength, no deficiency of DIP flexion

STUDIES
- Plain x-rays: true AP, lateral

> May see small avulsion fracture from dorsal tubercle of middle phalanx
> May have volar subluxation
> If chronic, PIP flexion, DIP hyperextension
- MRI not useful
- Arthrogram not useful

DIFFERENTIAL DIAGNOSIS
- Acute: hyperextension collateral ligament injury – PIP "sprain"
  > Digital block test of PIP extension
- Acute: reduced volar PIP dislocation
  > Difficult to differentiate without history or x-rays of dislocation
  > May be very swollen
- Late: isolated PIP contracture
  > PIP extension strength intact (test at similar position of flexion)
  > DIP flexion intact

TREATMENT
- Acute (no PIP flexion contracture)
  > Extension splinting PIP joint
  > May consider PIP pinning for select cases
  > Active and passive range of motion flexion of DIP joint
  > Maintain for 6 weeks
  > Start weaning program at 6 weeks
  > Out of splint fully at 10 weeks
- Subacute (with flexion contracture)
  > Dynamic extension PIP splinting until full correction of flexion contracture, then same program as acute
- Late (>3–6 months)
  > PIP release – staged or at same setting as extensor tendon reconstruction
  > Results fair to good, not good to excellent
  > Stress early recognition

DISPOSITION
N/A

PROGNOSIS
- Results depend on early recognition, treatment, patient compliance
- Functional results in most, full range of motion in few
- Return to play with protective splint at 6–8 weeks, without splint when extension strength restored

CAVEATS AND PEARLS
- Early recognition – Don't overlook in "jammed finger"
- Splint religiously
- First shot is your best shot

TRAUMATIC EXTENSOR TENDON DISLOCATION

JAMES B. BENNETT, MD

HISTORY
- Sports or work hand injury – closed fist
- Mechanism – direct trauma split tendon/forceful ulnar deviation subluxed tendon
- Subluxation of extensor tendons
- Rupture of extensor tendons
- Associated fracture dislocation of distal interphalangeal (DIP), proximal interphalangeal (PIP), and metacarpal phalangeal (MP) joint
- Painful, with inability to extend fingers
- Chronic instability
- Common sports: contact, boxing, karate
- Associated fractures
- Associated dislocations

PHYSICAL EXAM
- **Anatomy**
  - Extensor tendon MP extensor mechanism, PIP extension, DIP joint terminal extension
  - PIP joint central slip lateral bands
  - MP joint sagittal bands and extensor tendon mechanism
  - Acute subluxation and inability to extend the finger at DIP joint, mallet
  - PIP joint boutonniere with central slip rupture
  - MP joint radial or ulnar deviation with sagittal ligament tear and subluxation of extensor tendon
  - Split extensor tendon secondary to direct trauma and inability to extend
  - Associated ligament laxity
  - **R/O underlying fracture**

STUDIES

■ **Radiographs**
- ➤ AP and true lateral
- ➤ Rule out fracture
- ➤ Extensor tendon mallet fracture DIP joint
- ➤ Boutonniere fracture avulsion PIP joint
- ➤ MP joint associated fracture
- ➤ CT scan, MRI not required acutely
- ➤ **CT/MRI is indicated for chronic injury**

DIFFERENTIAL DIAGNOSIS

- ■ Mallet finger fracture vs. extensor tendon rupture
- ■ Boutonniere PIP joint fracture vs. extensor tendon rupture
- ■ Associated with volar dislocations PIP joint
- ■ Swan-neck deformity with dorsal position of lateral band and intact extensor mechanism
- ■ MP joint radial or ulnar collateral ligament injury
- ■ Fracture-dislocation MP, PIP, DIP joint

TREATMENT

■ **Acute**
- ➤ Mallet extensor tendon only: splint for 4 weeks full-time, 4 weeks part-time
- ➤ Splint vs. K-pin fixation for displaced fracture fragment
- ➤ Extensor tendon repair with laceration
- ➤ PIP joint boutonniere: extension splinting for 4 weeks full-time, part-time 4 weeks
- ➤ Extensor tendon repair with dislocation or laceration
- ➤ Lateral band reposition with swan-neck deformity
- ➤ MP joint sagittal band repair
- ➤ Sagittal band reconstruction with tendon graft through collateral ligament
- ➤ Sagittal band reconstruction with extensor tendon through base of proximal phalanx
- ➤ Split tendon repair longitudinally
- ➤ Split MP extensor hood 4 weeks full-time, part-time 4 weeks
- ➤ Conservative treatment with no fracture
- ➤ Open treatment with fracture displacement
- ➤ Open treatment of chronic dislocation/subluxation

Chronic

- ■ Reconstruction extensor tendon/extensor mechanism

DISPOSITION

- Return to function post splint 4–6 weeks non-operative, 6–8 weeks operative

PROGNOSIS

- **Nonsurgical**
  - ➤ Good prognosis if no displacement
- **Surgical treatment**
  - ➤ Good prognosis if no displacement and reconstructible
- **Return to Play**
  - ➤ Nonoperative
    - Splint for 4–6 weeks
    - Active participation with splint
  - ➤ **Reconstructive**
    - Splint 4–6 weeks
    - Return to play at 4–6 weeks with protection
- **Complications of treatment**
  - ➤ Failure of healing with chronic deformity, mallet finger at DIP level
  - ➤ Boutonniere deformity at PIP level
  - ➤ Chronic subluxation MP joint extensor tendon
  - ➤ Infection
  - ➤ Stiff finger deformity and joint extension contracture
  - ➤ Flexion contracture of joint

CAVEATS AND PEARLS

- Mallet finger deformity correction, conservative vs. surgical
- Boutonniere correction with K-wire fixation for 4 weeks
- MP joint ligament reconstruction with sagittal band reconstruction/collateral ligament/bone anchor
- Avoid tight repair that does not allow finger MP/PIP/DIP flexion
- Older individual spontaneous rupture due to attenuated ligaments at MP level
- Acute traumatic injury from sports participation with rupture longitudinally for repair (middle MP most common due to prominence)
- Buddy taping bracing for rehabilitation

TRICEPS TENDINITIS

CHRISTOPHER D. HAMILTON, MD

HISTORY
- Mechanism of injury
  - Forceful overload of triceps insertion on olecranon
  - Chronic overload of triceps
    - Leads to acute or chronic tendinitis
    - Onset of pain usually gradual, often insidious
    - Frequent in baseball pitchers
- Initial complaints
  - Recurrent pain during or after lifting activity
  - Ache with termination of activity
  - Forceful extension of triceps worsens pain
  - Pain at the extremes of elbow motion (i.e., full elbow extension and full flexion)
  - Occasionally wrist extension worsens pain
  - Decreasing performance in the gym
- Chronic cases
  - Deep elbow ache
  - Ache continues with activity
  - May be associated with anabolic steroid use
  - May predispose to rupture

PHYSICAL EXAM
- Acute
  - Initial exam may be benign unless process is active
    - Little deformity or swelling noted initially
    - Pain to palpation at triceps insertion
    - Pain elicited at extremes of motion
    - Flexion contracture not uncommon
    - Motion loss more highly associated with intra-articular pathology
- Chronic (and acute)
  - Loss of triceps strength
  - Elbow effusion may be present
  - Loss of elbow pronation and supination associated with arthritis

STUDIES
- Radiographs

➤ AP, lateral, and oblique (radiocapitellar) views helpful to rule out other bony causes of pain
- Traction spurs
- Loose bodies
- Calcification in tendon insertion indicative of chronicity
- Elbow arthrosis most common radiographic finding

■ Laboratory studies
➤ Rarely needed for routine cases, helpful in systemic diseases
➤ Renal osteodystrophy, hyperparathyroidism – calcium, PTH, alkaline phosphatase
➤ Marfan's syndrome – collagen typing
➤ Lupus – anti-DNA, sed rate, rheumatoid factor

■ MRI
➤ Study of elbow and distal humerus
➤ Can be used to locate partial tears or tendinosis
➤ Evaluation of MCL in throwers with tendinitis

■ CT scans (with or without intra-articular gadolinium)
➤ Useful for bony abnormalities and assessment of joint, especially spurs, arthritis, and loose bodies

■ Bone scan helpful in stress fractures or adolescents

DIFFERENTIAL DIAGNOSIS
■ Triceps tendinitis
■ Triceps tendon tears (partial or complete)
■ Elbow arthrosis
■ Posterior impingement and associated elbow instability medial collateral ligament (MCL)
➤ Baseball pitchers
➤ Javelin or other throwers
■ Olecranon stress fracture – bone scan may be needed
■ Olecranon physeal overload – seen in adolescent throwers
■ Extra-articular pathology – tumors, infection

TREATMENT
■ Must rule out other underlying factors (i.e., arthritis, instability)
➤ Treat first and often tendinitis resolves
■ Relative rest
■ Lighter weights with lower resistance
■ Avoidance of irritating activities
➤ Limited throwing
➤ De-emphasize triceps when lifting weights

- Ice after activity
- Anti-inflammatory medications
- Physical therapy
  - Modalities
    - Ice
    - Cross-friction massage
    - Iontophoresis
  - Restore normal flexibility of agonist and antagonist muscles
  - Eccentric strengthening of triceps
  - Slow return to activities as limited by pain
- Surgery
  - Rarely indicated unless partial tendon tears, calcifications, or osteophytes are present
  - Helpful for associated condition, ruptures, degenerative joint disease, loose body removal
  - In severe cases, may need triceps reattachment

DISPOSITION
N/A

PROGNOSIS
N/A

CAVEATS AND PEARLS
- Most cases of triceps tendinitis and partial ruptures are treated conservatively
- Recovery can be protracted in isolated tendinitis; may take up to 9 months
- Eccentric strengthening with soft tissue management may be most effective conservative management
- In throwers, have a high suspicion of valgus extension overload, MCL instability, and loose bodies
- Ruptures have bony avulsions present approximately 80% of the time on radiographs

TURF TOE INJURY

SCOTT A. RODEO, MD

HISTORY
- Sports injury to metatarsophalangeal joint (MTP) of great toe

- Most common in football and soccer
- Occurs on both artificial turf and natural grass
- Most common mechanism is hyperextension of great toe MTP joint
- Occurs with foot in dorsiflexion with forefoot on ground and heel raised
- Dorsiflexion injury results in disruption of volar joint capsule at attachment to metatarsal neck
- Hyperflexion mechanism can also occur – Results in injury to dorsal capsule
- More common in players wearing flexible shoes
- More common in offensive linemen, tight ends, wide receivers
- Player complains of pain, especially with dorsiflexion
- Pain with running, especially with push-off and cutting
- Chronic injury results in loss of motion at first MTP, especially dorsiflexion

PHYSICAL EXAM
- Tenderness over plantar aspect of first MTP joint
- Tenderness on dorsal aspect if hyperflexion mechanism (less common)
- Swelling and ecchymosis present with more severe injury
- Pain, especially with passive dorsiflexion of the MTP joint
- Chronic cases: loss of first MTP joint motion
- Rule out dorsal dislocation of MTP joint (rare)

STUDIES
- Radiographs
  - AP and lateral
    - Usually normal
    - Rule out small avulsion fracture, sesamoid fracture, separation of bipartite sesamoid, subluxation/dislocation of MTP joint
  - Dorsiflexion stress view can be used to detect separation of bipartite sesamoid – Will show increased separation compared with nonstress view
  - May consider axial (sunrise view) image of MTP joint to evaluate sesamoids
  - Chronic – Periarticular calcifications, dorsal metatarsal osteophyte, joint space narrowing
- Other tests
  - Other imaging tests uncommonly used

➤ MRI useful to assess joint capsule/plantar plate and sesamoid complex

➤ MRI may also show impaction injury to articular surface of metatarsal head.

➤ CT scan may show small avulsion fracture or sesamoid fracture.

DIFFERENTIAL DIAGNOSIS

■ Sesamoid fracture – Rule out with careful radiographs

■ Stress fracture of sesamoid – Detect with MRI or CT scan

■ Dislocation/subluxation of first MTP joint – May have spontaneously reduced

■ Hallux rigidus – See dorsal osteophytes at MTP joint, have loss of joint motion

■ Intra-articular fracture at first MTP joint

■ Intra-articular loose body

TREATMENT

■ Conservative treatment

➤ Treatment is generally conservative.

➤ Rest, ice, compression, elevation (R.I.C.E.)

➤ NSAIDs useful

➤ Early joint mobilization, but avoid extremes of dorsiflexion

➤ Taping to avoid dorsiflexion of MTP joint

➤ Consider crutches for 2–3 days for more severe injury.

➤ Use rigid shoe or rigid orthotic in shoe (i.e., spring steel insert) to avoid MTP dorsiflexion.

➤ Cortisone injection not recommended

■ Operative treatment

➤ Operative treatment rarely required

➤ Soft tissue reconstruction of plantar plate may be necessary for repeated episodes of subluxation/dislocation or chronic subluxation.

➤ Excision of sesamoid fragment indicated for sesamoid fracture or separation of bipartite sesamoid with persistent pain.

DISPOSITION

N/A

PROGNOSIS

■ Time to return to play quite variable, relates to severity of injury

■ Player may return to play when near-normal or normal pain-free range of motion present

- Loss of playing time ranges from 2 weeks to 6 months.
- Use rigid shoe or rigid orthotic to avoid dorsiflexion of MTP joint when returning to play.
- Return to play after surgery: minimum 3–4 months
- Complications
  - Most common complication is persistent pain when the athlete returns to play during same season
  - Hallux rigidus (loss of first MTP joint motion), progressive degenerative joint disease with recurrent injuries

CAVEATS AND PEARLS

- Morbidity and lost time can be significant with this injury.
- Coach and player often initially underestimate severity since it is "only" a toe injury.
- Persistent pain after return to play is common.
- Be wary of associated sesamoid injury.

ULNAR NERVE INSTABILITY AT THE ELBOW

CHAMP BAKER, MD
DAVID D. NEDEFF, MD

HISTORY

- May be normal; not always symptomatic
- Ulnar nerve shifts out of epicondylar groove with elbow flexion, returns to normal position with elbow extension
- Nerve irritated by repetitive friction over medial epicondyle
- Patient may present with numbness and paresthesias in ulnar distribution, medial elbow pain, or weakness of hand
- Palpate epicondylar groove as you flex the elbow
- Type A – nerve moves onto tip of epicondyle with flexion of 90° or greater
- Type B – nerve has more excursion and moves completely across the epicondyle with elbow flexion
- Must differentiate from asymptomatic hypermobility of the nerve, which is present in 15–20% of normal population
- Several possible causes
  - Congenital laxity of fibroaponeurotic covering over epicondylar groove
  - Traumatic tear in this covering

> Iatrogenic cause after simple decompression of ulnar nerve without transposition
> Congenital hypoplasia of trochlea (resultant cubitus varus)
> Associated with cubitus varus and dislocation of medial triceps
> Malunion of distal humerus with resultant cubitus varus

■ These patients are at risk for iatrogenic nerve injury from medial injections or elbow arthroscopy or direct trauma to the nerve while in the subluxated or dislocated position.

PHYSICAL EXAM
■ Clinical history may be the most important diagnostic tool
■ Physical exam should start at cervical spine
■ Detailed exam of elbow
> Carrying angle
> Range of motion
> Crepitus and/or tenderness
> Ligamentous stability
> Ulnar nerve subluxation with flexion
■ Detailed sensory exam (vibratory perception, monofilaments, two-point discrimination)
■ Wartenberg's sign (inability to adduct little finger)
■ Intrinsic motor weakness indicates chronic compression (weakness of thumb pinch – positive Froment's sign)
■ Subluxation often easily identified; may not be symptomatic

STUDIES
■ Plain radiographs
> AP, lateral, and tunnel or axial view
> Look for loose bodies, osteophytes, angular deformity, malunion, or congenital hypoplasia
■ MRI generally not necessary for diagnosis, although dynamic MRI may show nerve in subluxed or dislocated position
■ Electrodiagnostic studies (EMG, nerve conduction velocity) are not essential when diagnosis is obvious on history and physical exam

DIFFERENTIAL DIAGNOSIS
■ Medial epicondylitis
■ Ulnar compression at wrist
■ Cubital tunnel syndrome
■ Elbow instability
■ Cervical spine pathology
■ Medial triceps subluxation

TREATMENT

- Initial treatment includes avoidance of repetitive elbow flexion with activity modification or splinting
- NSAID
- Avoid local steroid injections around nerve
- Surgical indications
  - Persistent numbness, paresthesias, or pain after conservative management
  - Progressive muscle weakness
  - Persistent mild weakness for 3–4 months
  - Chronic neuropathy with weakness
- Several surgical options
  - Anterior transposition
    - Subcutaneous, intramuscular or submuscular
    - All procedures move nerve to more protected position
    - 2 to 3 cm of length is gained, which decreases nerve tension
    - All five sites of potential compression are addressed
    - Disadvantages include extensive manipulation of nerve and disruption of neural blood supply
  - Corrective osteotomy of distal humerus if significant cubitus varus
    - May need to perform concomitant excision of medial triceps
    - May be combined with anterior ulnar nerve transposition

DISPOSITION

N/A

PROGNOSIS

- Nonsurgical treatment successful in approximately 50% of patients
- Surgical results best in mild and moderate cases
- No significant differences between various types of anterior transposition
- Anterior transposition: 82–95% good or excellent results
- Short period (7 days) of immobilization in semiflexed position followed by gradual active extension
- Some authors favor immediate range of motion

CAVEATS AND PEARLS

- Careful clinical exam and history should be diagnostic
- Always look for this before injections or surgery to the elbow
- Usually bilateral in asymptomatic individuals

- Consider medial triceps subluxation
- Surgery indicated for persistent pain and paresthesia

VOLAR PLATE INJURIES

JAMES B. BENNETT, MD

HISTORY
- Sports or work hand injury
- Subluxation/dislocations distal interphalangeal joint, proximal interphalangeal joint, metacarpal phalangeal joint
- Dorsal, volar, rotatory subluxation/dislocation
- Associated fractures
- Associated collateral ligament injury
- Irreducible dislocation with inter-articular joint entrapment volar plate
- Instability: acute, recurrent, and chronic
- Common in all contact sports
- Chronic volar instability/swan-neck deformity

PHYSICAL EXAM
- Primary static restraint limiting joint extension/prevention of hyperextension
- Joint stability, articular contour, collateral ligament, accessory collateral ligament, volar plate
- Distal attachment fibrocartilage/proximal wing ligament attachment
- Avulsion fracture distally off the volar fragment of the base of distal phalanx, middle phalanx, proximal phalanx
- Strain, sprain, dislocation
- Deformity and instability
- Joint line tenderness/swelling
- Inability to flex and extend fully
- Laxity to stress – dorsal/volar
- Associated fracture with dorsal dislocation
- Extensor tendon avulsion injuries with volar dislocation
- Irreducible dislocation with volar plate interposition into joint
- Irreducible dislocation with collateral ligament interposition into joint

STUDIES
- Radiographs
  - AP and true lateral
  - Dorsal dislocation with volar joint fracture
  - Volar dislocation with extensor tendon disruption
- No CT or MRI required in acute injury
  - CT or MRI as indicated in chronic injury

DIFFERENTIAL DIAGNOSIS
- Hemarthrosis joint
- Ligament instability, acute vs. chronic
- Fracture dislocation
- Flexor/extensor tendon injuries
- Joint contracture

TREATMENT
- **Acute**
  - Closed reduction and tests for stability
  - Open reduction if irreducible and remove volar plate from inter-articular position
  - Volar plate arthroplasty if volar fracture involves greater than one third of the joint surface
  - Splinting if stable and small volar plate fracture 1–2 weeks
  - Extension block for dorsal dislocation to prevent full extension and instability at 30°
  - Extensor tendon repair with volar dislocation and instability
  - Rotatory subluxation with central slip and lateral band buttonhole
  - Collateral ligament repair if rotatory or lateral instability
  - Isolated volar plate repair rare
- **Chronic**
  - Reconstruction for chronic instability/swan-neck
  - Eaton volar plate arthroplasty
  - Flexor digitorum superficialis (FDS) volar tenodesis

DISPOSITION
- Return to function 2–4 weeks non-operative, 6–8 weeks operative

PROGNOSIS
- Poor with fracture dislocation
- Poor with extensor tendon disruption
- Poor with flexor tendon avulsion

- Early protected range of motion if stable, 1–2 weeks
- Protected extension blocking if unstable, 4 weeks
- K-wire fixation for 3–4 weeks if ligament or tendon injury
- Volar plate arthroplasty if fracture 30–50% of the articular cartilage
- Irreducible dislocation with volar plate interposition for surgical removal of volar plate
- Return to play with volar chip fracture fragment, small, 1–2 weeks
- Return to play after reconstructive surgery, 4–6 weeks with protective splinting
- **Complications of surgical treatment**
  - Recurrent subluxation
  - Recurrent instability
  - Traumatic arthritis
  - Infection
  - Joint contracture

CAVEATS AND PEARLS
- Volar dislocation, extensor tendon rupture with lax but intact volar plate
- Dorsal dislocation with intact extensor tendon but rupture of volar plate and collateral ligaments
- Volar plate arthroplasty for 30–50% fracture of the articular cartilage
- Irreducible dislocation with joint interpositioning of volar plate – open reduction
- Rotatory subluxation with interposition of lateral band – open reduction

---

VOLUNTARY SHOULDER INSTABILITY

JEFFREY ABRAMS, MD

HISTORY
- Patient can demonstrate subluxation
- Mechanism: atraumatic, minor traumatic, overuse
- Complaints: painful shoulder subluxation and reduction
- Weakness – possibly related to discomfort
- Useful classification
  - Positional – can sublux shoulder with arm in provocative position
  - Muscular contraction – sublux at side by selective muscular contraction
  - Habitual – psychological disturbance with minimal discomfort

PHYSICAL EXAM

- Patient can demonstrate glenohumeral subluxation and reduction
- Range of motion normal
- Abnormal scapular mechanics
  - Winging during elevation (subluxation)
  - Weakness of serratus
- External rotator weakness due to cuff dysfunction
- Translation stress testing of glenohumeral joint
- Inferior sulcus sign
- Anterior and posterior load-and-shift test
  - Positive results include reproduction of symptoms, increased translation compared to asymptomatic shoulder
  - Negative apprehension sign

STUDIES

- Radiographs – stress tests: can be done with fluoroscopy (C-arm)
  - Axillary views for anterior, posterior subluxation
  - Anteroposterior view for inferior subluxation
- MRI can identify labral tears, excessive glenoid retroversion
- EMG: normal extremity exam

DIFFERENTIAL DIAGNOSIS

- Missed dislocation
  - Generally posterior resulting in loss of passive motion, weakness and pain
  - Axillary radiograph confirms diagnosis
- Serratus palsy
  - Long thoracic nerve deficit can produce involuntary winging of the scapula, shoulder weakness, and pain
  - EMG can identify deficit
- Classify voluntary subluxation
  - Habitual
    - Minimal symptoms
    - Facial expression does not demonstrate pain with fixed subluxation
  - Positional
    - During arm elevation, shoulder may sublux posteriorly and with continued elevation spontaneously reduce
    - May start as voluntary and become involuntary
    - Abduction, external rotation can promote anterior subluxation

➤ Muscular contractions
  • Arm in slight flexion and abduction
  • Selective muscular contraction can drive shoulder posteriorly

TREATMENT
■ Establish diagnosis
■ Classify voluntary instability
■ All patients should be started on nonoperative program
■ **Nonoperative program**
➤ Avoidance of demonstrating subluxation
➤ Muscular re-education for proper movements without subluxation
  • Cuff strengthening
  • Scapular stabilizers
    • Trapezius, rhomboid, serratus, latissimus
➤ Habitual subluxators need additional psychological counseling
■ **Operative**
➤ Best opportunity in patients with positional instability
➤ These patients may be considered involuntary subluxators due to loss of control
➤ Many are variants of multidirectional instability
➤ Identify symptomatic directions of instability
➤ Inferior capsule shift
➤ Reduce inferior capsule redundancy
➤ Repair any labral detachments
➤ Reduce symptomatic translation posteriorly, anteriorly, or both
➤ Options
  • Anterior arthrotomy and inferior capsule shift with interval closure
  • Posterior arthrotomy and capsule shift
  • Arthroscopic capsular plication and interval closure
➤ Postoperative sling/immobilization:
  • 4–6 weeks
  • Position to reduce strain on capsule
  • Prevent inferior stress on repair
  • Slow rehabilitative program

DISPOSITION
N/A

PROGNOSIS
■ **Nonsurgical treatment**

> Best results in voluntary posterior subluxation due to muscular contraction
> Return to sports is good if scapular winging reversed
> Bracing has minimal impact
> Habitual subluxator needs multidisciplinary approach

■ **Surgical treatment**
> Preferred for symptomatic positional subluxators
> Best results when associated anatomic defect corrected (i.e., labral detachment)
> Stability success (85–92%)
> Patient satisfaction high – important postoperative restrictions
> Low success in habitual subluxators
> Lower success in muscular contraction group

■ **Follow-up**
> Monitor results every 4–6 weeks up to 6 months

■ **Return to play**
> Ability to control glenohumeral and scapulothoracic joints
> No shoulder pain
> Strength >85% normal
> Nonoperative program 6 weeks
> Surgical patients
  • Noncontact sport – 4 months
  • Contact sports – 6 months

■ **Complications**
> Recurrence 5–20%
> Stiffness 1–29%
> Hardware complications (suture anchors)
> Infection <1%
> Neurologic injury to axillary nerve
  • Open dissection of pouch
  • Thermal probes during arthroscopic shrinkage
> Degenerative arthritis – overconstrained joint

CAVEATS AND PEARLS
■ Identify direction and classification of instability
■ Discourage voluntary demonstration of subluxation
■ Work on muscular stabilizers
■ If minimal symptoms, can continue with sports
■ Best surgical results with:
> Traumatic onset

➤ Labral lesion on studies
➤ Positional subluxators
■ Worse surgical results with:
➤ Habitual subluxators
➤ Subluxations caused by abnormal muscular contraction

WRIST LIGAMENT INJURIES (RADIAL SIDE INJURIES)

ARTHUR RETTIG, MD

HISTORY
■ Mechanism of injury: fall on outstretched arm with wrist in dorsiflexion and ulnar deviation (intercarpal supination occurs)
■ Complaints
➤ Acute complaints
• Pain
• Swelling radial side of wrist
• May feel or hear pop
• Period of acute pain, swelling 7–10 days
• May not seek medical treatment acutely
• Frequently presents remote from injury
➤ Chronic complaints
• Pain, popping wrist, weakness, pain with dorsiflexion, paresthesias if associated carpal tunnel syndrome
• Postactivity aching

PHYSICAL EXAM
■ Acute
➤ Swelling, effusion
➤ Decreased range of motion
➤ Tenderness over scapholunate (SL) ligament
➤ Watson's usually negative acutely
➤ Test two-point discrimination, grip strength if possible
■ Chronic
➤ More frequent presentation
➤ Tenderness at SL joint
➤ Pain with dorsiflexion
➤ Positive Watson's (scaphoid shift) test – always compare to non-injured side
➤ Decreased grip strength
➤ Decreased range of motion

➤ Rule out bony tenderness distal radius
➤ Correlate tenderness to anatomy

STUDIES
■ Radiographs
  ➤ Five views plus flexion/extension dynamic studies
  ➤ May be normal in grade I and II SL injuries
  ➤ Widening of SL gap in grade III + ring sign
  ➤ Lateral most important
  ➤ Look for SL angle >70°
■ Arthrogram
  ➤ Traditional study to demonstrate perforation of SL ligament
  ➤ >50% normal + arthrogram in >40 years old
■ MRI
  ➤ Information regarding ligaments and bony structures
  ➤ Variable value depending on quality of study and interpretation
■ Bone scan
  ➤ Nonspecific
  ➤ May be helpful if normal radiographs
■ Arthroscopy
  ➤ In 2007, gold standard of diagnosis
  ➤ Quantifies degree of injury of SL ligament
  ➤ Evaluates chondral surfaces
  ➤ May combine with definitive treatment

DIFFERENTIAL DIAGNOSIS
■ Chronic tenderness at dorsal SL ligament
■ Scaphoid impaction syndrome: bone scan may show chondral lesion of scaphoid
■ Occult dorsal ganglion: MRI or arthroscopy
■ Dorsal carpal impingement syndrome: arthroscopy
■ Dynamic SL instability secondary to partial interosseous sprain: dynamic radiographs, arthroscopy

TREATMENT
■ Acute SL ligament injury
  ➤ If grade I or II (partial tear) may treat with splint, rest for 3–6 weeks
  ➤ Many acute partial tears become asymptomatic
  ➤ If grade III (<3 mm dissociation, <3 months from injury) may do arthroscopic-assisted internal fixation

- ➤ If acute grade III (static SL instability) recommend open repair (Blatt capsulodesis – pin SL and scaphocapitate joints)
- ➤ Postoperative – long-arm cast for 4 weeks, short-arm cast for 4 weeks, return to sport 6 months
- ➤ If grade IV (dorsal perilunate dislocation) must reduce dislocation, repair SL ligament (pin SL, lunotriquetral, and scaphocapitate joints)
- ■ Chronic SL dissociation
  - ➤ Many asymptomatic – leave alone
  - ➤ Chronic SL dissociation without degenerative changes
  - ➤ Blatt capsulodesis does not address SL ligament
  - ➤ Bone-ligament-bone reconstruction – source Lister's tubercle or cuboid-navicular bone-capsule-bone graft
  - ➤ Limited arthrodesis
  - ➤ Scaphotrapezial trapezoid fusion
  - ➤ Scaphocapitate fusion
  - ➤ With degenerative changes: arthroscopy with radial styloidectomy
  - ➤ Limited arthrodesis: Scaphoid incision with four-corner fusion (ulno-capitate-lunate-triquetral)
  - ➤ Scapholunate advanced collapse (SLAC) wrist: traditional wrist fusion

DISPOSITION
N/A

PROGNOSIS
- ■ Acute SL injuries
  - ➤ True natural history unknown
  - ➤ Grade I – probably good if treated with splint, rest
  - ➤ Grade II (dynamic) – may lead to arthrosis, > instability if not repaired
  - ➤ Grade III – good prognosis if anatomic repair achieved
  - ➤ Return to sport 6 months
- ■ Complications of treatment
  - ➤ Rest and splint
  - ➤ If ligament does not heal properly, may develop instability symptoms and ultimately
    - • Arthrosis
    - • Arthroscopy
    - • If ligament stability not restored, same as above

➤ Open repair: infection, stiffness, recurrent instability
- Partial arthrodesis: infection, decreased range of motion, decreased grip strength

CAVEATS AND PEARLS

- Acute grade III injuries rarely present to orthopedists
- Always compare exam (especially scaphoid shift test) to opposite side
- Dorsal wrist syndrome very common and probably represents chronic partial SL ligament injury
- Treatment with arthroscopy, debridement of dorsal wrist ganglion, and posterior interosseous nerve excision frequently curative
- Chronic SL instability – no ideal solution
- Must be sure wrist will be improved before recommending operative approach

Printed in the United States
by Baker & Taylor Publisher Services